# The Nursing Process in the Care of Adults with Orthopaedic Conditions

# The Nursing Process in the Care of Adults with Orthopaedic Conditions

· · · · · · · · · · · · · · · · · · · · · · · · · · · · · · · · · · · · · · ·

## Third Edition

**Leona A. Mourad, M.S., R.N., O.N.C.**

Associate Professor Emeritus, College of Nursing,
The Ohio State University, Columbus, Ohio

Nursing Consultant
Mourad Consultant Associates
Columbus, Ohio

**Millie M. Droste, B.A., R.N.**

Orthopaedic Nursing Consultant and former head nurse,
Orthopaedic Nursing Unit
The Ohio State University Hospitals,
Columbus, Ohio

Now Patient Education Coordinator

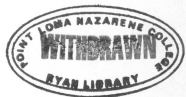
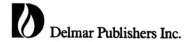
Delmar Publishers Inc.

## NOTICE TO THE READER

**Delmar Staff**
Administrative Editor: Patricia Casey
Project Editor: Cynthia Lassonde
Production Supervisor: Teresa Luterbach
Art Supervisor: Judi Orozco

For information, address Delmar Publishers Inc.,
3 Columbia Circle, Box 15–015
Albany, NY 12212–5015

COPYRIGHT ©1993
BY DELMAR PUBLISHERS INC.

Printed in the United States of America
Published simultaneously in Canada
by Nelson Canada
A Division of the Thomson Corporation

  2  3  4  5  6  7  8  9  10  XXX  99  98  97  96  95  94  93

*Library of Congress Cataloging-in-Publication Data*

Mourad, Leona A.
    The nursing process in the care of adults with orthopaedic conditions/
Leona A. Mourad, Millie M. Droste—3rd ed.
      p.cm.
    Includes index.
    ISBN 0-8273-4939-4 (textbook)
    1. Orthopedic nursing.   I. Droste, Millie M.   II. Title.
    [DNLM: 1. Nursing Process. 2. Orthopedics—nursing.  WY 157.6
M929n]
RD753.M68 1993
610.73'677—dc20
DNLM/DLC
for Library of Congress                                    92-22066
                                                           CIP

# CONTENTS

Preface................................................................................................ vii

Acknowledgments............................................................................. xi

List of Nursing Diagnoses ............................................................... xiii

Chapter 1    Orthopaedic Nursing Today................................................ 1

Chapter 2    Musculoskeletal Tissues: Anatomy and
             Physiology and Physical Assessment ................................ 28

Chapter 3    Nursing Process During Diagnostic Examinations................. 73

Chapter 4    Nursing Process in the Care of Patients with Trauma............ 110

Chapter 5    Nursing Process in the Care of Patients
             with Inflammatory Conditions...................................... 151

Chapter 6    Nursing Process in the Care of Patients
             with Degenerative Conditions...................................... 187

Chapter 7    Nursing Process in the Care of Patients
             with Bone Tumors...................................................... 202

Chapter 8    Nursing Process in the Care of Patients
             with Infections of Bone ............................................. 220

Chapter 9    Nursing Process in the Care of Patients
             with Metabolic Diseases ............................................ 231

Chapter 10   Nursing Process in the Care of Persons in Casts.................... 244

Chapter 11   Nursing Process in the Care of Persons
             in Traction or with an External Fixator......................... 278

Chapter 12   Nursing Process in the Care of Patients
             Having Orthopaedic Surgery........................................ 332

Chapter 13 Nursing During the Process of Rehabilitation.......................... 437

Chapter 14 Nursing Considerations in the Care of
Persons Having Complications Following
Trauma, Diseases, and Surgery.................................................... 466

Appendix A ANA/NAON Nursing Diagnoses............................................. 501

Appendix B Patient Education Guides............................................................. 504

Appendix C Universal Precautions to Prevent Occupational/
Nosocomial Transmission of HIV1............................................ 517

Glossary of Terms, With Generic Derivations.................................................... 519

Index ...................................................................................................................... 553

# PREFACE

Since the first two editions of this book were published, many changes have occurred in both the delivery of and payment for medical and nursing care. Now nursing services must provide skilled nursing care to patients to aid their recoveries within the economic restraints and time frames of DRGs. Nurses must aid in evaluating the patient's recovery in terms of preparation for self-care at home. Nursing care is most often based on standards of care and is being evaluated through continuous quality improvement programs.

The result of these economic and professional trends has been that nursing is now highly focused on providing both efficient and effective care. The third edition has been revised with this focus in mind. Information in the text is designed to quickly provide the nurse or student with clinical information that not only emphasizes safe, professional practice, but does so through a visually accessible, logical presentation. Specific detailed nursing diagnoses, with assessments, expected outcomes, interventions, and evaluations, are highlighted throughout Chapters 3 through 14. Orthopaedic procedures are also presented in a step-by-step format for easy retention and review. Discharge teaching and home care is included wherever appropriate, and the entire text has been reorganized and updated to reflect current orthopaedic nursing practice.

Chapter 1 provides an overview of the nursing process, the role of the nurse and of other members of the orthopaedic health care team. The impact of economic and demographic changes is noted, especially as it pertains to the physical requirements of an orthopaedic nursing unit. The last section in the chapter will be invaluable to head nurses or managers who will be involved in planning and equipping a newly opened orthopaedic unit.

Chapter 2 discusses the anatomy and physiology of the musculoskeletal tissues, information that all nurses who care for orthopaedic patients should know for safe practice and care. This chapter can serve as a basis for teaching patients and their families about the specific injury, disease, or condition being treated. The last part of Chapter 2 concerns physical assessment, with normal and abnormal findings commonly found when assessing orthopaedic patients. The data from the physical assessment are used to develop nursing diagnoses, care plans, and nursing interventions in the later chapters.

Chapter 3 is an exposition of the examinations commonly performed to aid in the diagnosis or treatments of orthopaedic patients. Tables contain descriptions of the specific examinations, normal findings, and the significance of the examinations for orthopaedic patients.

The remaining chapters have been separated into single focus chapters to ease presentation, reading, and study, and for exposition of pictures, illustrations, tables, and charts. All chapters incorporate the nursing process presentation of nursing care related to the condition or disease discussed in the specific chapter.

Chapter 4 contains current information related to trauma of musculoskeletal tissues. All areas of common injuries are explored with RICE (Rest, Ice, Compression, Elevation) highlighted as first aid of injuries. Fractures are discussed fully with the nursing process utilized for the nursing care.

Chapter 5 discusses inflammatory diseases with additions of ankylosing spondylitis, Lyme disease, bursitis, epicondylitis, and tendinitis. These additions greatly enhance this chapter.

Chapter 6 discusses degenerative conditions of musculoskeletal tissues, and contains a discussion of low back pain and its personal, economic, treatment parameters for the specific conditions causing the low back pain.

Chapter 7 contains current information related to the diagnosis and treatment of bone tumors. Even though bone tumors are rare, they must be accurately diagnosed and treated for the patient to have the most specific and beneficial treatment for the presenting tumor. Limb salvage procedures are discussed.

Chapter 8 discusses osteomyelitis as a severe infection of bones. Wound infections are also incorporated into this chapter.

Chapter 9 has current content related to metabolic diseases of musculoskeletal tissues. Since all persons are subjected to the development of osteoporosis, that content should be pertinent and useful for all health care personnel.

Chapter 10 updates care of persons in casts with home care information and care after removal of casts included.

Chapter 11 discusses the care of persons in traction and external fixators with nursing care factors incorporated.

Chapter 12 is an expanded discussion of surgical options for orthopaedic conditions. New sections are related to spinal and hand conditions and the Ilizarov technique for leg lengthening and other conditions. These additions add much strength to this chapter.

Chapter 13 recounts rehabilitation principles and practices. Current information for rehabilitation after orthopaedic trauma and diseases is presented.

Chapter 14 discusses commonly encountered complications after orthopaedic diseases, trauma, or surgery. Nursing factors are included with each complication.

The glossary of terms and index have been expanded to incorporate all the new vocabulary introduced in this edition.

Two new appendices have been added for use of nurses and health team members. Appendix A still has the NAON nursing diagnoses for orthopaedic nursing. Appendix B has many Patient Education Guides for home care to facilitate teaching. They can be copied for patient teaching and use. These guides are just some examples. Nurses should devise similar teaching guides for specific patients' conditions and home care. Appendix C contains the Universal Precautions from the Centers for Disease Control.

It is hoped that nurses will utilize this book for their own learning as well as for patient teaching activities. We wish you great success in your efforts at providing and improving patient nursing care.

Leona A. Mourad
Millie M. Droste

# ACKNOWLEDGMENTS

I wish to acknowledge the superb word-processing skills of Connie Prouty, and for her dedication in the preparation of this manuscript. It would not have been ready without her diligent attention. Thanks, Connie.

I also thank Millie Droste, coauthor, for her suggestions and excellent revisions of her chapters. They are powerful additions to the book.

I also again thank my long-suffering husband, George, for tolerating my evenings in my office to prepare the manuscript. I couldn't have done it without you, dear.

I also wish to thank Patricia Casey, administrative editor from Delmar Publishers, for her encouragement and welcome suggestions, even though she arrived on the scene during the latter days of the manuscript preparation.

Leona A. Mourad

I concur with my coauthor's sentiments and would also like to thank Dr. Robert Crowell, The Spine Clinic, Columbus, Ohio, for the generous use of x-rays and research materials. His support and knowledge of the spine contributed greatly to the addition of this material to the book.

Also I must thank Virginia Turner, former Director of the Allen Memorial School of Nursing, Waterloo, Iowa, for her support during my nursing education and her belief that I could someday be a nurse. Her curriculum of theory and extensive hands-on experience provided my strong foundation.

Lastly I again want to thank my family who endured the vacation days I took and spent at the computer, the meals that were never made and my less than desirable moods when in the throes of writing. My husband, who never wanted me to write again, nontheless provided the time needed by carrying on all the household chores, meal preparation, chauffeuring of children, and emotional support. Thanks, Galen! Finally, I want to thank my mother, who always believed that a person can do anything if there is determination. She has always said in times of doubt "just start walking with your right foot and drag your left one behind until you are walking with both." That motto works in everyday life and is certainly apropos for orthopaedics.

Millie M. Droste

# LIST OF NURSING DIAGNOSES

## Chapter 4

Impaired physical mobility related to fracture(s) of bone(s) and soft tissue trauma, **144**

Pain related to fractures and soft tissue trauma, **146**

Altered peripheral (pulmonary) tissue perfusion and impaired gas exchange related to fat embolism, **147**

Anxiety related to sudden injury and loss of mobility, **148**

## Chapter 5

Impaired physical mobility related to joint inflammation, tightened tissues, or deformities, **160**

Activity Intolerance related to tightened skin tissues, fatigue, anemia, and Raynaud's phenomenon, **162**

Pain related to joint tissue inflammation, deformity, and muscle/tendon involvement, **163**

Impaired gas exchange related to pneumonitis, pulmonary edema, and anemia, **164**

Self-care deficit related to joint deformity, inflammation, and presence of rheumatoid arthritis, systemic lupus erythematosus, or progressive systemic sclerosis, **165**

Potential for injury related to gastrointestinal distention, obstruction, or bleeding, **166**

Body image disturbance related to "pinched" facial appearance in PSS, rash with SLE, and deformity related to RA, **167**

**xiii**

Sleep pattern disturbance related to pain, muscle and joint stiffness, **168**

Altered role performance related to deformity and fatigue, **169**

Impaired physical mobility related to bursal inflammation, **172**

Pain related to bursal inflammation, **173**

Impaired physical mobility related to inflammation of vertebrae and major joints, **176**

Pain related to inflammation of spinal components and major joints, **176**

Alteration in body image and usual roles related to inflammatory changes and presence of abnormal, nonfunctional curvatures, **177**

Impaired physical mobility related to injury to a specific tendon area, **180**

Impaired physical mobility related to systemic and local infection in joint and joints, **182**

Hyperthermia related to systemic infection, **183**

Pain related to systemic infection, arthritis, or neurological signs, **184**

## Chapter 6

Impaired physical mobility related to osteoarthritis and limited range of motion, **191**

Pain (acute) related to degenerative joint changes and muscle spasms, **192**

Self-care deficit related to osteoarthritis, **193**

Impaired physical mobility related to pain and deformity, **196**

Body image disturbance related to deformity of foot or feet, **196**

Pain related to bunion and bursitis, **197**

## Chapter 7

Impaired physical mobility related to tumor mass, pressure, and pain, **214**

Pain related to pressure of enlarging mass on nerve(s), bone, or other tissues, **215**

Impaired gas exchange related to anesthesia, bed rest, and operative procedure (thoracotomy or forequarter amputation), **216**

## Chapter 8

Impaired physical mobility related to presence of osteomyelitis, **225**

Impaired skin integrity related to presence of purulent drainage or insertion of irrigating tubes at site of osteomyelitis, **226**

Pain related to bone infection and altered tissue perfusion, **226**

Knowledge deficit related to osteomyelitis, its treatments, and prognosis, **227**

## Chapter 9

Impaired physical mobility related to weakened bones from Paget's disease, osteomalacia, or osteoporosis, **235**

Potential for injury (risk of fracture) related to disease, less bone mass, and deformed mass, **236**

Pain related to abnormal bone growth and shape, nerve impingement, or degenerative arthritis, **238**

Pain related to joint inflammation and urate deposits, **240**

Altered nutrition related to incomplete purine metabolism, **241**


## Chapter 10

Potential for injury related to the presence of a damp cast, **253**

Impaired physical mobility related to injury and presence of a cast, **258**

Potential for impaired gas exchange related to a body or spica cast, **259**

Deficit in self-care, hygiene, toileting, or grooming related to a large cast, **260**

Alteration in comfort related to acute pain, **261**

Potential for alteration in skin integrity related to cast and decreased mobility, **263**

Potential for alteration in nutritional intake or utilization of foodstuffs, **267**

Potential alteration in bowel or bladder elimination related to the presence of the cast or back-lying position, **268**

Potential deficit in diversional activities related to cast limitations or participation in usual social activities, **269**

Knowledge deficit related to discharge and home care needs, **271**


## Chapter 11

Alteration in comfort related to muscle spasms or acute pain, **296**

Impaired physical mobility related to the presence of the skin traction, **298**

Actual injury to the musculoskeletal tissues and potential injury related to neurovascular compromise, **300**

Self-care deficit in hygiene and grooming related to pathology, bed position, and traction, **301**

High risk for impaired skin integrity related to imposed or prolonged bed rest, **302**

Potential for impaired gas exchange related to imposed bed rest, **303**

Inadequate nutritional intake, less than body requirements related to anorexia and inactivity, **304**

Potential impaired bowel elimination, constipation, and impaired urinary elimination, decreased urinary output, related to bed rest, decreased food intake, bulk or fiber or decreased fluid intake, **305**

Potential deficit in diversional activity related to bed rest and confined situation, **307**

Alteration in body image and self-esteem, role performance and socialization related to injury and traction, **308**

Actual injury to musculoskeletal tissues related to trauma (skeletal traction), **318**

Potential injury related to the presence of skeletal pins and traction, **320**

Alteration in comfort related to acute pain, injury, or muscle spasms (skeletal traction), **323**

Potential for impaired gas exchange related to pulmonary or fat emboli, **324**

Impaired physical mobility related to the skeletal traction and bed rest, **327**

Self-care deficit in hygiene and grooming; risk of impaired skin integrity related to imposed bed rest and skeletal traction, **328**

## Chapter 12

Potential for impaired skin integrity related to use of a brace or body cast, **355**

Potential for impaired gas exchange related to anesthesia, immobility, or bed rest, **356**

Alteration in tissue perfusion related to surgical trauma and immobility, **357**

Potential for alteration in bowel elimination related to anesthesia, immobility, bed rest and surgical trauma, **358**

Alteration in mobility related to the surgical intervention, **359**

Impaired physical mobility related to continued back pain or muscle spasms postoperatively (chemonucleolysis), **363**

Potential for injury related to the effects of anesthesia or chymopapain, **364**

Alteration in comfort related to acute pain, surgical trauma, and edema, **372**

Potential for injury related to displacement of a prosthesis, **384**

Potential for injury related to development of deep vein thrombosis, **388**

Potential for injury related to wound or joint infection, **390**

Impaired physical mobility related to weight-bearing limitations and use of ambulatory aids, **391**

Alteration in urinary elimination related to the presence of a urinary catheter and bed rest, **392**

Potential for impaired gas exchange related to immobility (total joint replacement), **401**

Potential alteration in peripheral tissue perfusion related to surgical intervention and immobility, **402**

Potential for impaired skin integrity (potential for skin breakdown) related to extended bed rest and presence of incision, **403**

Alteration in physical mobility related to surgical intervention, **405**

Alteration in comfort and acute pain related to surgical intervention, **409**

Alteration in tissue perfusion related to surgical trauma (arthrodesis or osteotomy), **414**

Alteration in comfort with acute pain related to the trauma of surgery, **415**

Disturbance in body image and self-concept related to loss of all or part of an extremity (amputation), **418**

Alteration in comfort related to acute surgical trauma or phantom pain (amputation), **420**

Alteration in skin integrity related to surgical incision (amputation), **421**

Impaired physical mobility related to the loss of an extremity (amputation), **424**

# 1

# ORTHOPAEDIC NURSING TODAY

Orthopaedic nursing has undergone many changes in the last 25 years, not only in the way in which nursing care is provided, but also in the makeup and interaction of the entire health care team and in the physical requirements of the orthopaedic unit. In addition, demographics and economic constraints have also had an impact on the structure and delivery of orthopaedic care. This chapter provides an overview of the nature and process of orthopaedic nursing, the orthopaedic health care team, and the physical layout of the modern orthopaedic setting.

## THE NURSING PROCESS

The nursing process, which is used throughout this book for the presentation of nursing care is a stepwise method of providing professional nursing care to patients using nursing assessment, nursing diagnoses, goal setting (expected outcomes), nursing interventions, and evaluation of goal achievement.

Assessment of the physical, psychological, cultural, spiritual, and economic influences on the patient's current condition begins upon his or her admission to the orthopaedic setting and continues until he or she is discharged.

Analysis of the nurse's assessment data provides the basis for nursing diagnoses; these are usually based on some alteration or potential alteration in the patient's functioning. Nursing diagnoses have been listed by the North American Nursing Diagnosis Association (NANDA) in many nursing texts and are used in this textbook as the basis for nursing care.

Planning involves goal setting with expected outcomes delineated for each nursing diagnosis. The plan gives priority to the more critical or serious alterations. The care plan must therefore be individualized for each patient although commonalities of care exist—especially those involving activities of daily living. The care plan should be developed from mutually determined goals of both patient and nurse when the patient's condition permits such input. The nursing plan is written on the patient's record, and its appropriateness and comprehensiveness are coordinated with the rest of the multidisciplinary team.

Nursing interventions needed to meet the patient's needs or accomplish the care goals are determined according to the priorities and nursing diagnoses. Interventions incorporate the physician's orders, and nursing activities are centered around these orders and nursing diagnoses. Nursing interventions are the means by which the goals and expected outcomes are achieved. Both the intervention and the results of the intervention must be recorded on the patient's chart, and the results are routinely analyzed as part of the evaluation of patient care.

Evaluation incorporates reassessment, replanning, goal restating or resetting, and new interventions as part of a cyclical pattern. Discussion with the patient and conferences with other health team members alerts everyone to changes in the care plan as they occur. Determining the patient's readiness for discharge is also part of evaluation.

The nursing process is widely acclaimed in theory but is sadly under-utilized in practice because it is so time-consuming to write and requires considerable thought to correctly word the nursing diagnoses, interventions, and expected outcomes. Nurses want and need to minimize paperwork and provide more "hands-on" nursing care time. If the care plan is too time-consuming it will not be completed.

To solve this problem of a lack of time versus a need for delineation of nursing care, generic forms were created. These specify certain nursing diagnoses applicable to specific nursing situations that are frequently found on nursing units. They are complete with interventions, expectations, and outcomes. The forms are then filled in with patient's name, date, and nurse initials. If the generic plan of care is utilized then it must be reviewed, modified, or enhanced to fit the patient's need.

Another solution may be to make the nursing care plan a more user-friendly, time-efficient form. It should be assumed that an intervention is specified because the nurse believes the expected outcome of this intervention will diminish or solve the nursing diagnosis problem. Requiring a nurse to explain all nursing interventions through writing rationale and expected outcomes should be reserved for the classroom, nursing care conference, and textbooks. In practice the nursing process should be followed step by step mentally in the formation of the care plan. Writing of the plan should be simplified to nursing diagnosis and interventions. Outcomes should be reviewed with other staff members as needed throughout the shift and interventions modified as needed to accomplish the goals. Nursing care conferences with health team members should include explanation of the entire nursing process as a teaching mechanism. This text will use the nursing process model to assist the nurse in the mental process of outlining optimal patient care.

## STANDARDS OF CARE

A standard is a guideline for nursing care that contains measurable goals. Appendix A contains orthopaedic standards developed by members of the American Nurses' Association (ANA) and the National Association of Orthopaedic Nurses (NAON). These two groups have developed standards for the care of orthopaedic patients using eight commonly seen nursing diagnoses: impaired physical mobility, high risk for ineffective coping, pain, self-care deficit, activity intolerance, pain management deficit, high risk for skin breakdown, and knowledge deficit regarding mobility skills. (See Figs. 1.1 and 1.2) In discussing the use of these selected diagnoses, the ANA and NAON state, "it is anticipated that use of [these eight diagnoses] will stimulate a dynamic process of validating and perfecting the diagnoses and criteria presented." In Chapters 3–14 the authors have attempted to meet this need for refinement by presenting clinically applicable nursing diagnoses with specific assessments, expected outcomes, interventions, and evaluation information drawn from years of orthopaedic nursing practice and clinical research. All diagnoses are based on the current NANDA list, as well as the ANA and NAON guidelines.

The specific format of a standard may vary in different areas of the country and by nursing specialty. Some standards may follow the categories of human functioning; others, such as the orthopaedic ones, may be oriented toward a specific nursing diagnosis. Some standards may include routine postoperative physician's orders—for example, the application of antiembolism stockings postoperatively—to familiarize nurses with common medical expectations. This type of standard may also include other routines for pre- and postoperative care, such as having the patient perform dorsiflexion/plantarflexion exercises every 2 hours. Standards also include patient teaching and discharge instructions, which for orthopaedic patients would include dietary orders; exercise programs for the specific joints, muscles, or extremities; and medication regimens for pain control, including possible side effects to be noted.

Standards written according to human needs begin as general subsystem assessments and expand to become specific for particular patients. A standard can include references to articles or books to make it more specific to the patient's need.

The use of a standard of care should serve to make patient care uniform, measurable, and evaluative all over the country. More standards still need to be developed to encompass the nursing needs of patients with various diagnoses, but when these are completed, accepted, and used by all nurses, the nursing profession will have taken a major step toward providing truly professional care.

---

*Etiology*
   The cause is decreased range of motion, imposed activity restriction, imposed mechanical restriction, decreased muscle strength, and/or pain.

*Defining Characteristics*
   The individual cannot move independently within the environment, in relation to such activity as bed mobility, transfer, and ambulation.
   The individual's movement is restricted by such means as casts, braces, traction, and imposed bed rest.

*Assessment Parameters*
   The nurse assesses the individual's—
      Ability to turn, transfer, or walk.         Coordination.
      Functional range of motion.                Gait pattern.
      Muscle strength.                           Comfort level.

*Process Criteria*
   The nurse assists the individual in maintaining limb function by—
      Instituting range-of-motion and strengthening exercises of all
         limbs, when appropriate.
      Positioning the individual in alignment.
      Scheduled turning, repositioning.
      Using mechanical devices, such as traction, braces, pillows, splints,
         exercise equipment, overhead trapeze, and ambulation devices.
   The nurse encourages the individual to progress with daily activities from bed mobility through ambulation, when possible.
   The nurse collaborates with the individual and other health professionals in developing and/or using safe and effective techniques for bed mobility, transfer, and ambulation.
   The nurse provides pain relief measures prior to and during activity if pain decreases the individual's ability to move.

*Outcome Criteria*
   The individual moves in the environment within imposed limitations, with or without assistive devices.
   The individual verbalizes and/or demonstrates safety measures to avoid injury associated with mobility.

---

**Figure 1.1** Standard of care for the nursing diagnosis: impaired physical mobility. (Used with permission of the American Nurses' Association, Kansas City, MO.)

**Figure 1.2** *Standard of care for the nursing diagnosis: pain. (Used with permission of the American Nurses' Association, Kansas City, MO.)*

*Etiology*
   The cause is inflammation, swelling, muscle spasm, and/or other musculoskeletal causes.

*Defining Characteristics*
   The individual reports pain.
   The individual demonstrates nonverbal indications of pain, such as moaning, massaging, guarding, wincing, and reluctance to move.

*Assessment Parameters*
   Assess pain characteristics, including—
      Location of pain and areas that are pain-free.
      Type, such as burning, stabbing, aching, pressing, and throbbing.
      Intensity, such as unbearable, severe, moderate, mild, or painful as measured on a pain scale (e.g., 0 = no pain, 10 = worst possible pain).
      Duration, such as minutes, hours, and days.
      Pattern, such as constant or intermittent.
      Precipitating or aggravating factors, such as movement, cold, stress, specific positioning, and lack of rest.
      Alleviating factors, such as rest, massage, relaxation techniques, exercise, specific position, heat, and cold.
   Explore the meaning of pain to the individual, including—
      Expectation of pain relief.
      Previous pain experiences.
      Beliefs that certain measures would be effective or ineffective in relieving pain.
      Ability and willingness to take an active role in pain control.

*Process Criteria*
   The nurse minimizes pain response associated with musculoskeletal injury by methods such as—
      Positioning the body to alleviate pressure, tension, edema, or spasm.
      Handling injured body parts smoothly and gently.
      Assisting the individual to exercise within the limits imposed by the pain or the orthopaedic condition.
      Promoting sleep by reducing environmental stimuli, providing comfort measures, and incorporating the individual's preferences and usual routine.
   The nurse considers and makes available alternate methods of pain relief based on individual needs, such as—
      Application of heat, cold, and massage.
      Relaxation exercises to decrease muscular tension.
      Diversional activity and techniques.

(Continued)

The nurse decreases the anxiety component of pain by interventions such as—
> Providing sensory and procedural information prior to any new and possibly painful procedure.
> Providing emotional support during a painful or frightening procedure.
> Acknowledging the individual's pain.

The nurse uses a preventive approach in alleviating pain.

The nurse collaborates with the individual and other health professionals in planning relief strategies.

The nurse monitors and reports, as indicated, any increase in pain or change in pain pattern.

The nurse reports and documents pain relief strategies and that prove most effective.

*Outcome Criteria*

The individual verbalizes that the pain is decreased, alleviated, or under control.

The individual's behavioral indications of pain (such as moaning, massaging, guarding, wincing, and reluctance to move) are reduced.

---

**Figure 1.2** (continued)

## CONTINUOUS QUALITY IMPROVEMENT

Standards of care are complemented by the presence of Continuous Quality Improvement (CQI) programs. CQI is a process of evaluation of the achievement of the process, expected outcomes, or goals set by and for the patient and health care team members. CQI is a continual process of evaluating current performance, levels of performance desirable, standards and critical pathways. Through CQI analyses, the quality and quantity of care is determined, and adjustments are made as needed. Thus, CQI is and must be ongoing and care changed as indicated by the CQI analysis.

A CQI outcome program would determine whether the expected outcomes have been achieved. For example, in evaluating the effectiveness of pain medications, the expected outcome would be that the patient would be able to control pain with oral analgesics by the time of discharge. The CQI evaluation would check the documentation of the patient's subjective data related to their effectiveness and the documentation of the objective data relative to the type of analgesic and the frequency of administration.

A nursing unit CQI committee is valuable in determining which issues should be or need to be addressed on a particular nursing unit. It also allows nurses to use creative and varied approaches to solve care problems specific to that nursing unit and encourages a commitment to find satisfactory solutions to the problems. It also provides immediate and direct feedback to the staff.

Unit committee members may be recruited by asking for volunteers interested in working on and finding solutions to a specific issue. Having committee members serve for issues that they are interested in rather than for a time period is a very effective way to maintain a high level of interest in problem solving and quality assurance.

## NURSING AND DIAGNOSTIC RELATED GROUPS

Use of the nursing process, standards of care, and CQI programs in nursing help to assure that the patient will receive the highest quality and most thorough care possible in these times of a major *outside* influence on nursing practice, namely, diagnostic related groups (DRGs), which began in 1981 in New Jersey and have become nationwide since 1983.

DRGs are groupings of related medical diagnoses with the corresponding number of days of hospitalization for the average patient and the types of diagnostic tests and treatments that are appropriate to a specific diagnosis. DRGs began as a cost containment measure for health care providers and hospitals and now influence medical and nursing practice throughout the United States. As a result of DRGs, a patient may be treated and cared for in a minimal care unit, "same day surgery" setting, and, if hospitalized, may be discharged before being fully recovered. Because of DRGs, the delivery of medical and nursing care has been permanently changed, and many patients are discharged to their homes requiring continuing medical and nursing care. The patient will have a quality of care that is more standard if nurses use the nursing process, nursing diagnoses, standards of care, and critical pathways and CQI programs.

## LEGAL CONSIDERATIONS IN NURSING

With all the changing internal or external factors that shape health care delivery, nurses must be continually aware of their professional, ethical, and legal obligations regardless of the setting.

Nurses' actions must be reasonable, prudent, and ordinary within the customary practices of the community. Nursing practice is governed by the state licensing laws outlining the specific actions included for practitioners within the discipline. Issues arise where nurses are confronted with equivocal situations involving the rights of more than one individual, the moral or ethical factors surrounding a particular situation, and their responsibility for safe, competent practice.

Professional nurses have many responsibilities in health care settings. They provide their care within the policies of the setting and with written physician's orders. Additionally, nurses base their care of patients on the knowledge and skills governing professional nursing practice. At times conflicts may arise concerning policies or orders that influence the nurse's actions and care. Nurses then are responsible for communicating their concerns to and with the persons involved and for trying to find solutions. Generally, solutions can be satisfactorily achieved and policies and/or orders modified or changed. If, after several attempts, solutions cannot be achieved, the nurse may have either to continue the efforts or to seek a change in the nursing or employment setting. Nurses exercise their rights within their professional skills and educational capacities, and their concern for the welfare of the patients in their care.

Nurse/patient relationships that are mutually determined emphasize personal rights and freedoms to privacy, personal control of one's body, and respect for the other's rights, and encompass the values to internal control by the nurse and patient.

Nurses do not have automatic, unimpeded access to the "person" of a patient just because of that patient's presence. Patient rights require that permission be explicitly granted in the mutually developed plan of care. Discussion and clarification of the strategies, timing, and roles of each participant provide the bases for the care. This type of care places a high value on the human qualities of reason and voluntary participation for decision making. It provides for ultimate goal achievement—the return to health of the patient.

## THE ORTHOPAEDIC HEALTH CARE TEAM

Just as orthopaedic patients require individualized, quality nursing care, so do they require specialized knowledge and expertise from other health care providers. Patients needs are best met by a multidisciplinary team of health professionals. Such a team is comprised of members of several disciplines with specialized services provided by the individual members; thus, members include orthopaedic physicians, nurses, physical therapists, occupational therapists, dietitians, social workers, and technicians such as the orthopaedic technician, the laboratory technician, or radiological technician. The major goal of the team members is to provide maximal care through coordinated, skilled care and to provide for discharge planning. Patient care conferences must be held with all members attending and contributing suggestions for care in their respective areas of expertise and according to the patient's condition. Tentative daily plans are discussed, and a projected discharge date is set. The number and length of the care conferences vary from patient to patient according to need. From the conferences, all team members learn of the patient's needs, the plans for care, and the best time and manner for the individual team member's specific contributions to the patient's care. This provides for continuity of care, with all members working toward the same goals (see Figure 1.3).

## The Primary Nurse

Primary nursing is a further step toward optimal care and nursing accountability. The primary nurse has the major responsibility for planning and coordinating the nursing care of a patient from admission to discharge. The primary nurse acts as liaison between all other members of the health team and the patient and family. A mutually derived plan of care is developed to meet the patient's goals (expected outcomes) for recovery and return to the community. Nursing diagnoses are determined from the assessments of the patient's condition, and appropriate nursing interventions are planned and provided as needed. Care is evaluated and revised in an ongoing fashion according to the goals or expected outcomes.

Second-generation primary nursing focuses on case management with the primary nurse coordinating and communicating with other health team members in planning patient care. The case manager may coordinate care with walking rounds in which other health care team members assist in evaluating and planning care through development of critical pathways.

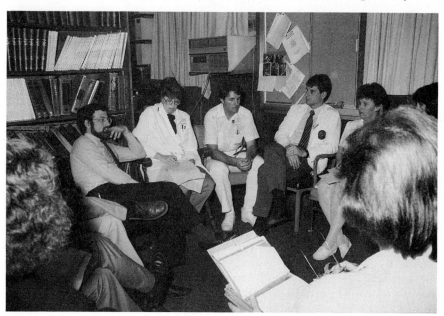

**Figure 1.3** Conference for patient discharge planning. Present are Head nurse, physician, social worker, staff nurse, resident physician, nurse, physical therapist, and dietitian. (Figures 1.3–1.16 used with permission of The Ohio State University Hospitals, Columbus, OH.)

Critical pathways is a patient care plan that specifies daily goals, interventions to help attain those goals, and a method of documentation. This is developed by the nurse, patient, significant other, and other members of the health team with the physician's plan of treatment and preferences kept in mind. A benefit of critical pathways is that it gives a concise treatment plan that also simplifies documentation for the nurse and is readily understood by any caregiver who reviews it.

A major benefit of primary nursing is that it provides a sense of continuity of care and a bond of empathy and responsibility between a nurse and a patient. Communications must be open, ongoing, and pertinent to specific patient needs so that the patient, the family, the primary nurse, and other health team members can maintain this continuity as the patient recovers and returns to the home and community.

## The Office Nurse

The office nurse has greater responsibility for preparation of the patient who is scheduled for surgery than ever before due to an increase in outpatient surgery, same-day admission for surgery, and decreased length of hospital stay. The luxury of admitting the person the day before surgery for perioperative teaching by the staff nurse and preadmission testing is gone due to third-party reimbursement constraints. Also because there is little time for the staff nurse to plan discharge for a patient with a shortened hospital stay, the office nurse must begin this process of discharge planning. If the patient has multiple health problems or a compromised home situation, discharge planning should be started before the day of admission to allow sufficient time to arrange for home care and equipment should they be needed.

Health education must begin in the physician's office and include instruction for the patient and significant others about scheduled testing procedures, preparation for surgery, and discharge instructions for outpatient surgeries. Teaching aids such as booklets and videotapes assist in this teaching and are now often developed for physician offices by nurses to provide information specific to that physician's preference and specialty.

The office nurse is the health care team member who is in the rewarding position of seeing the patient before, during, and after hospitalization during the acute, recovery, and well phase of health. This person is truly a primary nurse and as such should communicate with the hospital staff pertinent patient information as needed to enhance quality care. Communication is also directed to other health team members such as physical therapists, social workers, and public health nurses as is needed for both inpatient and outpatient care. This information will aid in the understanding of the patient and his/her home situation, which will assist in discharge planning.

## The Staff Nurse

Of vital importance are the units' nursing personnel, who provide the day-to-day, 24-hour expert care required by many orthopaedic patients. Staff nurses must be ready to care for patients who may have acute, intense, and often long-term pain. They must know and use multiple techniques beside drug administration to achieve relief of pain, including position changes, massage, relaxation techniques, imaging or visualization, and patient-controlled analgesia techniques and equipment. Staff nurses must be willing to care for the immobilized, dependent patient, who requires patient, intense, long-term care. The nurse must be able to flow with the patient's recovery efforts, yet be able to be firm and persistent during both regressive episodes and rehabilitative periods. A sense of humor helps ease the strain of such long-term relationships.

## The Occupational Therapist

The contribution of occupational therapists and their assistants involve helping a patient learn to cope with a particular condition or injury and to live with limitations. They maximize strengths and potentials. Occupational therapists help patients use exercises to strengthen muscles to enhance balance and ADL activities. They also design or prepare splints and adaptive devices to correct or maintain a specific muscular or joint condition, help patients adjust to using alternate muscles or joints when necessary, assist with patients' visual or perceptive exercises to enhance mental or special sense(s) functions, and help plan or teach recreational or diversional activities if needed. Occupational therapists also help patients make the transition from hospital to home.

## The Physical Therapist

Physical therapists assist orthopaedic patients to maximize their functional independence through gait and ambulation techniques and training, performing and teaching range of motion exercises with or without resistance, teaching exercises for rehabilitation, and using strengthening exercises to prepare patients for self-care and hospital discharge (see Figure 1.4).

## The Orthopaedic Technician

Technicians with specialized training, referred to as orthopaedic technicians, are valuable aides to assist with cast applications, inventory, and ordering the many and varied pieces of equipment needed for orthopaedic patients (see Figure 1.5). They may be a valuable asset to staffs on other nursing units in providing and setting up orthopaedic equipment needed for patients. Orthopaedic technicians also assist with the nursing care of orthopaedic patients.

## The Dietitian

The dietitian determines the patient's nutritional needs, monitors the patient's daily intake, suggests dietary changes to correct nutritional deficiencies, teaches dietary changes to patients or family, and assists in menu selection, considering both dietary preferences and the health status of the patient.

## The Social Worker

The social worker or RN discharge planner assists the patient, family, and other team members during the patient's hospitalization to handle the financial arrangements for home or extended care if needed. The social worker is a liaison for community services that might be needed after discharge. Because of the time required to locate and arrange for community services, the social worker's input to the patient's

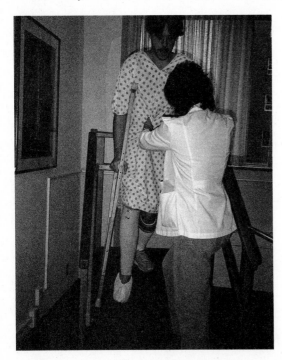

**Figure 1.4** Patient descending stairs in on-unit physical therapy room with the aid of the physical therapist.

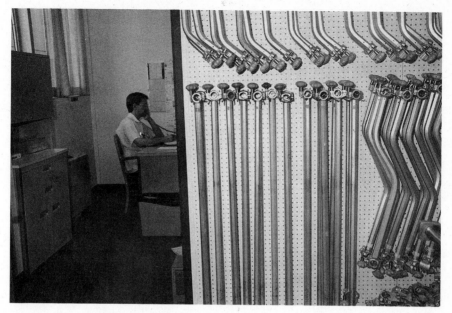

**Figure 1.5** *An orthopaedic technician assists with cast or traction applications, ordering and maintaining supplies, and patient care.*

interdisciplinary team provides for the best and most timely utilization of services. Continuity of care referrals are coordinated with all other members with or by the nurse and social worker for ease of patient transfer and care. Continuity-of-care forms are filled out and sent to the appropriate health agency to ensure uninterrupted patient care. Understanding insurance provisions, Medicare policies, and funding or reimbursement problems or possibilities are invaluable assets of social services for patient care.

## THE ORTHOPAEDIC NURSING UNIT

Because delivery of care to the hospitalized patient is so vital to the patient's recovery, the setting in which the care is provided must be conducive to the provision of top-quality care. The requirements of an orthopaedic unit setting and background demographics are discussed below.

The orthopaedic nursing unit should be designed with an understanding of the special, and sometimes unique, nursing care needs of a patient immobilized by the extent or nature of his or her injuries or by the particular treatment used for those injuries. The physical layout of the nursing unit should accommodate the patient's mobility limitations, provide for the patient's unwieldly cast or traction setup, and provide facilities for rehabilitation. Though some of the facilities, layout, and equipment on an orthopaedic nursing unit are similar to those of other nursing units, the particular equipment and care needed for orthopaedic patients require careful preplanning and incorporation of those specifications into the architectural designs and construction of the areas to be designated as the orthopaedic nursing unit.

Ideally, the physical layout of the unit should be determined by a formulating committee during the development of the architectural designs for a hospital or building expected to house patients with orthopaedic conditions. Members of the formulating committee should be those staff members who will be the "users" of the unit along with those with information about building codes, funding limitations, and the feasibility of incorporating suggested plans into the completed hospital or building. Thus, physicians, nurses, physical and occupational therapists, engineers, administrators, and architects should provide input as permanent or temporary members of the formulating committee. In addition, dietitians and social workers can provide vital input during the designing phase before construction begins. Each member brings to the planning meetings the knowledge or expertise vital to the development (or remodeling) of an orthopaedic unit that will be the most functional, cost effective, and satisfying to all concerned.

## Impact of Demographics

Before the blueprints for the unit are completed, members of the formulating committee must have an understanding of the demographics of the expected patient population correlated with health care trends, medical and surgical treatments of orthopaedic patients, and the nursing care and staffing considerations involved in the care and rehabilitation of orthopaedic patients.

Examination of the demographics of the expected orthopaedic patients should help determine the projected bed capacity of the unit, the number and qualifications of the staff, the type of patient rooms (whether private, semiprivate, or other), and auxiliary services needed.

Demographic information can be obtained from the admitting department or staff physicians and should include the average age of patients, the projected length of stay, the average daily census for persons with orthopaedic conditions, methods of payment, and the types and frequencies of various diagnoses.

The average age of patients depends on whether or not patients of all ages are to be admitted to a particular hospital. Children and adolescents may be cared for in "children's" hospitals, raising the age of patients in the projected orthopaedic unit. Also, the average age of patients must be considered when nurses are employed for specific nursing units; when the census reveals a high percentage of older or elderly patients, nurses with skills in gerontology would be the most cost effective, just as hiring nurses with skills in pediatric nursing would benefit pediatric patients.

The nature and design of educational materials are also influenced by the average-age data. Booklets and information sheets in larger print are more suitable for elderly persons; video cassettes may be more suitable for young people.

Just as the ages of patients must be taken into consideration during the planning of an orthopaedic unit, the number of beds assigned to the unit should be determined by the length of stay and average daily census for patients with orthopaedic conditions. If the average census is projected to be or actually is 20 patients, and the unit is planned for 40, the planners and administrators may design a smaller area or plan to place patients from other services on or next to the orthopaedic unit. A suitable "marriage" would be to combine orthopaedic patients with others requiring long-term rehabilitation, such as patients with neurological or neurosurgical conditions.

Payment policies and procedures influence both admissions to hospital units and nursing care because of some of their restrictive limitations. For example, Medicare, DRGs, insurance companies and specific policies all have requirements for payment of the patient's medical or hospitalization costs either to the patient or directly to the hospital. At times when patients are paying their bills with their own or insurance money, they may have covert expectations for amenities (private showers, suites, and the like) and although they may not make overt demands for such facilities, they may not accept readmission to a hospital lacking such facilities. Because of the current restrictions for payment of hospital and medical bills, patient expectations must be incorporated into the planning using the demographic data.

Another piece of the demographic "pie" concerns the type and frequency of the various orthopaedic diagnoses in patients on the orthopaedic unit. As was stated above, when hiring staff, the type and frequency of diagnosis—as for example, a large proportion of older persons admitted for total joint surgeries or following hip fractures—have an influence on the physical facilities to be constructed. Additionally, if sports injuries occur frequently in the proximity of the hospital, facilities must include equipment for the appropriate care and rehabilitation, including therapy facilities with strengthening and exercise equipment.

Following examination of the patient demographics, consideration must be given to the degree or extent of the patient's immobility, and facilities must be incorporated into the design of the unit to meet the patients' needs in the various stages of regaining mobility.

## Physical Requirements of the Unit

The physical placement of the unit should be based on ready access to other departments or units having services which are needed by those on the orthopaedic unit. Since most orthopaedic patients require physical or occupational therapies, the orthopaedic unit should be near enough to these departments for ease of consultation, transportation, and patient use of the services in these areas. Proximity enables the physician or nurse to more easily monitor the patient's condition or progress in rehabilitation.

Each nursing unit contains a nurses' station or nurses' center as the focal area on the nursing unit. Usually nursing stations have racks for patients' charts; unit manager or secretary spaces; assignment boards for nurses and patient listing by room or service; computers, desks or tables; and files, drawers, and shelves for nursing manuals or reference books and patient education materials. Nursing stations on an orthopaedic unit should also have x-ray viewboxes for ready x-ray viewing for diagnosis or teaching. Several viewboxes mounted securely on a wall permit viewing several x-rays simultaneously.

The layout of the patient's room on the orthopaedic unit must be thoughtfully planned and designed. Ideally, the rooms will have windows. Changes in climate and seasonal conditions provide orientation and reality to long-hospitalized patients, and efforts should be made for rooms with windows having unobstructed views of the outside world. Sunlight adds a cheery dimension not available with artificial lighting, whatever its intensity, although high-intensity lighting is necessary for good visibility during examinations, assessments of neurovascular status, and for wound examinations, irrigations, and dressing changes.

Each room should have a personal bathroom equipped with an unobstructed entrance for a wheelchair. The shower should have a hand-held removable shower head with flexible tubing. The soap shelf should be at waist level with a signal call light easily reachable from the shower or toilet. The sink should have bat-wing faucet handles for use by persons with limited small-muscle motor skills. If pipes project under the sink, they should be covered with insulation to protect the extremities of a wheelchair patient from being burned if they touch hot pipes (see Fig. 1.6).

Handrails in the shower or beside the toilet should be within easy reach (see Figs. 1.7 and 1.8). Rails next to the toilet are more functional if they are slanted downward and toward the base of the toilet and are as close to the toilets as practical. If handrails are too high, they are nonfunctional; they may even be hazardous if they are in the way of a wheelchair, cane, or crutches.

The toilet itself should be 23 inches in height from the floor. This is an optimal height to prevent a fall for a patient after a total hip replacement. The 23-inch height is higher than standard toilets, which also prevents

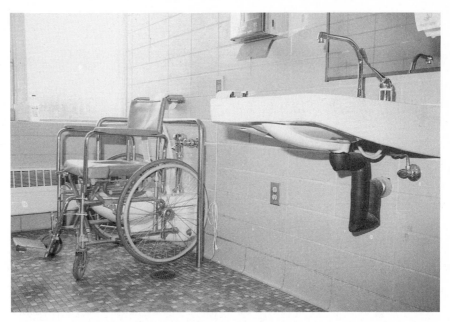

**Figure 1.6** Insulated pipes under sink to prevent burns in patients using a wheelchair.

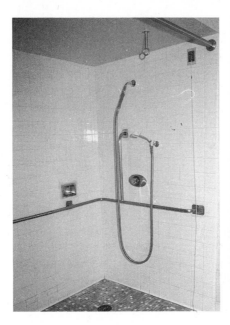

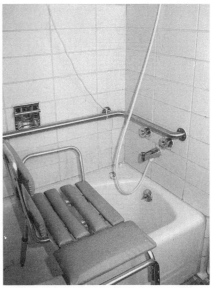

**Figure 1.7** Shower with wheelchair access and wall supports for patient safety.

**Figure 1.8** Tub and shower area with padded seat and chair for use of weak and injured patients. Note wall supports and signal cord within easy reach.

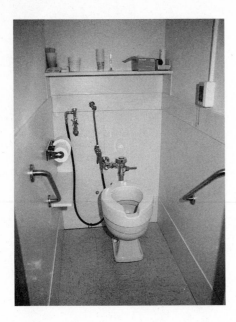

**Figure 1.9** Toilet seat raised to 23 inches to prevent hip dislocation.

overflexion of the operated hip, which could result in loosening or dislocation (see Fig. 1.9). For safety, the toilet seat should be permanently mounted or attached to the porcelain toilet to prevent its loosening. A temporary seat could be unsafe for orthopaedic patients, who are less mobile or weaker than some other types of patients. Heights of handrails, signal call lights, and sinks should be decided by using average heights of persons sitting in wheelchairs and actually using the attachments as the parameters for placement. Having a sink at wheelchair height is necessary for grooming, personal hygiene, and washing hair. Finally, the bathroom may not contain a bathtub, because limitations imposed by incisions, medical condition, weight-bearing limitations, or the presence of a cast makes a tub inaccessible to many orthopaedic patients. The door to the bathroom should be oriented so that opening and closing pose no difficulty or obstruction of easy passage in or out of the bathroom.

If the patient's room contains a television, it should be a small model suspended on a pull-out arm mounted near the head of the bed for easy access. Such mounting is space-preserving and is safer than mounting on the ceiling or at the foot of the bed. Stationary televisions may be caught by or in the overbed frame when the bed's height is adjusted, posing a hazard to the patient, to visitors, and to the set itself.

Sturdy, recessible hooks or arms can be mounted on the wall near the head of the bed (and in the bathroom beside the sink or toilet) to provide sites to hang intravenous bags. Such hooks or arms can also be used to support vertical slings used for elevating extremities.

The entire patient room size must allow for use of wheelchairs, walkers, crutches, canes, therapy equipment, or even a bedside commode. A room with insufficient space adds to a patient's frustrations when he or she is trying to manipulate unwieldly or unfamiliar apparatus while learning to ambulate with the equipment. The assisting personnel should be able to walk unobstructed alongside the patient for safety. The doors to the rooms (and the rooms themselves) should be large enough to permit passage of a cart (gurney) into the room for transporting patients (see Fig. 1.10). The width of doors should also then permit safe transfer of bedfast patients in casts or in traction with an overbed frame. Free passage of the bed and equipment is essential to prevent jarring the patient, which could cause additional pain or injury.

Designing the patients' rooms with a "toe-to-toe" arrangement of the beds allows for best utilization of available space (see Fig. 1.11). This design allows space on either side and at the foot of the bed, in contrast to typical semiprivate rooms, which have side-by-side placement of the beds. With toe-to-toe or foot-to-foot bed placement, the heads of the beds face each other for ease of patient interaction, and a curtain or folding door provides for privacy when desired.

Each side of this semiprivate room has its own phone and call system. A bulletin board or piece of plexiglass or plastic mounted on the wall provides space for cards or posters to personalize the room. This helps deter the taping of cards to the walls, which can damage them.

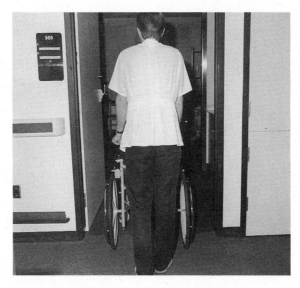

**Figure 1.10** Extra-wide doorway for easy access with a wheelchair or bed with traction frame.

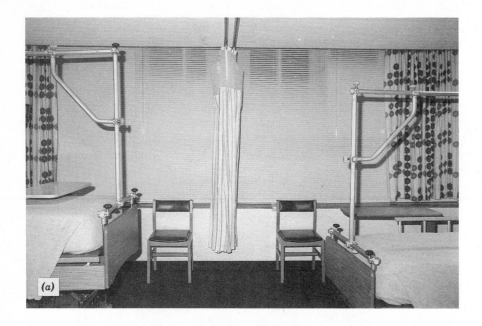

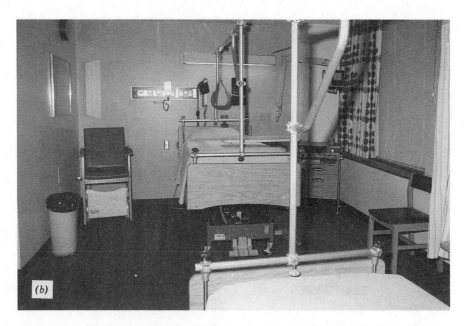

**Figure 1.11** (a) Toe-to-toe or foot-to-foot arrangement of patient beds to aid care and ambulation in unobstructed areas. (b) View from one end of the same room. Note recessed light, television, wall-mounted equipment, and chair with leg support.

Overhead or overbed lighting on the head wall should not protrude from the wall, because the light could be hit by the overbed frame when the height of the bed is adjusted. A loose fixture could be dangerous.

Just as patient rooms are designed to incorporate specific equipment or needs, the entire orthopaedic unit must be designed to provide sufficient space for equipment storage, application of casts, and on-unit physical and occupational therapy if feasible.

A specific room for cast applications, changing, or removal is vital. Such a room contains all the many materials needed for applications of any size or type of cast. Figs. 1.12 and 1.13 show the contents of a cast room. Because of physician preferences and cost containment, several (but not all) sizes and types of cast materials are available in the inventory of cast materials (see Fig. 1.14).

The cast room has a table for cast applications, with a part or parts that are removable and adjustable as needed. Cabinets contain the various skin coverings and padding used for skin protection when necessary. An overhead bar is built above the cast table to permit suspension of extremity(ies) during the application of the cast. The bar contains finger holds to support an upper extremity if needed. A sink is also near the cast table for water if plaster is used. Warming or drying lights or lamps are also readily accessible if needed for a specific cast material.

The equipment room provides storage for equipment, such as pulleys, splints, overhead frames, various parts of traction, walkers, and crutches. The need for such storage should be determined before space is designed on the unit (see Fig. 1.15).

On-unit physical and occupational therapy room or rooms offer proximity to the orthopaedic unit and utilization of equipment for maximal patient benefit. Having smaller on-unit rooms for these therapies lessens transportation time and conserves patient energy for specific therapies, as well as permitting close monitoring of patients' progress by the orthopaedic staff. The physical therapy room should have stationary ambulatory aids, such as parallel bars and a stairway; a full-length mirror for viewing a patient's posture and gait; and exercise or strengthening equipment, such as an exercise bicycle, and pulleys with weights and ropes for strengthening exercises. The room should be large enough for several patients to undergo simultaneous therapy and supervision by one therapist, when practical. The on-unit room does not replace the usual large, better supplied or equipped physical therapy room available in most hospitals for hydrotherapy or heat therapy not feasible in the on-unit room (see Fig. 1.16).

The occupational therapy section or on-unit room should have table space, counters, a sink, cabinets for equipment and supplies, and outlets for special equipment for patients to regain the use of weak or atrophied

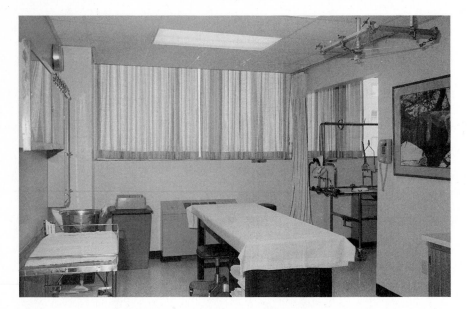

**Figure 1.12** Set-up of cast room for patients. Viewboxes are wall-mounted for viewing x-rays. Overhead bars are available for assistance with cast applications, and a Risser table is available (background, right) for application of spica casts.

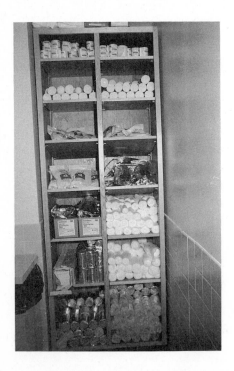

**Figure 1.13** Shelves holding materials for different types of casts including plaster, fiberglass, and casts with adhesive-backed tape.

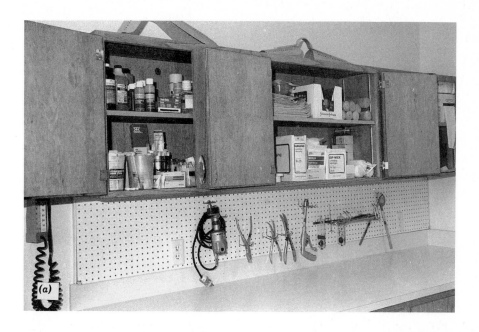

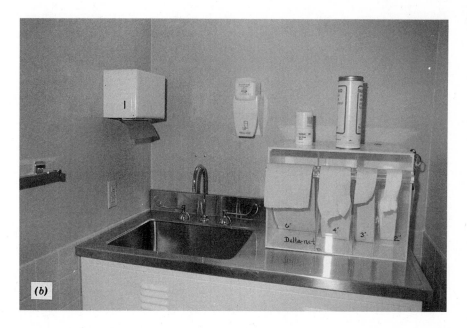

**Figure 1.14** (a) Shelves with accessory materials and equipment, including a cast cutter, for use with casts. (b) Sink for wetting plaster rolls, cleaning equipment and use by personnel; counter space for storage of cast padding materials and work space.

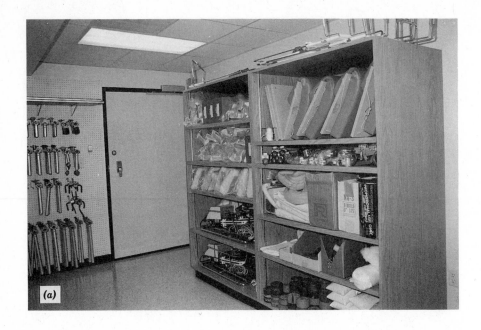

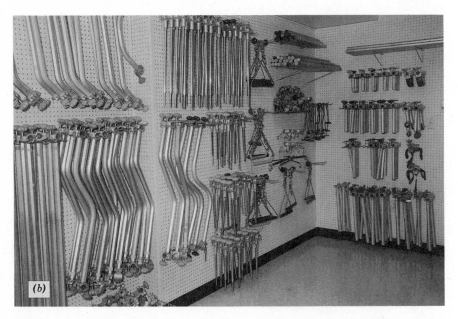

**Figure 1.15** Storage rooms for equipment for use in the care of orthopaedic patients.

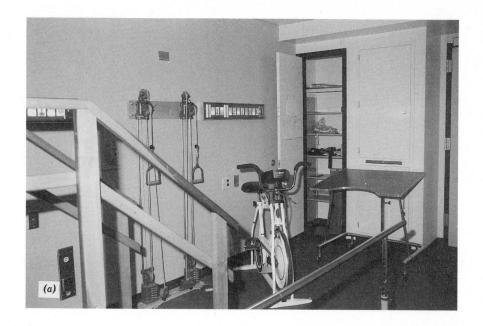

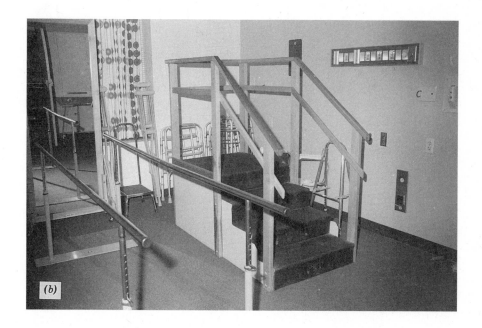

**Figure 1.16** On-unit physical therapy rooms showing (a) exercise bicycle and pulleys with weights and (b) parallel bars and stairs.

muscles and joints. Materials and an area for splintmaking and storage are valuable for the therapist to prepare and adjust splints to individual patient needs and specifications. The occupational therapy area may contain a tub and toilet to simulate a home environment to teach ADL when needed. No plumbing is needed, because the tub and toilet are used only to simulate transferring, toileting, and bathing. Home management techniques can be taught or learned with alternate muscles or joints in the simulated kitchen under the therapist's supervision.

Equipment used for strengthening or stretching exercises should be carefully mounted or stabilized for patient safety. Pulleys should be wall-mounted on a reinforced wall to prevent loosening. Pulleys, ropes, and weights should also be placed for use by patients in wheelchairs. Space should also be available for small-muscle activities, such as weaving, knitting, writing, or painting and for patient examination and record-keeping if needed.

The use of equipment for rehabilitation, and the layout and setting of the orthopaedic unit in general, are based on specific knowledge of the human body and of the patient's physical limitations in recovering from orthopaedic problems. As members of the health care team, nurses caring for patients with orthopaedic conditions must have a current, thorough knowledge of the musculoskeletal tissues, their anatomy and physiology, and methods of physical assessment in Chapter 2.

## BIBLIOGRAPHY

American Nurses' Association and National Association of Orthopaedic Nurses. (1986). *Orthopaedic nursing practice.* Kansas City, MO: American Nurses' Association.

Beckman, J.S. (1987). What is a standard of practice? *Journal of Nursing Quality Assurance, 1*(2), 1–6.

Fralic, Maryann, Kowalski, Patricia M., Llewellyn, Fay A. (1991, April). The Staff Nurse as Quality Monitor, *American Journal of Nursing, 91*(4): 40–42.

Gettrust, K.V., Ryan, S.C. & Engleman, D.S. (Eds.). (1985). *Applied Nursing Diagnosis.* New York: Wiley.

Haselford, Dianne. (1990). Patient Assessment, Association of Operating Room Nurses, 52(3):551–557.

Lucatorto, Michelle, Petras, Denise, Drew, Leslie. (1991, March). Documentation, *Journal of Nursing Administration,* 21(3):32–36.

Marker, C.G. (1987). The marker model: A hierarchy for nursing standards. *Journal of Nursing Quality Assurance,* 1(2), 7–20.

McClure, Margaret L. (1990). Shortage and Standards—an Incompatible Duo? *Journal of Professional Nursing,* 6(6):322.

Mosher, Cynthia, Cronk, Pamela, Kidd, Andrea, McCormick, Patricia, Stockton, Susan, and Sulla, Cynthia. (1992, January). Upgrading Practice with Critical Pathways, *American Journal of Nursing*, 41–44.

Tucker, S.M. (1984). *Patient care standards* (3rd ed.). St. Louis, MO: Mosby.

Zander, Karen. (1985, March) Second Generation Primary Nursing, *The Journal of Nursing Administration*, 18–24.

# MUSCULOSKELETAL TISSUES: ANATOMY AND PHYSIOLOGY AND PHYSICAL ASSESSMENT

To be healthy is a major goal of all people. Healthy, well persons are able to function through their daily activities with free and easy, pain-free movements. However, as people live and age, they encounter situations that affect their health and limit their easy, pain-free movements. Conditions involving the musculoskeletal tissues—including trauma, inflammations, infections, or tumors—cause discomfort and pain and limit easy mobility. At times, these conditions result in permanent health impairment, disability, and even death.

Nurses involved in the care of persons with orthopaedic conditions must have current knowledge and skills to help their patients regain as much health as possible and maintain a healthier state. Nurses, thus, must have basic understanding of the tissues that comprise the musculoskeletal system, the types of conditions affecting those tissues that they might encounter in their nursing activities, methods of treating these conditions, and the nursing considerations associated with orthopaedic health alterations. The remainder of this book focuses on the knowledge and skills necessary for expert nursing care.

## ANATOMY AND PHYSIOLOGY

Musculoskeletal tissues include bones, muscles, ligaments, cartilage, tendons, synovium, bursae, and collagen fibers.

### Bones

The skeleton is comprised of 206 bones shaped according to their function (Wolff's law). Fig. 2.1 shows the major skeletal bones, some of which are long (femur and humerus), short (ankle), flat (sternum or scapula), round (patella)

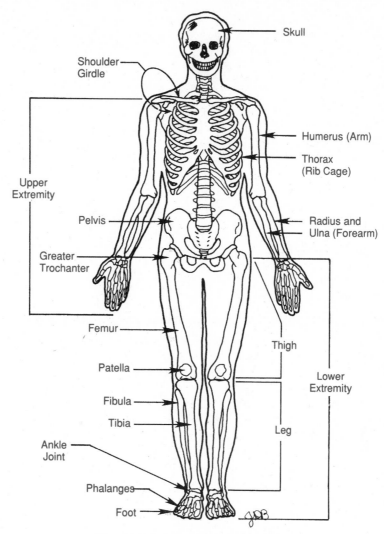

**Figure 2.1** Major bones of the body.

or irregular (ilium or vertebra). The 206 skeletal bones are arranged in two divisions: the *axial skeleton,* comprised of the bones of the skull, face, and auditory ossicles, ribs, vertebrae, sternum, and hyoid bone; and the *appendicular skeleton,* containing the bones of the upper and lower extremities, shoulders, and pelvis.

Divisional planes and directional terms are useful in describing anatomical locations in the body as shown in Fig. 2.2. The *transverse* plane divides the body into upper and lower halves, the *coronal* plane divides it into front and back

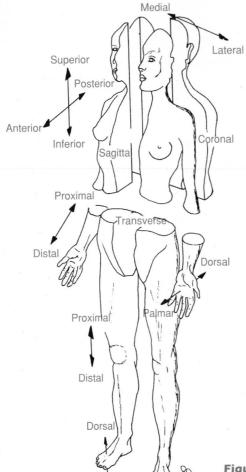

**Figure 2.2** Planes and directions related to the anatomic locations of the body.

parts, and the *sagittal* plane divides it into vertical quarters parallel to the vertical midline. Directional terms in Fig. 2.2 include *superior*, toward the cranial end of the body; *inferior*, toward the foot; *anterior*, toward the front; *posterior*, toward the back; *medial*, toward the center; *lateral*, toward the side; *proximal*, toward the midline; *distal*, away from the midline; *palmar*, toward the ventral (palmar) surface; *dorsal*, toward the posterior or back surface; and *plantar*, toward the sole of the foot.

Long bones consist of a shaft—the diaphysis—separated from the two ends—the epiphyses—by the growth plate and nutrient arteries of the metaphysis (see Fig. 2.3). Bones have a hard, dense outer surface (cortex) of

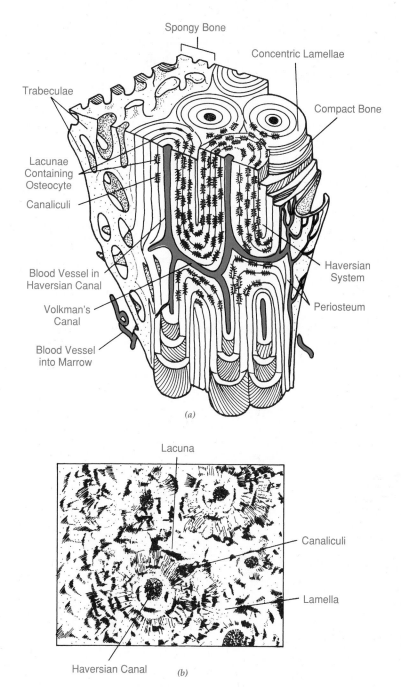

**Figure 2.3** (a) Bone showing haversian canal, cortical, and cancellous (spongy) bone. (b) Portion of compact bone showing lamella, canaliculi, lacuna, and haversian canal.

compact bone containing calcium to give them strength and rigidity. Approximately 99% of the calcium in the body is contained in the bony skeleton. The shafts of the long bones contain yellow bone marrow consisting primarily of fat cells giving it a yellow color. The yellow marrow has no identifiable function except in times of stress, when it can be converted to red marrow to assist in hematopoiesis, the process of blood cell formation in the bone marrow. The red marrow functions as the major hematopoietic tissue to produce red blood cells, white blood cells, and megakaryocytes, the cells that are essential for the production and proliferation of platelets in the bone marrow (megakaryocytes normally are not found in the circulating peripheral blood). Red bone marrow is contained in the ends of bones that are composed of softer, spongy areas of cells, referred to as cancellous bone. Cancellous bone is located in the ends of long bones, the crests of the iliac bones, the tibia, and the sternum.

Bones have a tough outer membrane, the periosteum, for protection and nutrition. Nutrient arteries in the periosteum bring oxygen and remove wastes. These arteries communicate with the haversian system in the central canal of bones.

Fig. 2.3 shows views of compact bones containing the haversian canals with their circular layers of compact bone cells (lamellae), penetrated by small passageways (canaliculi), which connect and open into tiny spaces (lacunae). The lacunae contain osteocytes, the bone-forming cells. Nutrient vessels course through the lamellae, canaliculi, and lacunae. These vessels carry nutrients for bone building and remove wastes and debris from bone resorption or bone growth. Osteocytes, the major bone-forming cells, develop from osteoblasts, spindle-shaped cells found under the periosteum and in the endosteum, the inner region of bones. Osteoblasts, in turn, are developed from fibroblasts.

Embryonic bone development and the formation of cartilage into bone is completed by the third month of gestation through two processes of ossification, either by intramembranous or endochondral ossification. Intramembranous ossification accounts for the majority of the flat bones plus the width and strength of bones. Endochondral ossification is directed or guided by a pattern of preformed, calcified cartilage matrix, which gives the length to cylindrical bones.

As shown in Figs. 2.4–2.6, the outer surfaces of bones contain prominences, ridges, grooves, depressions, and articulating surfaces, with each serving a specific purpose. Grooves or ridges provide indentations for nerves or blood vessels, whereas prominences provide attachment sites for ligaments, tendons, and muscles. Alveoli (sockets), sinuses (cavities), fissures (slits), and foramina (openings for nerves, blood vessels, or muscles) are also found on bones, as shown in Figs. 2.4–2.6.

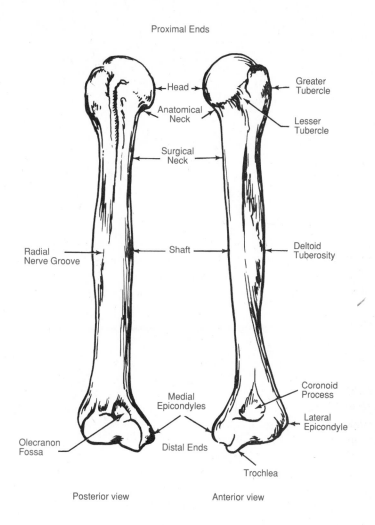

Proximal Ends

Head

Greater
Tubercle

Anatomical
Neck

Lesser
Tubercle

Surgical
Neck

Radial
Nerve Groove

Shaft

Deltoid
Tuberosity

Medial
Epicondyles

Coronoid
Process

Lateral
Epicondyle

Olecranon
Fossa

Distal Ends

Trochlea

Posterior view

Anterior view

**Figure 2.4** *Posterior and anterior views of the humerus showing the multiple grooves, depressions, and outgrowths common to bones.*

*Functions of Bones.* Bones have five functions:
- Support to permit erect posture
- Protection of internal organs
- Movement in coordination with muscles and nerves
- Hematopoiesis in the red bone marrow
- Storage of minerals, particularly calcium and phosphorus.

Bones are not inert structures. They are in constant processes of formation or resorption according to the particular needs of the person. Through those

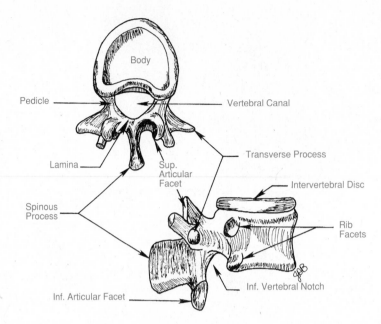

Body

Pedicle

Vertebral Canal

Lamina

Transverse Process

Sup.
Articular
Facet

Intervertebral Disc

Spinous
Process

Rib
Facets

Inf. Articular Facet

Inf. Vertebral Notch

**Figure 2.5** Views of a vertebra showing its irregularities and intervertebral disc.

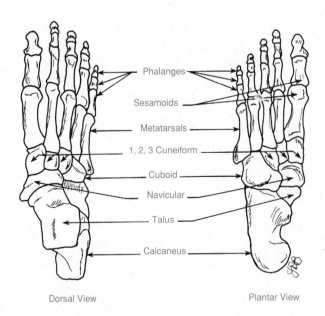

Phalanges

Sesamoids

Metatarsals

1, 2, 3 Cuneiform

Cuboid

Navicular

Talus

Calcaneus

Dorsal View

Plantar View

**Figure 2.6** Dorsal and plantar views of a normal foot showing the multiple irregular shapes and sizes of the bones.

processes, bones are prevented from becoming excessively thick and heavy or unhealthily thin and weak. Influences on bone formation and resorption include:

- *Serum calcium and phosphate levels.* Bone matrix is primarily made of calcium phosphate crystals. Low serum levels of either calcium or phosphate delay bone formation.

- *Vitamin D intake and activation.* Vitamin D stimulates absorption of calcium from the intestines; thus, low serum levels of Vitamin D result in less intestinal calcium absorption and, therefore, low serum calcium content for use in bone formation. For Vitamin D to be active in calcium absorption, it must be biochemically activated in the liver, then by the kidneys through the stimulation of parathormone from the parathyroid gland. Inadequate Vitamin D intake and activation causes rickets in children and osteomalacia in adults (see p. 232).

- *Immobility or inactivity.* Exercise and active muscle movements enhance bone retention of calcium; calcium is lost from bones from immobility and inactivity.

- *Infection.* Infection causes bone lysis or reduction through the processes of inflammation and infection.

- *Hypophosphatasia.* This metabolic condition is due to a lack of the enzyme alkaline phosphatase which is necessary for the normal mineralization of bone. Without sufficient alkaline phosphatase osteoid structures cannot accept and use mineral salts to form bone; this results in rickets in children and osteomalacia in adults.

- *Osteoporosis.* This condition occurs in both men and women, but it is more commonly found in women following menopause. It is characterized by a reduction in bone mass or quantity caused by a decreased rate of bone synthesis. Osteoporotic bones have thin cortices and trabeculae that are fine and sparse, making these bones more subject to fracturing, and deformation leading to pain and disability.

The bones form the skeleton, but bones need muscles in order to be moved.

## Muscles

Muscles of the musculoskeletal system are referred to as striated, as they are composed of layers or long bundles with light and dark bands. Muscles make up about 40% of one's body weight and provide contour and shape over bones (see Figs. 2.7 and 2.8).

Skeletal muscles are contained within a membrane, the sarcolemma. Inside the membrane is the muscle cytoplasm, the sarcoplasm. The muscle cells (myofibrils) are lined longitudinally within the sarcoplasm in alternating light and dark transverse bands, the striae.

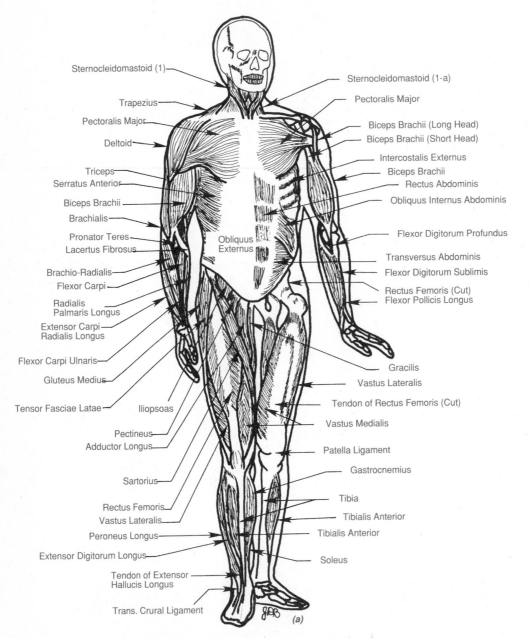

Sternocleidomastoid (1)

Trapezius

Pectoralis Major

Deltoid

Triceps
Serratus Anterior

Biceps Brachii

Brachialis

Pronator Teres
Lacertus Fibrosus

Brachio-Radialis
Flexor Carpi

Radialis
Palmaris Longus

Extensor Carpi
Radialis Longus

Flexor Carpi Ulnaris

Gluteus Medius

Tensor Fasciae Latae

Iliopsoas

Pectineus
Adductor Longus

Sartorius

Rectus Femoris
Vastus Lateralis

Peroneus Longus

Extensor Digitorum Longus

Tendon of Extensor
Hallucis Longus

Trans. Crural Ligament

Obliquus
Externus

Sternocleidomastoid (1-a)

Pectoralis Major

Biceps Brachii (Long Head)
Biceps Brachii (Short Head)

Intercostalis Externus
Biceps Brachii
Rectus Abdominis

Obliquus Internus Abdominis

Flexor Digitorum Profundus

Transversus Abdominis
Flexor Digitorum Sublimis
Rectus Femoris (Cut)
Flexor Pollicis Longus

Gracilis

Vastus Lateralis

Tendon of Rectus Femoris (Cut)

Vastus Medialis

Patella Ligament

Gastrocnemius

Tibia
Tibialis Anterior

Tibialis Anterior

Soleus

**Figure 2.7** Muscles of the body: (a) anterior view.

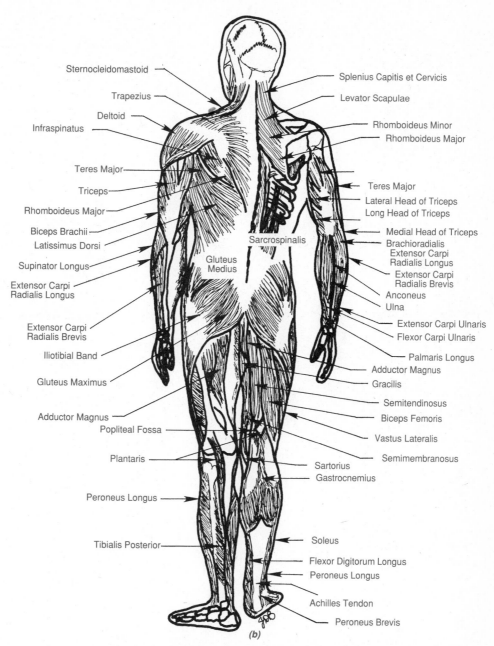

Sternocleidomastoid

Trapezius

Deltoid

Infraspinatus

Teres Major

Triceps

Rhomboideus Major

Biceps Brachii

Latissimus Dorsi

Supinator Longus

Extensor Carpi
Radialis Longus

Extensor Carpi
Radialis Brevis

Iliotibial Band

Gluteus Maximus

Adductor Magnus

Popliteal Fossa

Plantaris

Peroneus Longus

Tibialis Posterior

Splenius Capitis et Cervicis

Levator Scapulae

Rhomboideus Minor

Rhomboideus Major

Teres Major

Lateral Head of Triceps

Long Head of Triceps

Medial Head of Triceps

Brachioradialis

Extensor Carpi
Radialis Longus

Extensor Carpi
Radialis Brevis

Anconeus

Ulna

Extensor Carpi Ulnaris

Flexor Carpi Ulnaris

Palmaris Longus

Adductor Magnus

Gracilis

Semitendinosus

Biceps Femoris

Vastus Lateralis

Semimembranosus

Sartorius

Gastrocnemius

Soleus

Flexor Digitorum Longus

Peroneus Longus

Achilles Tendon

Peroneus Brevis

Sarcrospinalis

Gluteus
Medius

*(b)*

**Figure 2.7** Muscles of the body: (b) posterior view.

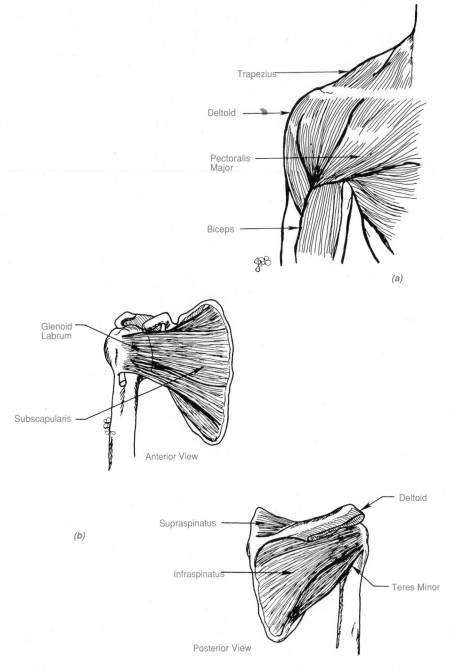

**Figure 2.8** (a) Muscles of the shoulder; (b) anterior and posterior views of the rotator cuff muscles of the shoulder.

Muscles have a large, fleshy section, the belly of the muscle, and taper at the ends into tough, dense fibers called *tendons.* Tendons attach the muscles to bones of the skeleton via the *origin,* the tendon attached to the more fixed, proximal bone, and at the other end via the *insertion,* attached to the more movable or distal bone. Some muscles have two or more origins, such as the biceps femoris, but there is usually only one tendon for insertion to concentrate the full force to one spot (convergence). Some muscles, such as those of the fingers, have several tendons for insertion to spread the action over several joints (divergence). Tendons called aponeuroses are flattened and broadened to serve large areas, such as the abdominal muscles (Fig. 2.7).

Each skeletal muscle sarcolemma is bound with others in bundles (fasciculi) by a connective tissue sheath (perimysium). The bundles of fasciculi are further bound by a stronger sheath (epimysium). These bundles of muscles make up the belly of the muscles, and the epimysium extends from the ends of the muscles to form the *tendon.* Each of the muscles of the extremities has a tough, silvery-looking covering called *fascia,* which helps bind the muscles to each other.

The layers of myofibrils within each sarcolemma form longitudinally through the length of the muscle. Transversely across the myofibrils are alternating bands of myofibrils in light and dark bands of a regular repeating pattern throughout the length of the muscle. Each repeating light, dark pattern of striations is called a *sacromere* which is the functional unit of the contractile system of the muscle.

*Functions of Skeletal Muscles.* Skeletal muscles move the bones of the body through muscle *contractions,* tightening and shortening of the fibers.

The *motor unit* brings about muscle contraction. Each motor unit is innervated by a single motor nerve axon and is composed of 100–200 muscle fibers. The motor nerve stimulates the motor unit of the muscle, which responds with the "all or none principle"—responding entirely or not at all to the stimulus. The strength of the muscle contraction is dependent upon the number of motor units contracting and the number of times per second each motor unit is stimulated. Through a series of interactions at the myoneural (muscle-nerve) junction, muscle contraction is induced. As the stimulus reaches the myoneural junction (motor end plate) of the muscle and synapses with the sarcolemma, acetylcholine is produced and released, bringing about muscle contraction by depolarizing the sarcolemma, allowing calcium ions to enter the muscle membrane to aid in the contraction. The entrance of calcium ions into the muscle cells serves as a catalyst to the energy-releasing processes, which bring about the sliding of actin along the myosin, thus shortening and contracting the muscle. The wave of depolarization spreads throughout the muscle fibers until it is stopped (deactivated) by the enzyme acetylcholinesterase, after which the fiber is again ready for reactivation.

The energy for muscle contraction comes from the hydrolysis of ATP into ADP + phosphate + energy. The energy is used to bring about the sliding of actin along the myosin bands. As needed, additional energy may come from phosphocreatine, a protein-energy source found only in muscle tissues, and from oxygen. Oxygen facilitates muscle contraction by oxidizing lactic acid formed by the anaerobic hydrolysis of the high-energy ATP bonds.

Following contraction, muscles must have a period of relaxation. If not allowed to relax, muscles may develop *spasms* and, possibly, a severe, sustained contraction called *tetanus. Spasms* are involuntary contractions of one or more muscles caused by activation of entire motor units from the repetitive firing of a motor nerve. Muscle spasms commonly occur secondary to trauma, fractures, and surgery. *Tetanus* is a sustained, summated contraction caused by a repetitive series of stimuli conducted along the sarcolemmal membrane.

Muscles are usually in a steady state of readiness (muscle *tone*) throughout the body, ensuring a rapid reaction to an external stimulus. Muscle tone may be increased or decreased, depending on the activity within the nervous system. Ironically, persons with well-toned muscles may have more muscle spasms following trauma or surgery because of the "all or none principle." Well-toned muscles respond to a lower stimulus (stimuli), and more motor units respond and contract. Following trauma or surgical incision in the muscle mass, muscle spasms may occur.

## Tendons

Tendons are the tough, long strands at the ends of muscles (see Fig. 2.9). They are nonelastic bands varying in length from 1 inch to approximately 1 foot (the Achilles tendon in the back of the leg at the heel). The arrangement of the fibers longitudinally in tendons bound together into fascicles gives them high tensile strength, which allows them to transmit forces from muscle to bone or cartilage while remaining undamaged themselves.

*Function of Tendons.* Tendons hold muscles to bones, serving as the origin or insertion of the muscle to bone.

## Ligaments

Ligaments are tough bands of fibers of collagen arranged in parallel bands to add strength. Ligaments are relatively long, depending on where they occur. Ligaments provide great stability to a joint when they are taut (tightened or contracted) by holding the bones in closer proximity to each other. Ligaments possess great tensile strength, but have limited extensibility. Generally, ligaments permit movements in some directions, whereas they limit move-

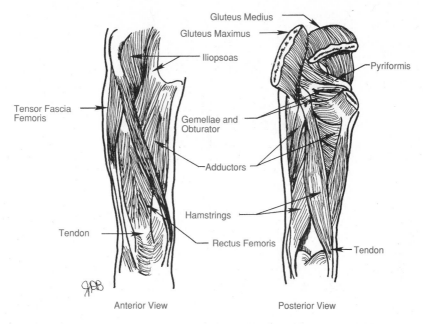

Anterior View          Posterior View

**Figure 2.9** Anterior and posterior views of the muscles of the thigh. Note tendon areas.

ments in other directions. They may encircle or be parallel or oblique to a specific joint (see Fig. 2.10).

*Functions of Ligaments.* Ligaments hold bones to bones as shown in Figure 2.10.

## Cartilage

Cartilage is a white or yellow layer of resilient tissue at the ends of bones. It is generally thought to have an even, smooth surface, but recent electron photomicrographs indicate that the surface may be undulating, with small depressions or rolling valleys (see Fig. 2.11). Thickness of the cartilage layer varies from 2–4 mm and may vary either from area to area within a joint or from joint to joint. Throughout adult life, the thickness of cartilage does not vary unless the cartilage is injured, which occurs frequently, as will be discussed later in this book.

Cartilage covers bones in layers referred to as the superficial, uncalcified layer, intermediate and deep uncalcified layer, and calcified layer. The calcified layer is attached to the underlying bones. Degeneration of hip, knee, and vertebral cartilage is shown in Fig. 2.11.

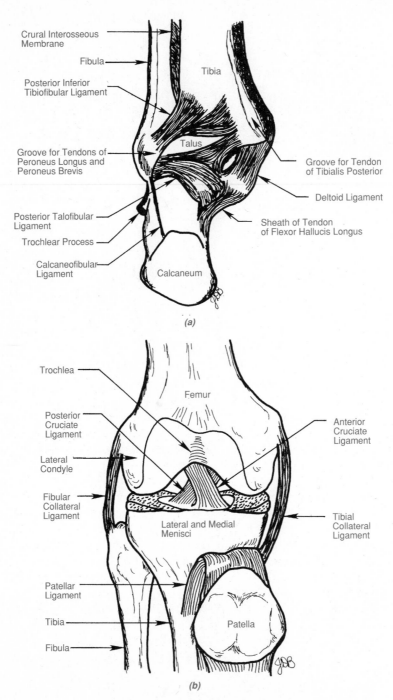

Crural Interosseous Membrane

Fibula

Posterior Inferior Tibiofibular Ligament

Tibia

Talus

Groove for Tendons of Peroneus Longus and Peroneus Brevis

Groove for Tendon of Tibialis Posterior

Deltoid Ligament

Posterior Talofibular Ligament

Trochlear Process

Sheath of Tendon of Flexor Hallucis Longus

Calcaneofibular Ligament

Calcaneum

*(a)*

Trochlea

Femur

Posterior Cruciate Ligament

Anterior Cruciate Ligament

Lateral Condyle

Fibular Collateral Ligament

Tibial Collateral Ligament

Lateral and Medial Menisci

Patellar Ligament

Tibia

Patella

Fibula

*(b)*

**Figure 2.10** (a) Ligaments of the ankle; (b) ligaments of the knee.

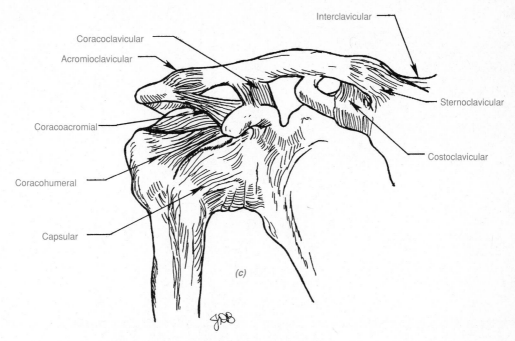

Interclavicular

Coracoclavicular

Acromioclavicular

Sternoclavicular

Coracoacromial

Costoclavicular

Coracohumeral

Capsular

*(c)*

**Figure 2.10** (c) Ligaments of the shoulder.

In most joints, the type of cartilage is referred to as hyaline (resembling glass) and differs from that found in skin, tendon, and bone. It is composed of Type II collagen fibers at its matrix with "filler" material between the matrix fibers; the filler is made of primarily protein-polysaccharide complexes interspersed with water, which gives hyaline cartilage its sponginess and elasticity. These characteristics are vital to prevent injury to either the cartilage or bone during the loading of weight bearing. The water content, for example, of adult patellar cartilage is about 75–80% of its net weight, with similar values in other joints. The water content does not change with aging. Extracellular water, however, increases after long periods of disuse. The water content of the cartilage is generally highest next to the articular surface.

Even in healthy adults, there is evidence that adult synovial joints almost invariably contain sites with local fraying of the articular cartilage interspersed with areas where the surface is intact, though undulating or elevated in spots. Severe fraying may lead to formation of scar (fibrous) tissue, lessening the elasticity of the cartilage.

It is generally thought that cartilage has no intrinsic blood supply, although the calcified layer does contain some intersecting blood vessels. Cartilage receives its nutrients and has waste removed through the synovial fluid forced

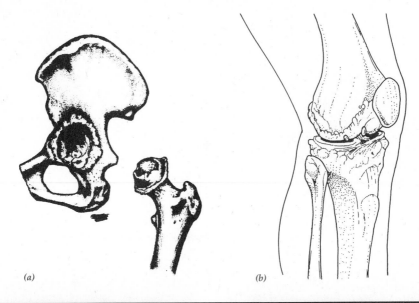

(a)  (b)

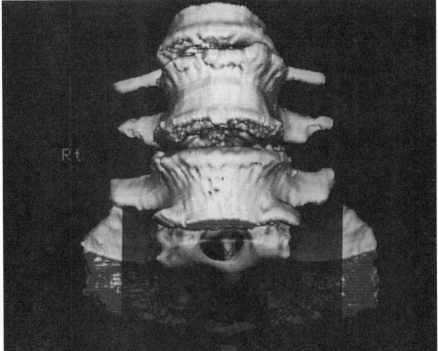

**Figure 2.11** (a) Fraying, cracking, and degeneration of cartilage of the hip.
(b) Degeneration of cartilage of the knee. (c) Degeneration of the annular cartilage
of vertebrae.

into its porous cellular matrix by the movements and weight bearing of the joints. Therefore, for cartilage to remain healthy, *movement and loading are mandatory.* Atrophy of the cartilage will occur if a particular joint ceases movement or weight bearing, leading to limitation of joint movements.

Hyaline cartilage is bluish white, and as well as covering the ends of bones making up synovial joints, it also is found in the ends of ribs, the nasal system, and the walls of the trachea. Fibrous cartilage is white and is particularly resistant to tension. It is found in the knee and symphysis pubis. *Yellow* cartilage is comprised of elastic fibers and is found in the epiglottis and pinna (outer ear).

*Functions of Cartilage.* Cartilage serves to dampen (cushion) the load placed upon it and bone in the process of loading or weight bearing. It absorbs weight through its sponginess and elasticity, and it absorbs shock, stress, and strain to promote movement and aid weight bearing and to prevent injury to joint tissues.

## Synovium

The synovium is a membrane that entirely lines the inside of some joints. It has villous folds which hold the blood vessels and lymphatic vessels to supply synovial fluid, the substance that bathes and lubricates articular cartilage. Synovial fluid also contains nutrients and phagocytes for joint functions.

*Functions of Synovium.* The synovium provides synovial fluid, supplies nutrients to joint tissues, and filters wastes and cells from the joint to protect and prevent joint injuries or infections.

## Bursae

Bursae are small sacs usually found in tendons around joints. Bursae are lined with synovium and contain synovial fluid (Fig. 2.12).

*Functions of Bursae.* Bursae act as cushions to reduce friction between tendons and ligaments to allow them greater freedom of movement. Some of the bursal fluid acts as a lubricant for the tendons and ligaments.

## Collagen

Collagen is a protein substance constituting approximately one-half the total body protein in adults. Collagen is composed of three strands of intertwined polypeptides aligned colinearly throughout the molecule.

Collagen strands are tightly coiled together in a left-handed (minor) helix. They then coil around a common central axis to form a right-handed (major) helix (see Fig. 2.13). This coiled-coil configuration is stabilized by interchain hydrogen bands.

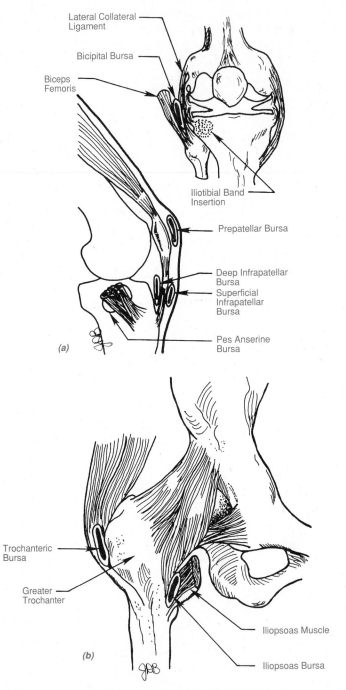

Lateral Collateral Ligament

Bicipital Bursa

Biceps Femoris

Iliotibial Band Insertion

Prepatellar Bursa

Deep Infrapatellar Bursa

Superficial Infrapatellar Bursa

Pes Anserine Bursa

(a)

Trochanteric Bursa

Greater Trochanter

Iliopsoas Muscle

Iliopsoas Bursa

(b)

**Figure 2.12** Bursae of the (a) knee; (b) hip.

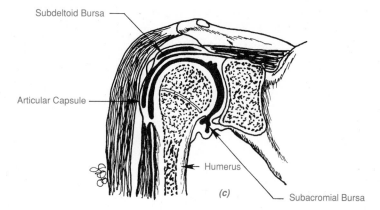

**Figure 2.12** *Bursae of the (c) shoulder.*

Collagen molecules are commonly referred to as Type I, II, or III. Type I collagen fibers are found in all major connective tissues (bones, tendons, dentin, and fibrocartilage) and in some organs. Type I collagen fibers play a major role as support for tissues that normally exhibit very little distensibility under mechanical stress. Type II collagen is found primarily in hyaline cartilage, where it aids in maintaining the mechanical strength of cartilage. Type III collagen is found in tissues that are most distensible, such as the skin, blood vessel walls, and uterine wall. Each type of collagen develops under the control of separate and distinct structural genes, which makes it most suited to its specific tissue and distribution in the body.

*Functions of Collagen.* Collagen gives strength and structure to connective tissues. It also plays an active role in cell attachments, chemotaxis, and the binding of antigen-antibody complexes. "Collagen diseases," now referred to as connective tissue diseases, are inflammatory conditions that can occur in any collagen tissues and frequently are systemic diseases.

## Joints

Joints are connections between bones formed when bone surfaces come together and articulate; they are classified according to their degree of move-

**Figure 2.13** *Strand of collagen showing its helical shape.*

ment. Immovable (synarthrotic) joints found in the skull are held together by fibrous tissues called sutures. Slightly movable (amphiarthrotic) joints of the pubic symphysis and radioulnar joints allow slight movement through their fibrocartilaginous disc or fibroligament, respectively. Freely movable (diarthrotic) joints are the majority of joints, also called synovial joints, because they are lined with synovial membrane. Diarthrotic joints are also identified by their major form of movement, such as ball and socket (hip, shoulders), hinge (elbow, knee), pivot (atlas, axis), gliding (intervertebral), condyloid (wrist), and saddle (first metacarpal and trapezium).

*Function of Joints.* Joints function to bring about movements of other musculoskeletal tissues or to maintain relative immobility between bones, as stated above. Joint movements are referred to as their range(s) of movements.

The range of motion of a joint varies with its movability. Table 2.1 presents the movements of joints. Figs. 2.14–2.19 illustrate many of the movements.

The preceding discussion has focused upon normal growth and development of musculoskeletal tissues. In order to determine the condition of the tissues making up the musculoskeletal system, assessment of the specific tissues is required.

**Table 2.1** Types of Movements of Joints

| | |
|---|---|
| Abduction | Movement away from the midline (see Fig. 2.14a) |
| Adduction | Movement toward the midline (see Fig. 2.14a) |
| Circumduction | Movement in a 360° arc to complete a circle (see Fig. 2.14b) |
| Dorsiflexion | Movement of foot up toward the leg (see Fig. 2.15a) |
| Eversion | Movement of the ankle turning the sole of the foot away from the opposite foot (see Fig. 2.16a) |
| Extension | Straightening or lengthening the angle between two bones (see Fig. 2.17) |
| Flexion | Movements to shorten the angle between two joints (see Fig. 2.17) |
| Inversion | Movement of the ankle turning the sole of the foot toward (facing) the opposite foot (see Fig. 2.16b) |
| Pronation | Movement of forearm and hand to turn the palm down (see Fig. 2.18a) |
| Rotation | Movement of turning one bone or another without changing the angle between the two bones (see Fig. 2.19) |
| External rotation | Rotating the limb outward |
| Internal rotation | Rotating the limb inward |
| Supination | Movement of forearm and hand to turn the palm up (see Fig. 2.18b) |

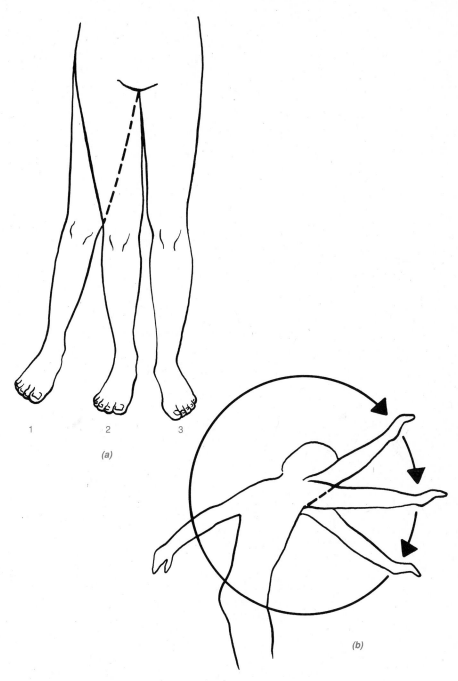

**Figure 2.14** (a) Movements of the hip: (1) abduction, (2) adduction, and (3) neutral position; (b) circumduction of the shoulder and arm.

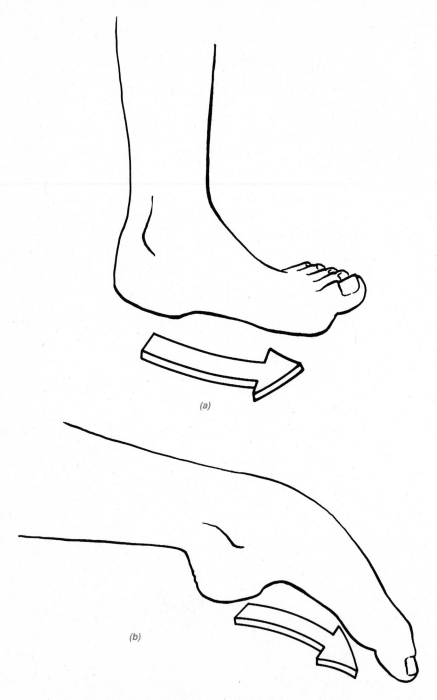

**Figure 2.15** (a) Dorsiflexion; (b) plantarflexion of the foot.

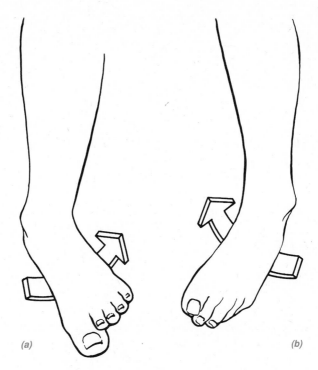

**Figure 2.16** (a) Eversion; (b) inversion of the foot.

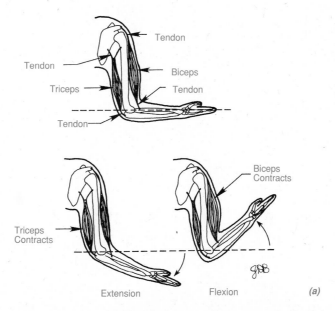

**Figure 2.17** (a) Flexion and extension of the forearm.

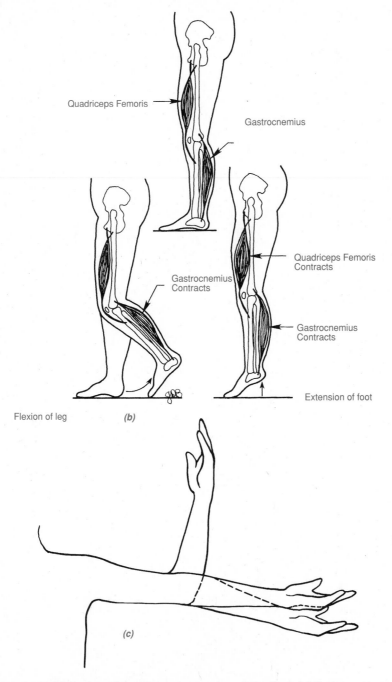

Quadriceps Femoris

Gastrocnemius

Quadriceps Femoris
Contracts

Gastrocnemius
Contracts

Gastrocnemius
Contracts

Extension of foot

Flexion of leg

*(b)*

*(c)*

**Figure 2.17** (b) Flexion of the leg and extension of the foot; (c) flexion, extension, and hyperextension of the forearm.

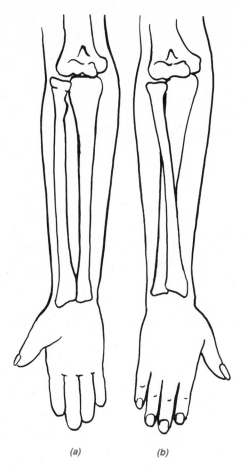

**Figure 2.18** (a) Supination and (b) pronation of the hand and forearm.

(a)          (b)

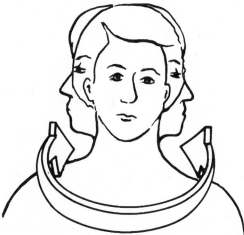

**Figure 2.19** Rotation of the neck.

## Procedures

### Physical Assessment

The purpose of a physical assessment is to determine the current physical status or condition of the person's musculoskeletal tissues and the associated skin areas as a step in diagnosis. Physical assessment may provide evidence to corroborate a patient's complaints and symptoms.

Physical assessment procedures should be done systematically and thoroughly in sequence to ensure that nothing will be overlooked.

The following information provides guidelines for an in-depth assessment. In-hospital physical assessment is usually defined by the specific health care facility.

*Assessment Features*

- Securing a patient history
- Observing the patient's movements and actions
- Examining the patient from head to toe
- Checking reflexes and dermatomes
- Assessing joint movements and ranges of motion
- Inspection and palpation of skin and musculoskeletal tissues plus other areas as indicated by patient's complaints or symptoms
- Auscultation of bruits, breath sounds, and heart sounds as deemed necessary

*Equipment Needed*

- Tape measure to measure extremity circumferences and lengths for bilateral comparisons
- Pin or paper clip for determining discrimination of sharp/dull perceptions
- Reflex hammer for testing reflexes
- Goniometer for measuring angles of joint range of motion (see Fig. 2.20)
- Cotton ball for discrimination of touch
- Sphygmomanometer for determining blood pressure
- Stethoscope for auscultations of blood pressure, bruits, and other sounds
- Thermometer for temperature determination
- Flashlight for pupillary reactions and oral/pharyngeal assessments

*Techniques of Physical Examination*
The examiner:

- Introduces self and states the purposes of the visit.
- Provides for privacy and positions the patient as comfortably as possible.

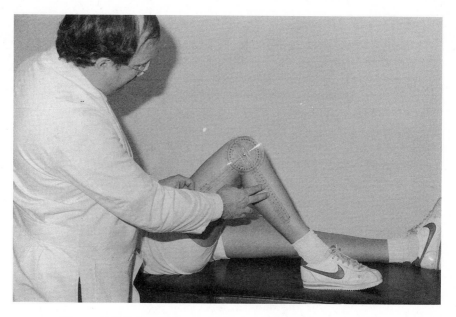

**Figure 2.20** *Measuring joint movements with a goniometer.*

- Obtains the history by interviewing the patient, relative, or significant others and by reviewing previous records. The health history includes gathering data about the patient's:
  - age, sex, ethnocultural and racial data
  - present complaint
  - symptoms of the current condition or illness
  - development, progression, and associated symptoms
  - past medical and surgical conditions with associated dates of each condition or operation
  - childhood diseases and immunization history
  - family health history, with past and present health states, and causes of death elicited and diagrammed
  - social history, including occupation, employment history, hobbies, and recreational history
  - intake of alcohol, tobacco use, and medications (prescribed, over the counter, and other drugs)
  - living arrangements and home layout as they affect or are affected by the patient's present and past health states

- other factors the patient considers to be related to the present condition, such as recent stressors and injuries.
- Performs a systemic "review of systems":
  - verbally goes through the body systems (circulatory, musculoskeletal, neurological, renal, etc.) to determine possible intersystem correlations
- Performs a complete physical examination:
  - Inspects the patient's tissues from head to toe to determine normal or abnormal conditions, such as presence of skin lesions, deformities, and masses.
  - Palpates the tissues to determine their condition, temperature, presence of edema, masses, tenderness, or pain (injured or diseased tissues are examined last to prevent unnecessary discomfort except in life-threatening situations).
  - Auscultates breath sounds, bowel sounds, cardiac sounds, and arterial bruits
  - Percusses for the gastric bubble, thoracic/lung sounds, and the abdominal organs and their sounds
- Asks about the patient's usual activities of daily living, energy levels, ability to do self-care, hygiene, grooming, dressing, bathing, eating, getting in or out of a car, bed, chair, or bathtub, and sleep history
- Observes the patient walk (if condition permits), checking gait, coordination, posture, walking rate, and rhythm or abnormalities (see Table 2.2)
- Measures the active and passive joint ranges of motion (ROMs) (see Table 2.3), and measures joint angles with a goniometer (see Fig. 2.20)
- Rates muscle strength (see Table 2.4)
- Checks skin sensory dermatomes for sharp/dull and 2-point discrimination
- Checks reflexes (see Table 2.5) and does bilateral neurovascular assessments of the tissues comparing their color, temperature, edema, motor and sensory functions, peripheral pulses, capillary refill, and presence of pain
- Measures lengths and circumferences of extremities (variations of less than 1 inch may be related to the "handedness" of the patient or to repetitive activities involving one hand, arm, or leg)
- Performs specific tests of particular joint, muscles, or other tissues (see Tables 2.6 and 2.7 and Figs. 2.21 and 2.22)
- Checks the patient's vital signs and weight (may use the admitting data if recent)
- Clarifies any questions or concerns from the client, as able
- Correlates findings with laboratory data such as hematologic, radiologic, urologic, or other studies

**Table 2.2** Abnormal Gaits

| Gait | Abnormalities | Interpretation |
|------|---------------|----------------|
| Antalgic | Patient has pain or discomfort on weight-bearing; has a short stride and wants to stay on the unafffected limb longer. May have facial or verbal expressions of pain. | May be due to muscle, joint weakness or pathology. |
| Ataxic | Uncoordinated, staggering gait with sway at times; may have accompanying foot slapping or foot stomping. | May be due to cerebellar pathology. |
| Festinating | Patient holds trunk rigid and leaning forward while taking short, quick, shuffling steps without bending knees. | Frequently due to loss of fine motor movement due to Parkinson's disease. |
| Quadriceps | Patient uses hand on thigh to assist lifting up. | May be due to loss of nerve or muscle function. |
| Senile | Patient holds onto person or support to get started, then takes short, quick steps; turns self "en bloc." | Usually associated with aging. |
| Spastic | Patient takes short steps while dragging or scraping foot; may have crossed knee or scissors gait; jerky, uncoordinated steps. | Usually due to cerebral palsy or secondary to cerebral vascular damage. |
| Steppage | Patient must utilize increased hip and knee flexion to clear foot off floor. | May be due to injury to the peroneal nerve. |

**Table 2.3** Active Ranges of Motion for Major Joints

| Joint | Movements | Ranges (Degrees) |
|---|---|---|
| Shoulder | Elevation through abduction | 170–180 |
|  | Elevation through forward flexion | 160–180 |
|  | Lateral rotation | 80–90 |
|  | Medial rotation | 60–100 |
|  | Extension | 50–60 |
|  | Adduction | 50–75 |
|  | Circumduction | 200 |
| Elbow | Flexion | 135–150 |
|  | Extension | 0–10 |
|  | Supination of forearm | 90 |
|  | Pronation of forearm | 80–90 |
| Wrist | Flexion | 80–90 |
|  | Extension | 70–90 |
|  | Radial deviation | 10–15 |
|  | Ulnar deviation | 30–45 |
| Fingers | Flexion | 0–90 |
|  | Extension | 0–45 |
|  | Abduction | 20–30 |
|  | Adduction | Fingers touch each other |
|  | Thumb abduction | 60–70 |
|  | Thumb adduction | 30–100 |
| Hip | Flexion (with knee flexed) | 110–120 |
|  | Extension | 10–15 |
|  | Abduction | 30–50 |
|  | Adduction | 30 |
|  | Lateral rotation | 40–60 |
|  | Medial rotation | 30–40 |
| Lumbar spine | Forward flexion | 135 |
|  | Extension | 15–20 |
|  | Side flexion | 15–20 |
| Knee | Flexion | 135 |
|  | Extension | 0–15 |
|  | Hyperextension | 0–10 |
|  | Medial rotation of the tibia on the fermur | 20–30 |
|  | Lateral rotation of the tibia on the fermur | 30–40 |

**Table 2.3** (Continued)

| Joint | Movements | Ranges (Degrees) | |
|---|---|---|---|
| Ankle | Dorsiflexion (walk on heels) | 20 | |
| | Plantarflexion (walk on toes) | 50 | |
| | Inversion (walk on outer sides of feet) | 45–60 | |
| | Eversion (walk on inner sides of feet) | 15–30 | |
| Toes | | Extension | Flexion |
| | Lateral toes—metatarsal phalangeal joint | 40 | 40 |
| | Proximal interphalangeal joint | 0 | 35 |
| | Distal interphalangeal joint | | 60 |
| | Great toe MTP joint | 40 | 45 |
| | IP | 0 | 90 |
| Cervical spine | Flexion | 80–90 | |
| | Extension (backward) | 70 | |
| | Side flexion (ear to shoulder) | 20–45 | |
| | Rotation to side | 20–45 | |

**Table 2.4** Ratings of Muscle Strength

| Grade | Value | Movement |
|---|---|---|
| 5 | Normal | Complete ROM against gravity with maximal resistance |
| 4 | Good | Complete ROM against gravity with moderate resistance |
| 3+ | Fair+ | Complete ROM against gravity with minimal resistance |
| 3 | Fair | Complete ROM against gravity |
| 3– | Fair– | Some but no complete ROM against gravity |
| 2+ | Poor+ | Initiates motion against gravity |
| 2 | Poor | Complete ROM with gravity eliminated |
| 2– | Poor– | Initiates motion if gravity is eliminated |
| 1 | Trace | Evidence of slight contractility but no joint motion |
| 0 | Zero | No contraction felt or palpated |

**Table 2.5** Reflexes Tested During Physical Examination

| Name of Reflex | Procedure for Testing | Interpretation |
| --- | --- | --- |
| Abdominal | Have patient supine abdomen uncovered; stroke each quadrant with a pointed object in a triangular pattern around the umbilicus. | Normal: umbilicus is drawn in; Abnormal: absence of reflex may indicate an upper motor neuron lesion. |
| Achilles | Have patient's ankle at 90° or slightly dorsi-flexed; tap reflex hammer over Achilles tendon. | Normal: foot "twitch"; Abnormal: no reflex may indicate $S_1$ nerve root pathology. |
| Anal | Examiner strokes perianal regions. | Normal: contraction of the external and anal sphincter muscles; Abnormal: no contraction may indicate $S_2$–$S_4$ pathology. |
| Babinski | Examiner strokes outer sole of foot from heel to under toes with pointed object. | Normal: absence of reflex; Abnormal: great toe extends down and lateral toes splay out indicative of corticospinal pathology (children under 6 months have a Babinski). |
| Biceps | Examiner percusses tendon of biceps brachii muscle in the antecubital fossa over examiner's thumb. | Normal: forearm jerk; Abnormal: no jerk may indicate $C_6$ pathology. |
| Brachioradialis | Examiner percusses the brachioradialis tendon or muscle at the lateral wrist. | Normal: hand jerk; Abnormal: no jerk; may indicate $C_6$ pathology. |
| Chaddock | Examiner strokes lateral surface of foot with pointed object stroking toward toes. | Normal: no response; Abnormal: great toe extends; may indicate $S_1$ pathology. |

**Table 2.5** (Continued)

| Name of Reflex | Procedure for Testing | Interpretation |
|---|---|---|
| Cremasteric | Examiner strokes inner surface of upper thigh toward scrotum with pointed object. | Normal: scrotal sac draws up; Abnormal: absence may indicate upper motor neuron lesion. |
| Gordon | Examiner exerts sudden pressure on the deep flexor muscles of the calf of the leg. | Normal: no response; Abnormal: great toe draws up; may indicate pyramidal tract pathology. |
| Hamstring | Patient lies prone with leg resting in examiner's arm; examiner places thumb over hamstring tendon in posterior patellar fossa and taps thumb with reflex hammer. | Normal: leg jerk; Abnormal: lack of jerk may indicate $L_5$ pathology. |
| Jaw jerk (temporomandibular) | Examiner places thumb over midpoint of chin and taps thumb. | Normal: chin draws up; Abnormal: lack of response may indicate pathology of cranial nerve V (trigeminal). |
| Oppenheim | Examiner strokes fingernail over crest of tibia. | Normal: no response; Abnormal: great toe extends indication of $S_1$ pathology. |
| Patellar | Have patient sitting with leg hanging off table; examiner taps patellar tendon at knee. | Normal: leg jerks forward Abnormal: no response may indicate $L_3$ pathology. |
| Pectoralis major | Have patient supine; examiner taps thumb placing tension on pectoralis tendon in front of axilla on inner shoulder. | Normal: muscle contraction; Abnormal lack of response may indicate $C_7$–$C_8$ pathology. |
| Triceps | Have patient sitting; examiner holds arm flexed at elbow and hanging loosely; examiner taps triceps tendon on posterior arm just above elbow. | Normal: forearm jerks; Abnormal: lack of jerk may indicate $C_7$–$C_8$ pathology. |

**Table 2.6** Physical Examination Tests of Musculoskeletal Tissues*

| Test or Sign | Technique | Interpretation of Findings |
|---|---|---|
| Adson test | Locate and continue to palpate radial pulse while abducting, extending, and externally rotating patient's arm; have patient take a deep breath and turn head to arm being tested. | Pulse should remain strong. If marked decrease or absence of radial pulse is noted, there is occlusion of the subclavian artery, which may be from an extra cervical rib or from tightened neck muscle. |
| Belvor sign | Have patient do a ¼ sit-up with arms crossed on chest; observe the umbilicus for movement. | Normal: no umbilical movement. Abnormal: movement up, down, or laterally indicates some problem in the anterior abdominal or paraspinal muscles. |
| Chvostek's sign | Lightly tap the facial nerve over the cheek in front of the ear (facial nerve enters face). | Normal: no twitching of face or cheek. Abnormal: twitching or contracting of cheek and lip caused by hypocalcemia. |
| Drop arm test | Have patient abduct and slowly lower arm. | Normal: should be able to slowly and evenly lower arm to side. Abnormal: arm may be dropped suddenly or unevenly, indicative of a tear in the rotator cuff. |
| Drawer test | Anterior: have patient lie on back with knee flexed (block foot from sliding forward). Cup examiner's hands around knee with thumbs on medial and lateral joint lines, and draw tibia forward (see Fig. 2.21a). Posterior: same as for anterior position; gently | Normal: tibia will not easily slide forward. Abnormal: tibia will slide forward, indicative of a torn anterior cruciate ligament. Normal: tibia doesn't move back. |

| Test | Procedure | Findings |
|---|---|---|
| Drawer test (continued) | push tibia backward (see Fib. 2.21b). | Abnormal: tibia can be moved back, indicative of a torn posterior cruciate ligament. |
| Fabere (Patrick) test | Have patient supine; abduct the hip and place the foot on the opposite knee. Press down on the flexed knee while stabilizing the opposite anterior superior iliac spine. | Normal: no pain in hip or knee. Abnormal: patient may experience inguinal pain if hip is involved or may have sacroiliac area pain if sacroiliac joint is involved. |
| Finkelstein test | Have patient make a fist with the thumb inside the first; deviate the wrist toward the ulnar side while holding the forearm still. | Normal: can do without pain. Abnormal: patient may feel sharp pain in the anatomic "snuff box" indicative of stenosing tenosynovitis (DeQuervain's disease). |
| Gaenslen test | Have patient lie supine; ask patient to flex both knees to chest; assist patient to side of table so one buttock extends over edge; ask to extend unsupported leg while keeping other leg flexed. | Normal: no pain when leg is extended. Abnormal: may have pain in sacroiliac area indicative of pathology in that area. |
| Hoover test | If patient says, "I can't raise my leg," as patient tries, cup your hand under opposite heel. | Normal: if patient is really trying to raise leg, you will note increased pressure in your hand. Abnormal: if no pressure is felt from patient's bearing down to raise leg, patient may not be genuinely trying (may be malingering). |
| Kernig test | Have patient lie supine; have patient place hands under head to flex head forward. | Normal: no complaints of pain. Abnormal: patient may have pain along |

(continued)

**Table 2.6** (Continued)

| Test or Sign | Technique | Interpretation of Findings |
|---|---|---|
| Kernig Test (continued) | | spinal column into legs, indicative of meningeal irritation. |
| McMurray test | Have patient lie supine, legs extended; cup heel in hand and flex leg fully; place other hand on knee joint with fingers on medial joint line and thumb on the lateral joint line; rotate leg internally and externally; push lateral side to apply stress to the medial side, while rotating the leg externally; gently extend the leg as you feel the medial joint line (see Fig. 2.22). | Normal: no sounds or clicks. Abnormal: if hear "click" within the knee joint, there is a probable tear in the medial meniscus. |
| Milgram test | Have patient lie supine; ask to raise straight leg about 2 inches off table. | Normal: can hold both legs up for about 30 seconds. Abnormal: cannot maintain elevation indicative of possible cord pressure from herniated nucleus pulposus. |
| Naffziger test | Have patient lie supine; compress jugular veins about 10 sec (face will flush); have patient cough. | Normal: no pain noted. Abnormal: may have pain if there is abnormal pressure on cord from tumor or disc herniation. |
| Ober test | Have patient lying on side with affected leg uppermost; abduct the leg as far as possible; flex the knee to 90° with hip neutral; release the abducted leg. | Normal: thigh should drop to the adducted position. Abnormal: if leg remains abducted there is a likely contracture of the fascia lata. |

| | | |
|---|---|---|
| Oppenheim test | Have patient lie supine; scratch fingernail along crest of the tibia. | Normal: no reaction. Abnormal: extension of great toe with plantar flexion of other toes and splaying (spread out) indicative of reflex pathology. |
| Ortolani test | Have baby lying supine; abduct and externally rotate the flexed thigh. | Normal: no sounds or clicks. Abnormal: click may be heard or felt as the femoral head slides over the acetabular rim indicative of congenital hip dislocation or dysplasia. |
| Patrick test | Same as Fabere test described above. | |
| Phalen test | Have patient flex wrists tightly against each other at right angles and hold position for 1 min. | Normal: no tingling or discomfort. Abnormal: may experience tingling of thumb or fingers indicative of carpal tunnel syndrome. |
| Thomas sign | Have patient lie supine and stabilize the pelvis; have patient flex uninvolved leg to chest. | Normal: opposite leg stays flat. Abnormal: opposite leg moves off table indicative of a flexion contracture. |
| Tinel sign | Tap area between the olecranon and the medial condyle (for ulnar nerve) or tap the volar surface of the center of the wrist (for the median nerve). | Normal: no tingling. Abnormal: tingling along ulnar nerve pathway if neuroma is present and tingling of fingers if median nerve is compressed as with carpal tunnel syndrome. |

(conntinued)

**Table 2.6** (Continued)

| Test or Sign | Technique | Interpretation of Findings |
|---|---|---|
| Tennis elbow test | Have patient make a fist and extend the wrist while you stabilize the forearm; apply pressure with your other hand to attempt to force the wrist into flexion. | Normal: no pain with flexion. Abnormal: severe pain may occur at the lateral epicondyle indicative of lateral epicondylitis (tennis elbow). |
| Trendelenberg test | Stand behind patient and observe the dimples over the superior iliac crests and observe patient walking and shifting weight from side to side. | Normal: dimples appear level when weight is evenly distributed and when standing erect, the gluteus medius muscle should contract as soon as leg is off ground and the pelvis is elevated on the unsupported side (muscle is functioning). Abnormal: pelvis on unsupported side remains in position or descends. |
| Yergason test | Have patient flex elbow at 90° while you cup the elbow in your hand, externally rotate the arm with your other hand on the wrist and pull down on the elbow. | Normal: no pain. Abnormal: there may be pain if the biceps tendon has popped out of its bicipital groove. |
| Valsalva test or maneuver | Have patient hold breath and bear down. | Normal: no pain. Abnormal: pain along spinal cord indicative of increased pressure. |

*These tests are usually performed by physicians or clinical nurse specialists.

**Table 2.7** Examination of Musculoskeletal Tissues

| Area of Body | Inspected For | Normal Findings | Abnormal Findings |
|---|---|---|---|
| Posture | Overall posture while standing; alignment of extremities; spinal alignment or curvatures. | Upright posture; no lateral listing or leaning; no kyphosis, lordosis, or scoliosis except natural spinal curves. | Listing or leaning unilaterally; exaggerated kyphosis (dowager's hump); Scheuermann's disease (excessive kyphosis in teenagers); scoliosis with varying degrees of curvature or rotation. |
| Gait | Length of steps, rhythm and speed of steps, push off, heel, and toe strike, phases of gait (gait cycle). | Step length is 35–41 cm (females take smaller steps than males, taller persons take longer steps); smooth rhythm, lateral pelvic shift of 2.5–5 cm with step; vertical pelvic shift up to 5 cm; foot entirely off floor with step; heel strikes floor first; hip flexion of 20–30° with steps; initial, midswing and terminal swing phases of gait cycle. | Abnormal gaits are listed in Table 2.2. |
| Head and neck and shoulders; temporomandibular joint; mouth opening | Relationship with neck and shoulders; symmetry; muscle spasm; "winged" shoulder blades and shoulder level; movements; symmetry. | Head in midline of shoulders; dominant shoulder/arm side slightly lower than nondominant side; shoulder blades equal with no winging; movements on Table 2.3*. | Wry neck (torticollis); winged scapula (Sprengel's shoulder); TMJ syndrome with accompanying headaches and other symptoms. |

(continued)

**Table 2.7** (Continued)

| Area of Body | Inspected For | Normal Findings | Abnormal Findings |
|---|---|---|---|
| Facial expression | Wincing, grimacing, frowning; symmetry. | Calm expression; can wince, grimace, or frown on request; cervical spine nontender; no temporomandibular joint pain or limitation of movements. | Expressions of pain, sadness, anxiety, frowning. |
| Joints of shoulder, elbow, wrist, and each joint of fingers | Elevation, abduction, adduction, pronation, supination, circum-duction, flexion, extension, opposition of thumb with fingers; tenderness, heat, edema, crepitus; muscle tone, joint laxity; each joint's ROM with resistance; shrug shoulders; palmar creases; thenar eminence on palm; deformities of fingers. | See Table 2.3 for movements; each joint should have no redness, edema, pain, tenderness, or crepitus; joints should have close attachments without laxity; should have no joint or subcutaneous nodules; no deviation at wrists; no finger deformities (see Table 2.4 for muscle strength norms). | Pain and limitation of movements (could be related to bursitis, rotator cuff tears; arthritis, or degenerative joint disease; subcutaneous nodules and Bouchard's nodes (enlargement of the MP and PIP joints of fingers) are seen in rheumatoid arthritis; Heberden's nodes of the DIP joints are seen in osteoarthritis; ulnar deviation occurs in rheumatoid arthritis. |
| Spine | Curvatures; lateral, forward and backward bending; rotation. | Normal cervical, thoracic, and lumbar curves; normal ROM in spinal segments as on Table 2.3. | (As previously given under posture.) |

| | | |
|---|---|---|
| Thorax | Rib expansion and contraction with breathing; anterior-posterior diameter; rib-sternal relationships; use of accessory muscles for breathing. | Ribs and intercostal muscle move easily with breathing; no rib or sternal deformities; no increased A/P diameter; no use of accessory muscles. | Increased A/P diameter (barrel chest); pigeon chest (pectus carcinatum funnel chest (pectus excavatum); use of accessory muscles with asthma and emphysema. |
| Hips and pelvis | Sacroiliac joints; iliac crests; hip movements; gluteal folds; tenderness or pain and deformity in joints; edema. | No tenderness in joints; level iliac crests; hip movement on Table 2.3; gluteal folds level; no pain, edema, or tenderness in joints. | Deformity of hip as in rheumatoid arthritis or osteoarthritis; pain and limitation of movements in hips or sacroiliac joints; gluteal folds can be uneven in muscle wasting or tumor presence. |
| Thigh/leg | Length of limbs; rotation; movements at hip; femur and tibia/fibula relationships. | Lengths equal bilaterally; no rotation or tibial torsion; movements on Table 2.3. | Leg length inequality; can have tibial torsion with genu varum (bowlegs) or genu valgus (knock knees). |
| Knee and patella | Edema, pain, soreness; movements; ligament stability; patella—relationship to femur and tibia/fibula; posterior swelling. | No edema, pain, or soreness of knee; no muscle or ligament wasting (see knee tests); patella should be in midline (no medial or lateral deviation); no posterior swelling. | "Squinting" patella (medial deviation); frog's eye patella (facing up), grass-hopper's patella (out and away from each other); Baker's cyst is |

(continued)

**Table 2.7** (Continued)

| Area of Body | Inspected For | Normal Findings | Abnormal Findings |
|---|---|---|---|
| Knee and patella (continued) | | | posterior swelling behind knee. |
| Ankle, foot and toes; toenails | Relationship of foot, heel, and toes with ankle; pain, edema, color; arch of foot; flat foot; calluses, corns; plantar warts; splaying (widening) of forefoot. | No equinus of toes or heel related to ankle; pink color; no edema or pain; normal arch of ankle and metatarsal area; no corns, calluses, or warts; no splaying; no toe abnormalities. | Equinovarus or valgus; toeing medially or laterally may be present flat foot (pes planus); excessively high arch (pes canus); splaying of metatarsals; hammer toe (flexion deformity of PIP joint of toe); mallet toe (flexion of DIP joint of toe); bunion; hallus valgus (deformity of head of first metatarsal bone of great toe and lateral deviation of the head in relation to the center of the foot). |

General observations to be made by examiner in examining each area and tissues:

- signs of inflammation: redness, heat or hot areas, edema, pain, soreness or tenderness, changes in function, color of tissues with bilateral comparison in each area
- deformity: bumps, lumps, bulges, nodes
- sensory changes: complaints of numbness, tingling, pins and needles, anesthesia, or hyperesthesia
- motor changes: limitation of movements, muscle tone, weakness, laxity, strength against resistance or gravity (see Table 2.4)
- affect of limitations (if present) on activities of daily living, job performance, hobbies, or recreational activities
- number and anatomic relationships of contiguous tissues with one another
- use of an ambulatory aid: cane, crutches, or walker
* Joint ranges of motion for each area are listed on Table 2.3 to conserve space in this table.

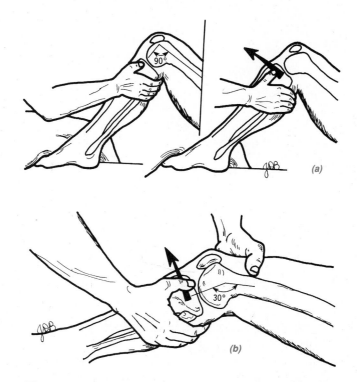

**Figure 2.21** (a) Anterior drawer test; (b) Lachman drawer test.

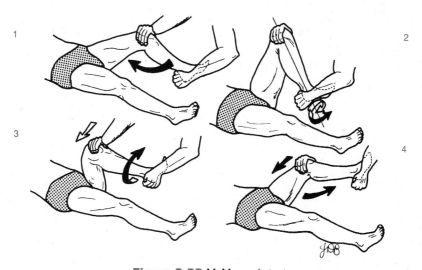

**Figure 2.22** McMurray's test.

Using knowledge of anatomy and physiology of the musculoskeletal tissues correlated with the patient's history and physical examination, the physician attempts to arrive at the most accurate diagnosis of the patient's orthopaedic condition or disease.

## BIBLIOGRAPHY

Galli, R.L., Spaite, D.W., & Simon, R.R. (1989). *Emergency orthopedics: The spine.* Norwalk, CT: Appleton & Lange.

Guyton, A.C. (1986). *Textbook of medical physiology* (7th ed.). Philadelphia: Saunders.

McRae, R. (1990). *Clinical orthopaedic examination* (3rd ed.). New York: Churchill Livingstone.

Magee, D.J. (1987). *Orthopaedic physical assessment.* Philadelphia: Saunders.

Post, M. (1987). *Physical examination of the musculoskeletal system.* Chicago: Year Book.

Salmond, S.W., Mooney, N.E., & Verdisco, L.A. (Ed.). (1991). *Core curriculum for orthopaedic nursing* (2nd ed.). Pitman, NJ: Janetti.

Sculco, T.P. (1985). *Orthopaedic care of the geriatric patient.* St. Louis: Mosby-Year Book.

Seidel, H.M., Ball, J.W., Dains, J.E., & Benedict, G.W. (1991). *Mosby's guide to physical examination* (2nd ed.). St. Louis: Mosby-Year Book.

Shipman, P., Walker, A., & Bichell, D. (1985). *The human skeleton.* Cambridge, MA: Harvard University Press.

Simon, R.R., Koenigsknecht, S.J., & Stevens, C. (1987). *Emergency orthopaedics: The extremities* (2nd ed.). Norwalk, CT: Appleton & Lange.

Sullivan, J.D., Olha, A.E., Rohan, I. & Schulz, J. (1986). The properties of skeletal muscle. *Orthopaedic Review, 15*(6),349–363.

# 3

## NURSING PROCESS DURING DIAGNOSTIC EXAMINATIONS

Persons who experience an orthopaedic injury or disease usually undergo multiple diagnostic laboratory studies. The studies may only be required to aid in making the diagnosis or may be repeated frequently over time to monitor the recovery or healing process. Many persons undergoing any laboratory study are unfamiliar with the purpose of the study, the study procedure, and the significance of the study findings. They must receive sufficient explanation about the nature and purpose of the study so that they can be as cooperative and comfortable as possible throughout the procedure and can understand the meaning of the results as they might influence current or future care.

Nurses must also fully understand each laboratory study so that they can best inform and prepare the patient and family members. If they do not have full understanding, nurses might omit information, which could add to a patient's discomfort or necessitate a repeat of the test or study. Mutually satisfying results are usually the outcome of well-understood, well-administered laboratory studies.

Orthopaedic patients frequently have studies of samples of blood serum, urine, stool, and other discharges. They also have radiologic studies of their bones, joints, organs, blood vessels, and other tissues with the use of x-rays alone or with the addition of radioisotopes or dyes to outline or delineate the tissues more specifically. Studies might involve scanning of the whole body or a region with "slices" via computerized tomography or MRI. Tests may not only be physical, but may also be the patient's psychological responses. When the results of the tests are compiled, they should provide valuable information to aid the physician in arriving at the most logical and correct diagnosis.

Chapter 2 listed multiple physical examination tests useful while examining the patient. The reader is referred to that chapter for that information.

## SEROLOGIC STUDIES

Table 3.1 contains the common serologic studies useful in diagnosing orthopaedic problems. These studies include a complete blood count, hematocrit, hemoglobin, white cell differential, platelets, blood sugar, blood urea nitrogen, alkaline and acid phosphatase, serum glutamic oxaloacetic transaminase and glutamic pyruvic transaminase, creatophosphokinase, lactic dehydrogenase, serum amylase, total protein and albumin/globulin ratio, and electrolyte (sodium, potassium, and calcium) levels. These studies are generally considered part of the admission "battery" for use in diagnosis or to establish baseline data. Additional serologic tests—including antistreptolysin titer, c-reactive protein, rheumatoid factor, antinuclear antibodies, immunofluorescence, and serum electrophoresis—might be required for persons with rheumatic or arthritic conditions. Bleeding and clotting times give vital information for diagnosis of adequacy or deficiency in those areas.

### Patient Education and Preparation for Serologic Studies

The patient may have had positive or negative prior experience of having blood samples drawn. Past experiences contribute to the patient's present attitude about the upcoming venipuncture. Teaching should include information about when the venipuncture will be done, why it is necessary, the fact that one or more vials of blood will be taken, and the reasons for careful cleansing before insertion of the needle and application of pressure following removal of the venipuncture needle. Efforts should be made to determine whether the patient fears having a venipuncture, because some persons react by closing their veins involuntarily. The patient may also be able to state sites that are better than others from past experience, and may or may not want to watch when the needle is inserted.

The majority of venipunctures for serological studies are performed by hematologic technicians; however, nurses also should be able to perform venipuncture, because they usually initiate intravenous solutions.

### DIAGNOSTIC EXAMINATIONS OF URINE

Urine has been examined microscopically and chemically for its contents, which may give indications of renal function or evidence of the presence of a systemic disease or condition.

**Table 3.1** Studies of Serum and Blood Commonly Ordered for Diagnosis

| Test | Normal Values | Significance for Orthopaedic Patients | Nursing Observations/ Care Strategies |
|------|---------------|---------------------------------------|---------------------------------------|
| Complete blood count (CBC)<br>• Red blood cells (RBC) | Men: 5,000,000/cu mm<br>Women: 4,500,000/cu mm | Increases could signify hemoconcentration (dehydration), polycythemia. | Monitor fluid intake and output closely; watch for clotting and hypoxic manifestations; note constipation if dehydrated. |
| • Hematocrit (Hct) | Men: range 43%–48% (average 45%)<br>Women: 42% ± 5% | Correlated with RBC count; lower in anemias and hemorrhage. | Note signs of hemorrhage in urine (hematuria); stool (occult blood); vomitus (coffee-ground or bright red colors); sputum (rusty or blood-streaked); site of injury (hematoma).<br>Note skin color: pale lips, pale conjunctivae are indicative of anemia. |
| • Hemoglobin (Hgb) | Men: 14–16 gm/100 ml<br>Women: 11.7–14 gm/100 ml<br>Children: 12–14 gm/100 ml | Carries oxygen to the cells; levels are lower in anemias. | Same as above.<br>Note signs of dyspnea and increased respirations. |
| • White blood cell (WBC) count total | 5,000–10,000/cu mm (range 4,000–11,000) | Increased in bacterial infections, stress response, blood dyscrasias, anesthesia, rheumatic menstruation. | Check drainage from orifices for signs of infection; check for systemic signs of infection, such as fever, increased pulse, and respirations; |

(continued)

**Table 3.1** (Continued)

| Test | Normal Values | Significance for Orthopaedic Patients | Nursing Observations/ Care Strategies |
|---|---|---|---|
| White blood cell (continued) | | | note any disorientation and symptoms or signs related to each bodily subsystem— e.g., neurological: neck stiffness, etc. Check menses onset and flow. |
| | | Decreased in viral infections, drug reactions, blood dyscrasias. | Note signs of viral infections, such as cold symptoms, swelling of parotid glands (mumps), sore throat, and enlarged glands (infectious mononucleosis). |
| | | Drugs such as sulfonamides, antibiotics, bone marrow depressants, and anti-thyroid drugs decrease WBC counts. | Note drug therapy and effects on total WBC count. |
| ▪ WBC differential: Segmented neutrophils | 40%–60% of total WBC count | Increases in neutrophils occur in inflammatory and infectious conditions, acute hemorrhage, poisonings (with liver damage), neoplastic conditions, and blood dyscrasias. | As above, check for signs of systemic or local inflammatory and/or infectious conditions: redness, swelling, fever, drainage, etc. Check history for intake of possible toxic fluid, fumes, or drugs. |
| | | Decreases in neutrophils occur when bone marrow is affected by radiation or | As above, note signs or symptoms of long-term infections or therapy with medications |

| WBC differential (continued) | | radiation. Note deficiency conditions of GI surgery and pernicious anemia, as affecting vitamin $B_{12}$ and folic acid. |
| | chemotherapy; and in vitamin $B_{12}$ or folic acid deficiency. | |
| Band neutrophils (unsegmented, juvenile) | 0%–5% of total neutrophils | Increase in acute infections. | Check for signs of local or systemic infections such as appendicitis, abscess formation. |
| ▪ Lymphocytes | 20%–40% of total WBC count | Increase in lymphocytes in febrile diseases; viral diseases (herpes zoster or shingles, hepatitis, infectious mononucleosis); lymphatic leukemia. Decreases in lymphocytes may occur in lupus erythematosus, radiation syndromes. | Check for exposure to viral diseases from children and others. Note signs of fever, increased pulse and respirations; look for local signs of infection, such as rash, tenderness, skin reactions. |
| ▪ Monocytes | 4%–8% of total WBC count | Increases in monocytes in tuberculosis, Gaucher's disease, monocytic leukemia, typhoid, infectious mononucleosis. | Check skin test results for positive tuberculosis; check chest x-ray exam results. Check for evidence of local or systemic infections as given above. |
| ▪ Eosinophils | 1%–3% of total WBC count | Increases in allergies, parasitic infestations, psoriasis, neoplasms and blood | Check for known allergies; note reactions to drugs and therapy, such as rashes, |

(continued)

**Table 3.1** (Continued)

| Test | Normal Values | Significance for Orthopaedic Patients | Nursing Observations/ Care Strategies |
|---|---|---|---|
| • Eosiniphils (continued) | | dycrasias, radiation therapy, menstruation. | hives, asthma. Note picking of lips, biting nails, and itching or rectal irritation as signs of parasitic infestations (more common in children than adults. |
| • Basophils | 0%–1% of WBC count | Decreases in acute infections. Increases in polycythemia, colitis, Hidgkin's disease, myxedema. Decreases in allergies, hyperthyroidism, stress. | Check for signs of clotting manifestations; check for diarrhea, cramping, or abdominal tenderness. Note thyroid function results. Check for rashes, hives, asthma. Check for hyperthyroid symptoms, such as intolerance to temperature extremes, elevated pulse, blood pressure, cardiac arrhythmias. |
| • Platelets | 1500,000–450,000/cu mm | Vital for blood clotting. Increased in trauma, hemorrhage, menstruation, | Check for clotting manifestations with each condition. |

| | | | |
|---|---|---|---|
| | | thrombocythemia, polycythemia. Decreased in bone-marrow depression, anemias, some leukemias, transfusion reactions, infectious mononucleosis. | Check for prolongation of clotting mechanisms or increased bleeding tendencies, easy bruising, bleeding of gums, and following injections. |
| Blood sugar (glucose) | 80–100 mg/100 ml (Folin-Wu units) 65–95 mg/100 ml (Nelson-Somogyi units) | Increased glucose levels (hyperglycemia) occur in diabetes mellitus, stress response, acute pancreatitis, Cushing's syndrome, obesity, eclampsia. Decreased glucose levels (hypoglycemia) occur in insulin overdose, pancreatitis, liver disease and pancreatic islet cell tumors. | Check for signs of hyperglycemia such as thirst, dry skin, frequency of voiding, itching of labia; check urine for sugar and acetone AC* and HS**. Check blood sugar levels with glucometer. Check for signs of hyperinsulinism: hunger, sweating, nausea, clammy skin. |
| Blood urea nitrogen (BUN) | 5–25 mg/100 ml | Increased in renal diseases, starvation, bleeding ulcers, diabetes. Decreased levels are rare, but may occur in severe liver failure. | Check intake and output carefully; check for cerebral function with sudden elevations of BUN. May have uremia with acute renal failure. Note liver function test results. |

(continued)

**Table 3.1** (Continued)

| Test | Normal Values | Significance for Orthopaedic Patients | Nursing Observations/ Care Strategies |
|---|---|---|---|
| Alkaline phosphatase | 1.5–4 Bodansky units<br>5–13 King-Armstrong units | Increases in osteoblastic activity (bone tumors, fractures); liver diseases and inflammatory conditions; infectious mononucleosis; pulmonary infarcts. | Check results; levels may remain elevated throughout hospitalization. Check for localizing signs in bone, liver, and lungs if indicated by marked elevation. |
| Acid phosphatase | 0.5–2 Bodansky units<br>1–5 King-Armstrong units | Increased in metastatic carcinoma of prostate, and in Paget's disease (osteitis deformans). | Check for signs of metastatic disease such as bone pain, low back pain, pathological fractures. |
| Serum glutamic oxaloacetic transaminase (SGOT) | 5–40 Karmen units | Normally high amounts are found in heart, liver, skeletal muscles, and brain. Sudden increases occur in death of heart cells and liver conditions. Muscular distrophy, intestinal trauma, and radiation cell damage may also cause elevations. | Check for evidence of cardiac trauma: e.g., elevated pulse, arrhythmias, chest pain, dyspnea. Left-sided chest pain is usually of cardiac or pulmonary origin. Pain in upper right quadrant (RUQ) of abdomen may signify liver disease. |
| Serum glutamic pyruvic transaminase (SGPT) | 5–40 Karmen units | Normally high amounts are found in liver, kidney, | Check, as above (for SGOT) for signs of liver, cardiac, renal, |

| | | | |
|---|---|---|---|
| Serum glutamic pyruvic transaminose (continued) | | heart, and skeletal muscles SGPT more elevated in liver than heart diseases. SGOT more elevated in heart diseases. | or skeletal conditions. Check for elevated temperature, increased pulse, and respiratory rates, dyspnea, tenderness in RUQ (liver); in costoverbral angle (CVA) for kidney, and left side of chest for cardiac. Skeletal injury is noted in involved area. |
| Creatophosphokinase (CPK) | 0–12 Sigma units/cc 0–50 IU | Normally high in striated or skeletal muscles, heart, and brain. Injury or death to skeletal, cardiac, or brain tissues cause serum elevations, such as necrosis or atrophy of skeletal muscle, acute myocardial infarct, progressive muscular dystrophy, and traumatic muscle injury. Levels may elevated for 2 to 3 weeks. | Check for localizing signs of injury to tissues named. Note signs of inflammation in specific tissues. Note subsequent levels in serial testing. |
| Lactic dehydrogenase | 50–400 units/100 cc | Normally found in significant levels in kidneys, liver, heart, skeletal muscles, | Check levels: note increasing levels during early postinjury period with gradual return |

(continued)

**Table 3.1** (Continued)

| Test | Normal Values | Significance for Orthopaedic Patients | Nursing Observations/ Care Strategies |
|---|---|---|---|
| Lactic dehydrogenase (continued) | | and erythrocytes. Serum levels are increased following damage to any of these tissues. Peak elevations are 10–14 days postinjury. May also be elevated after pulmonary embolism. | over time to normal levels. Note increases: if sudden may signify new injury to cardiac, lung, or kidney tissue from infarct. Isoenzyme studies may be done for specificity of site and injury. |
| Serum amylase | 80–150 Somogyi units | Normally in high concentrations in pancreas, liver, and salivary glands. Increase in acute pancreatitis, perforated ulcer, pancreatic duct obstruction, mumps, surgical parotitis, acute gallbladder disease, intestinal obstruction. Amylase is decreased in severe pancreatic or liver destruction. | Check for localizing signs of inflammation in glands or organs named. Note signs of peritoneal irritation; abdominal distention, tenseness, nausea, vomiting irritability, lack of bowel movements, etc. Sudden elevations may be indicative of "acute abdomen" Check sugar and acetone AC and HS; check vomitus for blood; check abdominal girths. |

| | | | |
|---|---|---|---|
| Total protein, albumin/globulin (A/G) ratio | 6–8.5 gm/100 ml Albumin 3.5–5.5 gm/100 ml Globulin 2.5–3.5 gm/100 ml A/G ratio = 1:2.5 | Relatively increased in dehydration, vomiting, diarrhea. Albumin is produced by the liver; decreases signify liver disease. Albumin is the chief regulator of colloid-osmotic pressure of blood and tissue fluids. Globulin fractions consist of alpha 1 and 2, β and γ globulins; they increase in infectious diseases because they are antibody fractions. | Check intake and output: Note abnormal losses; decreased intake. Check for signs of liver disease. Malnutrition may lead to decreased albumin production, leading to ascites, edema, or loss through the kidneys. Check for signs of acute infections. Decreased amounts of γ (gamma) globulins may accompany antirejection therapy. |
| Electrolytes Potassium | 3.5–5.5 mEq/l | Intracellular ion. Serum levels increased in hypooventilation, severe cell destruction or damage, acute renal failure, metabolic acidosis. Decreases occur in diarrhea, stress, malabsorption. Fluctuations in potassium levels cause cardiac arrhythmias and muscle weakness. | Check serum level results daily. Note muscle strength and stress response of each particular patient. Encourage deep breathing to increase ventilation. Check apical pulses for regularity with radial pulses. Check sugar and acetone for signs of acidosis. |

(continued)

**Table 3.1** (Continued)

| Test | Normal Values | Significance for Orthopaedic Patients | Nursing Observations/ Care Strategies |
|---|---|---|---|
| Sodium | 135–150 mEq/l | Detects gross changes in water/salt balances. | Increase in Na⁺: check for adequate urine output (30 cc/hr), lung congestion, edema, and elevated B/P. Decrease in Na+: diuresis. |
| Chloride | 100–110 mEq/l | Serum levels increased in dehydration, renal failure, and cystic fibrosis. Levels decreased in vomiting, diarrhea, diuresis, intestinal fistulas, etc. | Check serum levels of chlorides with sodium or potassium levels (chlorides accompany either loss or retention of those ions). Check for sources of loss: vomiting, diarrhea, etc. |
| Calcium | 4.5–5.5 mEq/l | Serum levels are increased in conditions of immobility, and bone demineralization, such as bone cancer, bed rest (prolonged), multiple myeloma. Serum levels are decreased in malabsorption, and malnutrition. Pancreatitis also decreases serum levels. | Check serum level results. Observe for signs of lowered levels such as tetany and tingling of fingers and around mouth. Check Chvostek's sign (see glossary). Keep patient as active as possible within limits of condition to keep calcium in bones. |

| | | |
|---|---|---|
| Antistreptolysin (ASO) test | Up to 150–160 Todd units | High values indicate recent streptococcal infection. Values above 500 units are found in acute rheumatic fever, glomerulonephritis. Rising titer does not indicate whether infection is past or ongoing. | Observe for signs of acute illness: fever, joint pains, weakness, change in urinary output, hematuria, etc. |
| C-reactive protein | Negative | Test is positive if an α globulin precipitates the c-polysaccharide of pneumococcus. Nonspecific test. Can be positive in persons with lupus erythematosus, active streptococcal infections, cancer, etc. | Persistently elevated results indicate continuing infection: observe for temperature elevations, localizing signs, etc. |
| Rheumatoid factor | Positive if titers are in the 1:10060 range | Primarily the expression of antiIgG activity. Can be positive in rheumatoid arthritis, lupus erythematosus, sarcoidosis, cirrhosis, etc. May be negative in some persons with rheumatoid arthritis who are hypoglobulinemic. False positives in 5% of general population. | Observe for signs of rheumatoid arthritis; check protein electrophoresis for globulin levels. |

*(continued)*

**Table 3.1** (Continued)

| Test | Normal Values | Significance for Orthopaedic Patients | Nursing Observations/ Care Strategies |
|---|---|---|---|
| Antinuclear antibodies | Positive in 80% of persons with active lupus erythematosus. | If positive, there is a high probability of presence of active lupus. | Observe for presence of symptoms in skin, urinary output, joints, |
| Immonufluorescence | Pattern of fluorescence varies with specific condition: may be homogeneous, speckled throughout, nucleolar flourescent, and peripheral stains more pronounced. | If done carefully, can yield 95%–99% positive results for active lupus erythematosus; the most reliable diagnostic exam for this disease. | |
| Hepatitis-associated antigen (HAA—formerly called Australia antigen) | Positive for past and/or present serum hepatitis (may remain positive for extended periods in serum). Positive for persons with chronic hepatitis. | If positive for HAA, carries 40%–70% risk of causing hepatitis (if blood used for transfusion). Test can be positive for persons on immunosuppressive medications. | Observe for symptoms of present disease such as jaundice, dark urine, fatigue, loss of appetite and loss of desire to smoke—a highly correlated symptom. Use caution in handling secretions and excretions, and in needle and syringe techniques, to prevent transfer. |
| | | Bleeding/Clotting Times | |
| Prothrombin time | 9.5–12 sec | Prolonged by coumadin or aspirin anticoagulation therapy. | Anticoagulation therapy may by used as prophglaxis for PE or DVThrombosis. Check |

| | | | |
|---|---|---|---|
| Prothrombin time (continued) | | | urine and stool for blood. Apply pressure to all venipunctures for 5 min. Caution patient about using safety razor for shaving and to use pressure for any for any cuts to lessen bleeding. |
| Activated partial thromboplastin time (aPTT) | 35–45 sec | Done to help regulate heparin dosages in pulmonary embolism or to prevent deep vein thrombosis. | Watch for any bleeding from gums or cuts. Observe urine and stool for blood; use electric razor for shaving. |
| Partial thromboplastin time | 20–45 sec | Prolonged by coumadin or aspirin anticoagulation therapy. | Monitor daily PT/PTT levels. |
| Factor VIII assay | 50%–200% | Deficient in classic hemophilia. | Monitor levels and give Factor VIII or IX as necessary. Follow above anticoagulation precautions. |
| Factor IX | 60%–140% | Deficient in pseudophemophilia (Christmas Disease). | |
| Myoglobin | Up to 85 mg/ml serum | Increases indicate muscle necrosis or myocardial infarction | Check for blackened, injured tissues, movement pain, sensation of injured limb. |

\* AC before meals (ante cibum).
\*\* HS = upon retiring (hora somni).

## Patient Education and Preparation for Securing a Urine Specimen

The majority of adults have had the experience of supplying a voided urine sample. They may not have prior experience with providing a "clean voided" specimen. Therefore, instructions should be thoroughly explained so the patient can provide the best sample possible. The reasons why the clean voided specimen is preferred over either the straight voided or, sometimes, over the catheterized specimen should be given.

Once the specimen is obtained, it should immediately be sent to the laboratory for analysis. Any delay could adversely affect the results; for example, bacterial counts can change, and the pH may change after long standing. After dispatching the urine specimen, the nurse records the transaction on the patient's chart. Table 3.2 contains results of studies on urine samples.

## DIAGNOSTIC RADIOLOGIC EXAMINATIONS

Multiple radiologic examinations may be done to aid the diagnostic process, including chest x-rays; flat plates of the abdomen and pelvis; views of one or more extremities and parts of the hands, fingers, feet, toes, spinal vertebrae, and skull. The above x-rays are external and noninvasive, as are the CT scan and the MRI. Other radiologic studies are invasive, with needles or catheters introducing contrast media or radioisotope solutions into the body.

### Noninvasive Examinations

Generally, preparing patients for noninvasive x-ray studies centers around the fact that the procedure will be painless (unless the patient has one or more fractures or soft tissue trauma, and moving the part or parts will be somewhat painful) and will take very little time. The patient should be told that eating and drinking will not affect the results. The examination will be scheduled to avoid having long waiting periods, which could tire or excite the patient. Also, the patient should be told that results of the x-rays may be known in a relatively short time, so that definitive care can then be given. If the x-ray is taken on an emergency basis, it is read usually as soon as the film is processed.

Following the noninvasive examination the patient is returned to his/her room and positioned comfortably. The completion of the examination and the patient's reaction, if any, are recorded on the patient's record. Table 3.3 contains noninvasive examinations commonly ordered for orthopaedic patients.

## Invasive Diagnostic Examinations

Invasive procedures may be required to outline a specific area or areas of the body to provide a more definitive diagnosis. Some invasive examinations involve the use of a contrast medium as a radiopaque substance to provide a contrast in density between the tissues or organs being filmed and the medium. The contrast substance aids in outlining the interior of the hollow organs, including blood vessels, the heart, gastrointestinal organs, gallbladder, respiratory passages, and spinal canal. The patient should be told how the contrast medium will be introduced—whether through a catheter or needle into the tissues or organs to be filmed.

Radionuclide skeletal scans referred to as bone scintigraphy or skeletal imaging are invasive examinations utilizing the gamma rays emitted by the injected radioisotope (radionuclide) to provide an "image" of the skeletal tissues being studied. Bone scintigraphy is discussed later in this chapter. Table 3.4 lists common invasive examinations performed on orthopaedic clients.

*Patient Education and Preparation.* Prior to undergoing the examination, the patient should receive information about the examination from the physician and signs the consent form for the examination. During the "informed consent" discussion, the physician explains the purpose of the test, how it will be done, the benefits and risks; the physician also answers patient's questions. The physician might draw or point out on the patient's body the area that will be involved. From the fear either of the examination itself or its risks, or of the language, the patient might be unduly anxious about the test and may require additional explanations or additional time to adjust to the need for the examination; sedation might be required. Nurses should devote time to all patients about to undergo invasive procedures to help them understand the test and to clarify any questions when possible.

If possible, the patient showers or is bathed to rid the skin of transient organisms. The patient is dressed in a gown that opens with ties or snaps easily for ready access to the test area and is transported to the proper laboratory. The skin is shaved, if necessary, just prior to the test at the site of needle or catheter insertion, and the site is carefully and thoroughly cleansed with a long-acting antiseptic, such as povidone-iodine. The patient is positioned for optimal access to the site, and might be given a mild sedative or narcotic to relieve discomfort. The radiopaque substance, dye, or radioisotope is injected, and the examination proceeds. The physician or assisting personnel keep the patient informed of the progress of the examination and offer encouragement; efforts are made to keep the patient quiet, calm, and still.

**Table 3.2** Diagnostic Studies on Urine

| Test | Normal Values | Significance for Orthopaedic Patients | Nursing Observations/Care Strategies |
|---|---|---|---|
| Urinalysis | | | |
| ▪ Color | Straw-colored, yellow | Variations in color occur from bleeding, drugs, presence of hemoglobin, red cells, bilirubin. | Check for signs of hemorrhage, drug reactions, jaundice, liver disease—such as hepatitis, cirrhosis, etc. Fluids may be increased or decreased depending on cause of color change. |
| ▪ pH | 4.6–8 range average pH = 6 | Normally acid; acidity increased in acidosis, diabetes, chronic nephritis, acidic drugs. Alkalinity of urine increases with intake of alkaline substances such as antacids and bicarbonate of soda; with vomiting, prolonged cold, and leaving sample standing. | Check pH with nitrazine paper or stick. Send urine to lab immediately to avoid delay before pH checked. |
| ▪ Sugar/acetone | Sugar: Trace Acetone: 0 | Present in diabetes mellitus, toxemia of pregnancy, starvation, malnutrition, some digestive disturbances. | Check sugar and acetone in voided specimens AC and HS or as ordered. Record promptly. |

| | | | |
|---|---|---|---|
| ▪ Protein | 25–75 mg/24 hr | Elevated in renal diseases infections of kidney, diabetes, tubular damage, hemorrhage, incompatible blood. | Check for proper typing and cross-matching for transfusion. |
| ▪ Cells | 0 | RBCs may be present in inflammatory or traumatic conditions or organs of urinary tract. | Check color of urine for hematuria; hemistix urine for occult blood; note menses as sources of blood in urine. Note signs of urinary tract infection such as fever, malaise, urgency, frequency, burning, etc. |
| ▪ Casts | Hyaline casts normal if protein. Epithelial casts not normal. | Casts (cylinduria) are shed from tubules of kidney. Epithelial or waxy casts occur in acute and/or chronic glomerulonephritis, pyelonephritis, fatty degeneration of kidney. | Check for clarity of urine for sediment—may be indicative of casts. |
| ▪ Specific gravity | 1.003–1.030 range | Increased in diabetes mellitus, dehydration, glomerulo-nephritis, vomiting. Decreased in increased fluid intake, diabetes insipidus, aldosteronism | Check specific gravity on early morning specimen; overnight; concentration may indicate renal function to concentrate urine. Check urinometer for accuracy |

(continued)

Table 3.2 (Continued)

| Test | Normal Values | Significance for Orthopaedic Patients | Nursing Observations/ Care Strategies |
|---|---|---|---|
| ▪ Specific gravity (continued) | | (NaCl retention and water reabsorption). | in water (specific gravity of water is usually 1.000). |
| ▪ Bacteria | Absent | Present in urinary tract infections or from contaminated specimen. | Instruct patient in clean techniques or use cath. specimen if ordered. Ask patient about burning on urination or frequency. |
| ▪ Myoglobin | Absent | Present in muscle necrosis. | Can be detected as positive on some products that test for blood in urine. Monitor affected tissues for neurovascular changes. |

**Table 3.3** Common Noninvasive Examinations for Orthopaedic Patients

| Name of Examination | Purpose | Normals | Significance for Orthopaedic Patients | Nursing Observations/ Care Strategies |
|---|---|---|---|---|
| Flat plate of abdomen | To ascertain GI and urinary conditions. | Anatomic locations of GI and urinary organs; no excess or loops of gas; no obstructions; no masses or foreign bodies. | Gives evidence of abdominal organs, whether intact or interrupted; shows size and shape of organs. | Inform patient that eating or drinking do not disturb exam. Inform patient x-rays will be taken with the patient flat on his/her back, standing or sitting when necessary. |
| Chest x-ray | To aid in diagnosis of chest pathology, such as tumors, metastasis, pneumonia, and others. | Normal size and shape of lungs, heart, and vessels.<br><br>lungs, tuberculosis | Gives evidence of pressure or absence of fat or pulmonary emboli, presence or absence of pneumonia, primary or metastatic tumors to the<br><br>fractured ribs or pneumothorax. | Inform the patient that the x-rays will be taken back-to-front and side-to-side, that the patient will be in the room alone and will be asked to take a deep breath and hold it briefly; and will be asked to wait while film is checked for adequacy and will then be returned to the nursing unit. |
| Electrocardiogram | To record the electrical activity of the heart. | Recordings are within normal limits for the rate and rhythm with | Aids in diagnosis of cardiac capacity and output to the systemic vessels. Gives evidence of heart size, | Inform the patient that electrodes will be placed on 8–12 places on the chest around the heart and |

(continued)

**Table 3.3** (Continued)

| Name of Examination | Purpose | Normals | Significance for Orthopaedic Patients | Nursing Observations/ Care Strategies |
|---|---|---|---|---|
| Electrocardiogram (continued) | | waves and peaks. | arrhythmias of myocardial infarct, or congestive heart failure. | breast areas, that the electrodes will be connected to a machine which will record the activity of the heart, and the test will be painless and take 3–5 minutes. |
| Tomograms of lungs, kidneys, or other organs | To determine presence or absence of tumors by viewing slices of the organ. | No tumors noted; normal size of organs examined. | To aid in diagnosis of primary or metastatic tumors. | Inform patient that test will last 30–45 minutes; that x-rays will be taken from various positions around the chest, kidney, or other organ. |
| Pulmonary function tests | To determine lung capacity or disorders as COPD, or others. | Lung capacity: 5500 cc. Vital capacity: 4000–4800 cc. Residual volume: 1200–1500 cc. Expiratory reserve: 1200–1500 cc. Inspiratory capacity: 2500–3600 cc. | Aids in diagnosis of lung capacities to aid recovery. | Inform patient tests will be done in special pulmonary lab; that his/her breathing will be measured and checked. |
| Ultrasound or Echograms | To aid in diagnosis of | Ultrasonic images show normal | Gives evidence of organ trauma or intactness. | Inform patient that sound waves will be used to |

| | | | |
|---|---|---|---|
| | presence or absence of pathology in various organs, as the spleen, bladder, kidneys, heart, or liver. | size, position, or structure. | penetrate the organs to be examined and they will be viewed on a special machine from the echoes the sound waves produce to show the size, shape, and location of the organ examined. |
| Guaiac test | To determine presence of blood in stool. | No evidence of presence of blood. | Aid in determination of bleeding associated with anti-inflammatory medications, anemias, colitis, or GI malignancy. | Inform patient that test will be done and that a stool sample will be needed, preferably saved in a bedpan. The sample is tested with reagents to determine if blood is present. (False positives may be associated with intake of iron, salicylates, steroids, and thiazides.) |

**Table 3.4** Invasive Examinations for Orthopaedic Patients

| Name of Examination | Purpose | Normals | Significance for Orthopaedic Patients | Nursing Observations/ Care Strategies |
|---|---|---|---|---|
| Anthrogram | To visualize the interior of a joint. | No erosions or hemorrhage within the joint; ligaments intact. | Aids in diagnosis of joint, cartilage or ligament pathology (see Fig. 3.1) | Inform patient that the joint will be cleansed with an antiseptic and a local anesthetic may be injected to lessen pain. There will be some pain when the radiopaque solution is injected. X-rays will be taken. The exam may take over an hour. Postexam: observe joint for redness, edema, or increased pain; pain medication may be given to ease soreness. |

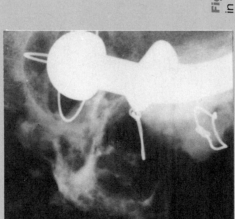

**Figure 3.1** Fistulogram showing infection in a hip joint following total hip replacement.

| | | | | |
|---|---|---|---|---|
| Body scans<br>Brain<br>Bone<br>Kidney<br>Liver<br>Spleen<br>Lung | To determine presence or absence of tumors by concentration of a radioisotope in the area of pathology (tumor, increased bone activity, fracture osteomyelitis), function of organ scanned. | Normal uptake and distribution of the radioisotope. | Aids in diagnosis of primary or metatastic tumor in the organ(s) scanned, fracture, osteomyelitis, function. | Inform the patient that a radioisotope will be injected into a vein followed by scanning of the organ(s) or body by a special camera that will pick up the radioisotope emissions. The patient should be told the test will take 1–2 hours, and that he/she must lie quietly. Assess patient for allergies to iodine or seafood prior to scheduling this exam Postexam: check for adverse reactions to the radioisotope. Iodine and barium will interfere with scans. therefore tests using these two substances should be scheduled after scans when possible. |
| Lumbar puncture | To secure fluid for examination to detect pathological conditions. | Spinal fluid should be clear; contain 0–8 cells per cu. mm.; have 15–45 mg/dl of | Aids in diagnosis of cranial hemorrhage, brain tumors, or meningitis. | Inform patient that the lumbar area of the back will be cleansed with antiseptic and a local anesthetic will be injected, followed by the |

(continued)

**Table 3.4** (Continued)

| Name of Examination | Purpose | Normals | Significance for Orthopaedic Patients | Nursing Observations/ Care Strategies |
|---|---|---|---|---|
| Lumbar puncture (continued) | | protein; have a pressure of 75–180 mm $H_2O$; have 45–85 mg/dl of glucose; have 118–130 mEq/l of chloride and have 7–15 mg/dl urea. | | insertion of the needle into the spinal canal below the area where the spinal cord ends. The needle is removed and the site is covered with a small dressing. The patient should understand he/she may have to remain flat for at least 8 hours after the test and that fluids will be forced (when possible) to replace the fluid withdrawn. The patient should be observed for changes in the level of consciousness, for headache, restlessness, or confusion during checks. |
| Electromyogram | To check muscle action and strength of contraction. | Normal functions of muscle with normal nerve conduction. | Aids in diagnosis of peripheral nerve damage or muscle diseases. | Inform patient that a small electrode will be inserted into the muscle to be tested and its activity will be seen on an oscilloscope. The muscles will be checked at rest and during contraction. |

| | | | | |
|---|---|---|---|---|
| Discogram | To determine integrity of intervertebral disc(s). | Intact disc. | Aids diagnosis of low back pain pathology. | there is very little pain when the needle-electrode is inserted into the muscle. Inform patient that a local anesthetic will be injected into area to be examined, then small amount of contrast agent will be injected into disc area, then x-rays will be taken to determine condition of disc. If disc is abnormal, there will be pain on injection of the contrast agent. |
| Computed tomogram scan (CT scan and 3-D scan) | To determine condition of structures, 3-D scan provides results in a new format or picture. | Intact structures. | Provides specific findings to determine extent or type of injury. | Inform patient that x-rays will be taken from various views, and that patient must remain still during procedure. |
| Wound Culture | To determine the presence and type of organisms in a wound. | Normal flora should be present. | Aids in diagnosis of superficial or deeper wound infections. | Inform the patient that a small amount of drainage will be removed with a sterile swab for analysis. |
| Intravenous Pyelogram | To determine condition of the kidneys, | Normal size, shape, and | Aids in diagnosis of renal or urinary | Inform the patient that a dye will be injected intravenously |

(continued)

**Table 3.4** (Continued)

| Name of Examination | Purpose | Normals | Significance for Orthopaedic Patients | Nursing Observations/ Care Strategies |
|---|---|---|---|---|
| Intravenous pyelogram (continued) | ureters, and bladder. | location of all tissues with no obstruction. | sites of tumors or infections or metastasis to the skeleton | and x-rays will be taken at intervals over 5–60 minutes. After the exam the patient should be observed for iodine sensitivities. |
| Bone marrow aspiration | To determine bone marrow cells and if marrow is producing cells. | Active production of erythroid, myeloid, and megakaryocytes with no "blast" cells or metastatic cells. | Aids in diagnosis of multiple meyloma and other blood dyscrasias and anemias. | Inform the patient that the aspiration will be done in\ the breast bone (sternum) or iliac bone (iliac crest), that the skin will be cleansed, and a local anesthetic will be injected. The aspiration will be done following insertion of a needle into the bone and the cells will be aspirated. It may take up to 1 hour to complete the test. the site is covered with a sterile dressing. |

When the examination has been completed, the patient is returned to his/her room and placed in the required position. The patient is observed for allergic or unusual reactions to the radiopaque substance, dye, or radioisotope used. The site is observed for leakage, and neurological or neurovascular checks may be performed. Reactions to the examination are recorded on the patient's record. Vital signs and temperature are monitored as indicated or as ordered.

Several examinations frequently performed on orthopaedic patients require more extensive discussion than can be summarized in a table. These examinations are arthroscopy, magnetic resonance imaging, myelogram, joint aspiration and arteriogram, and bone scintigraphy.

## ARTHROSCOPY

Arthroscopy may be used as part of the diagnostic work-up. Diagnostic arthroscopy is the direct visualization of the interior of a joint through a specially designed fiberoptic instrument called an arthroscope. With the advent of this technology, the ability to accurately diagnose joint injuries has dramatically increased. Arthroscopy may be performed on the shoulder, elbow, ankle, or wrist, but it is most commonly performed on the knee.

Arthroscopy is useful in detecting injuries to the cruciate ligament, meniscal tears, articular cartilage damage, or synovial defects. Visualization of the posterior cruciate ligament, the posterior capsule, and the inferior or most anterior aspects of the menisci is not as good as that of other structures.

Surgical arthroscopy is performed to repair cruciate or meniscal tears, obtain biopsies, and visualize loose bodies. With the advent of this procedure, the need for arthrotomy has decreased, as has the rehabilitation time.

The procedure includes shaving the knee, draping the knee with surgical drapes, and reducing bleeding potential. A pneumatic tourniquet is applied above the knee, and an irrigating solution of epinephrine and normal saline to distend the knee, and an irrigating solution of epinephrine and normal saline may be inserted to distend the knee and minimize bleeding. The knee is flexed 45°, and a local anesthetic is injected prior to insertion of the arthroscope. One or more "ports" may be needed for full examination.

Preparation of the patient includes education, nothing by mouth past midnight, and shaving and scrubbing the knee. Posttest care involves frequent neurovascular assessment, assessment of the arthroscopy site, elevation of the leg to heart level, and application of ice.

Benefits of arthroscopic surgery include decreased postoperative immobility, decreased hospitalization time, decreased blood loss, and more rapid rehabilitation. Complications are infrequent following arthroscopic knee surgery, although infection, hemarthrosis, and thrombophlebitis can result.

## MRI (Magnetic Resonance Imaging)

Formerly called nuclear magnetic resonance, MRI analyzes electromagnetic waves released from atoms in the cell nucleus that have been exposed to a magnetic field. Polarized atoms will tend to line up with the magnetic field. Radiowaves are broadcast into the body's cells, altering the alignment of the atoms. When the radiowaves are stopped, the atoms realign into their original positions and release absorbed energy in the form of radio signals that can be picked up by an antenna. The signals are then projected into an image with the use of a computer.

The magnetic resonance machine consists of a very powerful magnet that must be housed in a facility designed to protect the machine from disturbance of external radio or magnetic waves. The usual facility has thick concrete walls and a copper roof to lessen interference.

## Patient Education and Preparation

Prior to entering the magnet area or room, all persons must remove all articles that could be attracted to the magnet, including watches, coins, hairpins, keys, credit cards (the magnetic line will be erased), pens, scissors, and other objects. Some patients pass through metal detectors similar to airport metal detectors to be certain all metallic objects have been removed. Pacemakers or metallic orthopaedic internal fixation devices may prevent the patient from having MRI.

Patients should be taught that they will lie on a softly padded table and will gradually move through the hole in the center of the magnet. They must be cautioned that they must lie very still and assured that they can be heard if they call for assistance during the examination. They should be asked about claustrophobic feelings which, if intense, could preclude their having the examination. They should also understand that they might be asked to lie with their arms extended above their heads as they move through the magnet. When the examination is completed, the patient is returned to his/her room.

The MRI is very sensitive to tumors, avascular necrosis, disruptions of ligaments, and presence of infection. The signals visualize different tissues as light, dark, or bright areas. Generally, and depending on the "strength" of the signal, air, cortical bone, flowing blood, cerebrospinal fluid, fluid-filled cysts, and ligaments give darker images; brighter images come from fat, cancellous bone, and bone marrow. Light or intermediate intensities come from muscle and the spinal cord. Because of these sensitivities, the MRI is a valuable diagnostic examination for orthopaedic and neurological examinations and may replace the myelogram as the technique is perfected over time. (see Fig. 3.2).

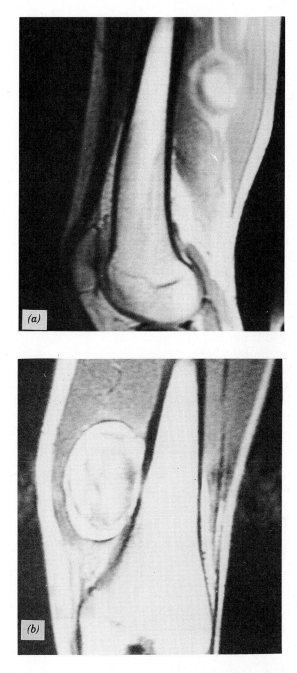

**Figure 3.2** Magnetic resonance images of an arterial aneurysm of the distal thigh. Images clearly show no bone attachments to aid in differentiation of this arterial aneurysm and an aneurysmal bone cyst.

## MYELOGRAM

A myelogram is a radiologic examination of the spinal canal to determine presence of herniated intervertebral discs, tumors, and congenital or degenerative conditions that put pressure on the spinal cord or the spinal nerves as they exit the spine. Most often a lumbar myelogram is performed; however, thoracic or cervical myelograms may also be done.

To visualize the area radiologically, a radiopaque solution (or air) is injected into the subarachnoid space. The solutions most commonly used are iophendylate (Pantopaque), which is an oil-based solution, or metrizamide (Amipaque), which is a water-soluble solution. The decision to use the water-soluble or oily solution is mutually made by the physician and patient because of the advantages and disadvantages of each solution.

Advantages of iophendylate are that its viscosity provides a good contrast density for examination of the spinal nerve coverings and pathways to demonstrate pressure or obstruction from a herniated nucleus pulposus, tumor, or other lesion in the spinal canal and that it remains in the desired areas for the duration of the examination. Disadvantages of iophendylate are that it must be removed as completely as possible to avoid irritation to the meninges, and it can cause severe headaches if small quantities are retained (see Fig. 3.3).

Advantages of metrizamide (Amipaque) are that it is less viscous than iophendylate, permitting better visualization of smaller areas, and that it is absorbed into the cerebrospinal fluid, so it need not be removed following the examination. However, its major disadvantages are that it can cause seizures, nausea, and vomiting from 4–8 hours following the myelogram. If metrizamide is to be used, the patient must avoid medications such as amphetamines, tricyclic antidepressants, and phenothiazides, which lower the seizure threshold. The patient must be kept well hydrated prior to the myelogram.

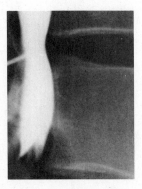

**Figure 3.3** Myelogram showing obstruction to flow of the contrast agent from a herniated nucleus pulposus.

## Patient Education and Preparation

A thorough explanation of the myelogram as an outpatient procedure is vital for full patient participation and understanding. Patients may be anxious or fearful about having a needle and dye inserted in the spinal canal. The physician should explain the procedure and use pictures to clarify what will be done before, during, and after the myelogram. A patient history of allergic reaction to previously used contrast agents would necessitate performing this myelogram with air contrast. A myelogram is not repeated within 14 days of a previous myelogram or lumbar puncture because of the risk of mixing contrast agents.

On the morning of the examination, the patient may be allowed a clear liquid breakfast; nothing is administered by mouth for 4–6 hours before the myelogram. Narcotics and muscle relaxants are usually withheld, although a sedative or antiemetic may be ordered for a very tense or anxious patient. As was stated above, medications that lower the seizure threshhold should be withheld for 12 hours before the examination when a water-soluble contrast agent is to be used.

The myelogram is performed in the radiology department. Approximately 10 cc of cerebrospinal fluid is withdrawn (and usually sent for laboratory analysis), and the contrast agent in injected. The table is tilted to allow the contrast material to fill the spinal canal areas desired, while serial x-ray films are taken. If iophendylate was used as the contrast agent, it is removed as completely as possible, to avoid causing inflammation of the subarachnoid or arachnoid membrane. The agent is removed under fluoroscopic guidance.

Water-soluble metrizamide diffuses into the cerebrospinal fluid easily; therefore, the table rarely needs to be tilted. This agent also diffuses and fills nerve sheaths more completely and more easily flows through narrow canals.

Following completion of the myelogram, the patient is returned by gurney to his or her room and is kept flat in bed for 6–8 hours or longer if iophendylate was used. Fluids are forced to replace the cerebrospinal fluid removed, and a normal diet can be resumed. With metrizamide, the patient is kept on bed rest for 6–8 hours with the head of the bed elevated 30°, followed by putting the bed flat for 8–16 hours, to decrease the risk of seizures. Fluids are forced and the patient's diet is resumed.

A headache can occur after the use of either contrast agent. Generally, lowering the head of the bed or placing the patient flat will lessen the headache. Neurologic checks are performed to determine any untoward reactions to the contrast agent.

Other postmyelogram complications can occur with either contrast agent. Other common complications with iophendylate include radicular pain, adhesive arachnoiditis, and a severe reaction to the contrast agent. With metrizamide, nausea and vomiting are the most common complications, although seizures, visual or speech disorders, and arrhythmias may occur.

## ARTERIOGRAM

Arteriography is done to determine the arterial circulation into or around a tumor and to determine the adequacy of distal circulation in an extremity. A radiopaque agent is injected, followed by serial x-ray films to observe the arterial flow through the tissues. Because the thigh and lower extremity are frequent sites for neoplastic growths, the femoral arteriogram is the one most often done in orthopaedic patients and will be discussed below (see Fig. 3.4).

### Patient Education and Preparation

The patient should be given an explanation about the purpose(s) of the arteriogram and the benefits of the examination in making an accurate diagnosis. Using pictures of the circulation in the area under study helps to clarify the procedure for the patient. A history of allergic reactions or hypersensitivity to contrast agents or iodine is a contraindication for arteriography. Other risks include bleeding into the tissues and (rarely) vasospasm leading to arterial clot formation.

The patient is given nothing by mouth for 8–12 hours prior to the examination and is given a sedative before being transported to the radiology department. The patient is placed in a back-lying position on the x-ray table. The groin area over the femoral artery is cleansed with povidone-iodine, and a local

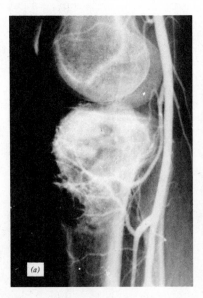
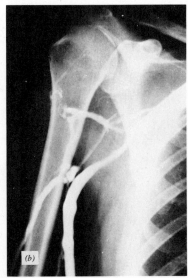

**Figure 3.4** (a) Arteriogram. (b) Venogram.

anesthetic is injected. The femoral artery is punctured with a large-bore needle, and a guidewire and catheter may be threaded into the artery toward the area to be examined; then the guidewire is removed. The contrast agent (usually diatrizoate sodium [Renographin]) is injected while serial x-rays are taken as the arterial flow proceeds through the thigh and leg. As the dye is injected, the patient may feel hot and flushed and should be prepared for those transitory feelings by the radiologist performing the examination. The length of time for the examination varies with the purpose and the adequacy of the x-ray films. Once adequacy is assured, the radiologist removes the catheter and holds pressure on the site for 5–10 minutes to prevent bleeding and formation of a hematoma. A small, sterile dressing is applied over the arterial puncture site, and the patient is transported to his/her room. The patient is maintained on bed rest to avoid bleeding. Neurovascular checks are performed, and the groin site is checked carefully to note signs of bleeding, clot formation, or vasospasm. Clot formation or severe vasospasm are noted by the absence of peripheral pulses, and a cool, pale extremity that becomes painful with burning, sharp pain from anoxia. An embolectomy may need to be performed to remove the obstruction.

## BONE SCINTIGRAPHY (RADIONUCLIDE SCANS)

Bone scintigraphy involves the intravenous injection of a measured amount of radioisotope (radionuclide)-containing solution, which has a high affinity for localization in skeletal tissues. Following a specified waiting period of 2–6 hours (usually 3 hours) to allow skeletal localization, the distribution of the radionuclide is imaged through the use of a scintillation camera. The image is a localized and total body picture of "hot" spots of high concentration of the radionuclide in a specific area. The radiologist's interpretation of the meaning of the high concentration is based on the patient's clinical history and the radiographic findings.

Skeletal imaging has been possible because of the development of the Anger scintillation camera, the radionuclide generator for technetium 99m, and the bone-localizing diphosphonate complexes of technetium 99, the radionuclide used for skeletal imaging. Gallium-67-citrate is also now used for skeletal imaging.

Bone scintigraphy is now a commonly used tool to aid in diagnosis of bone infection, avascular necrosis, degenerative disease, fracture, or metastatic bone disease. The radionuclide has a low radiation dose and provides good image resolution at a relatively low cost compared to, for example, MRI. Good resolution is achievable even on an extremity in a cast.

### Patient Education and Preparation

The physician explains the purpose of the particular scan planned, the radionuclide injection procedure, the need for the specified waiting period, and the imaging steps. The patient signs the informed consent form for this invasive procedure.

The only preparation is to provide the proper gown for this radiologic procedure, one which is long, loose-fitting, and easily opened if needed. When in the nuclear medicine department, the patient is "screened" before the injection site is chosen to determine any areas that will require special attention during the imaging process. Care is taken by the technician to be certain that the radionuclide is injected intravenously and not inadvertently intraarterially, which could create confusing scintigraphic findings.

Following the intravenous injection of the radionuclide, the patient must wait the selected time interval determined by the specific study to be done, the patient's age, renal and cardiac function, and the scheduling needs of the department. The patient may eat and drink fluids during the waiting period, and in fact, should consume at least 100 cc of fluid preinjection and a minimum of an addition 500 cc postinjection until imaging is begun to initiate frequent urination, to reduce the radiation dose to the bladder and reproductive organs. If the patient has a catheter or urine collection bag, these are drained to eliminate interference from high concentrations of radionuclide in the bladder. Following voiding, the patient's perineal area should be carefully cleansed to avoid skin contamination with the radionuclide.

The length of time for the skeletal imaging varies with the amount of information or "counts" to be made with the imaging camera. The patient must understand the long time period necessary for the entire examination to be completed.

## BIBLIOGRAPHY

Beltran, J. (1990). MRI *musculoskeletal system.* Philadelphia: Lippincott.

Berquist, T.H. (1986). *Imaging of orthopedic trauma and surgery.* Philadelphia: Saunders.

Billings, F.T., Jr. (1986). An evaluation of the usefulness of routine preoperative tests. *Surgical Rounds, 9*(12), 54–61.

Braunstein, E.M., Vydareny, K.H., Louis, D.S. & Hankin, F.M. (1986). Cost effectiveness of wrist fluoroscopy and arthrography in the evaluation of obscure wrist pain. *Orthopaedics, 9*(11), 1504–1506.

Cohen, M.D., Weetman, R.M. Provisor, A.J., Grosfeld, J.L., West, K.L., Cory, D.A., Smith, J.A., & McGuire, W. (1986). Efficacy of magnetic resonance imaging in 139 children with tumors. *Archives of Surgery, 121*(5),522–529.

Eisenberg, R.L. (1987). *Diagnostic imaging in surgery.* New York: McGraw-Hill.

Fraser, R.D. Osti, O.L., & Vernon-Roberts, B. (1987). Discitis after discography. *Journal of Bone and Joint Surgery, 69B*(1), 26–35.

Hendee, W. R. & Davis, K.A. (1985). Magnetic resonance imaging: Part II. Musculoskeletal applications. *Contemporary Orthopaedics, 11*(3), 45–58.

Hendee, W.R. & Davis, K.A. (1985). Magnetic resonance imaging: Part I. Theory and principles. *Contemporary Orthopaedics, 11*(2), 48–55.

Hughes, J. (1984). Techniques of bone imaging. In Silberstein, E.B. (Ed.), *Bone scintigraphy* (pp. 39–50). Mount Kisco, NY: Futura.

Iraci, J.C. (1986). Diagnostic and therapeutic procedures: Central venous access. *Surgical Rounds, 9*(8), 110–112.

Lange, T.A. Austin, C.W., Seibert, J.J., Angtuaco, T.L., & Yandow, D.R. (1987). Ultrasound imaging as a screening study for malignant soft-tissue tumors. *Journal of Bone and Joint Surgery, 69A*(1), 100–105.

Lotysch, M. (1986). Scrutinizing knee joints with MRI. *Diagnostic Imaging,* 8(8), 90–94.

Mandell, G.A., & Alavi, A. (1984). Scintigraphic evaluation of bone trauma. In Silberstein, E.B. (Ed.), *Bone scintigraphy* (pp. 95–130). Mount Kisco, NY: Futura.

McBride, K. (1986). Can ventilation-perfusion scans accurately diagnose acute pulmonary embolism? *Archives of Surgery, 12*(7), 754–757.

Mourad, L. (1991). Orthopedic disorders. St. Louis: Mosby.

Ramsey, R.G. (1986). MRI shows spinal defects without artifacts. *Diagnostic Imaging, 8*(8), 74–79.

Rothschild, B.M. (1986). Thermographic assessment of bone and joint disease. *Orthopaedic Review, 15*(12), 765–780.

Silberstein, E.B. (Ed.). (1984). *Bone scintigraphy.* Mount Kisco, NY: Futura.

Solomonov, M. Baratta, R., Zhou, B.H., Shoji, H. & D'Ambrosia, R. (1986). Historical update and new developments on th4e EMG-force relationships of skeletal muscles. *Orthopaedics, 9*(11),1541–1543.

Sundaram, M. McGuire, M.H., Herbold, D.R., Wolverson, M.K., & Heiberg, E. (1986). Magnetic resonance imaging in planning limb salvage surgery for primary malignant tumors of bone. *Journal of Bone and Joint Surgery, 68A*(6),809–819.

# 4

## NURSING PROCESS IN THE CARE OF PERSONS WITH TRAUMA

Trauma is any injury resulting in physical or psychological changes. Orthopaedic trauma may be minor or severe, multiple injuries that require extensive care and long-term rehabilitation. Orthopaedic trauma may affect soft tissues, bones, muscles, ligaments, tendons, bursae, or joints.

Depending on the exact tissues involved and the specific injury or injuries, the person may have pain, edema, bleeding, and hemorrhage, and usually will have some alteration in function. Hospitalization is frequently required. Trauma is the leading cause of death in the age group 16 to 34 years from automobile and motorcycle injuries.

### FIRST AID MEASURES FOR TRAUMA

There are four commonly used first aid measures easily recalled by the mnemonic RICE:

**R** = Rest to the part. May be short-term or more prolonged nonuse or nonweight bearing, depending on the injury.

**I** = Ice. Ice applications lessen bleeding and edema formation. Ice is applied for 48–72 hours or longer, again depending on the severity of the injury and extent of trauma to the surrounding tissues.

**C** = Compression. Accomplished by use of elastic bandages or at times application of a circular cast. Elastic bandages are applied to compress the *venous* vessels and should be applied firmly, but not so snugly that arterial blood flow is compromised. The bandages should also be applied distally to proximally to aid venous constriction and venous return.

**E** = Elevation. The injured part should be elevated to at least heart level to aid venous return to lessen edema. Care should be taken to avoid elevating *too* high (or above the person's central venous pressure*), which could impede arterial flow and increase, rather than decrease, edema. Upper extremities may be held in a sling for elevation.

## Trauma Management

Certain principles govern the care of persons with trauma. Centers around the United States have been designated as level 1 trauma centers so that treatments of injured persons can be expedited with the greatest speed and thoroughness. Level 1 trauma centers have teams of personnel, and all the various types of equipment and facilities to provide the care necessary for persons with different types of orthopaedic trauma. Rescue personnel know which hospitals are level 1 trauma centers and transport patients to such centers for optimal care.

The principles of emergency care involve primary and secondary assessments of the injured person or persons while maintaining immobilization of head, neck, or bones to prevent additional injury. The ABC's (*a*irway, *b*reathing, and *c*irculation) are priority assessments followed by neurological, musculoskeletal, gastrointestinal, endocrine, and genitourinary. Each treatment team member carries out his or her required care, under the supervision of one or more physician team leaders. Once assessments are finished, decisions are made regarding transfer of the person to the operating room, intensive care unit, or appropriate nursing unit. Some injuries may be x-rayed in the Emergency suite and casts, splints, or joint immobilizers may be applied prior to transfer. Serologic blood samples also may be drawn and intravenous fluids begun, as well as oxygen therapy to aid circulation and cellular oxygenation.

## SPECIFIC MUSCULOSKELETAL INJURIES

### Definitive Care for Musculoskeletal Injuries

Table 4.1 lists the various types of musculoskeletal injuries. There is always soft tissue trauma with each type of injury.

*Contusion.* This soft tissue injury can occur anywhere in the body. It is usually from a fall, bump, or direct blow to the part, which breaks capillaries and other

---

* Normal central venous pressure (CVP) ranges from 6–13 cm $H_2O$ pressure. When there is no CVP line for measuring the exact CVP, the limb may be elevated up to 5 inches above the heart (2.5 cm = 1 inch; 5 inches = 13 cm). Since the CVP may not be at the highest level, the limb should be elevated no higher than 5 inches. Elevation above the CVP places added stress on the heart and arterial side of the vasculature.

**Table 4.1** Types of Musculoskeletal Injuries

| | |
|---|---|
| Contusion | A bruise that does not break the skin; bleeding into tissues causes "black and blue" discoloration. |
| Strain | An injury to a muscle, tendon, or ligament resulting from excessive force or pull. Severity of strain is referred to as first, second, or third degree. |
| Sprain | An injury to a tendon, ligament, or muscle around a joint with partial or complete tearing of the tissues from their attachments. As with strains, severity of sprains is referred to as first, second, or third degree. |
| Subluxation | A partial dislocation of a bone from its joint. |
| Dislocation | The displacement of a bone from a joint. |
| Fracture | A break in a bone; it can be a partial or complete break. |

blood vessels, leading to bleeding into the tissues, resulting in the development of a "black and blue" area. Extensive bleeding can produce a hematoma. Edema is also noted because of disruption of venous return (see Fig. 4.1).

Small contusions usually require no treatment, but those with more bleeding, edema, or pain may be treated with external pressure and ice applications to lessen bleeding. Applications of heat or immersion in hot water should be avoided as heat causes vasodilation and increased bleeding. Generally, no limitations to use of the affected tissue are imposed. External pressure may be applied by manual pressure or by use of elastic wraps. Contusions usually become less sore or painful in 24–48 hours, with the edema and discoloration

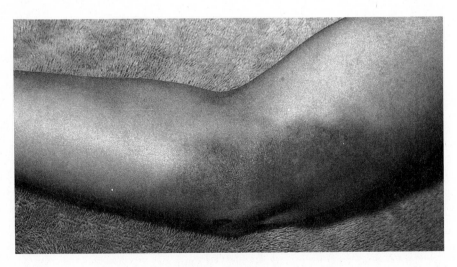

**Figure 4.1** Contusion of the forearm and elbow.

gradually resolving over 3–5 days as the extravasated blood is absorbed. No permanent scarring or evidence of the previous contusion will occur.

*Charleyhorse.* A "charleyhorse" is a quadriceps or hamstring contusion caused by a direct blow to the muscles, causing bleeding and some tearing of muscle fibers. Symptoms include pain over the anterior, lateral, or posterior aspects of the thigh (vastus lateralis, intermedius, or hamstring muscles) followed by edema and hematoma formation. Treatment includes RICE for 24–48 hours. Complications may include development of myositis ossificans.

A charleyhorse can also refer to muscle cramps of the lower leg (gastrocnemius) caused by dehydration, depletion of electrolytes, and from heat. Mobility is severely limited during these cramps. Treatment includes dorsiflexion of the foot and replenishing of fluid and electrolytes. If the cramp or contraction has lasted several minutes, the person will experience a dull ache for several days.

*Strain.* A strain is a pull or excessive stretch of a muscle, ligament, or tendon leading to transitory weakness, numbness, and soreness and some bleeding into the strained tissues. Although the numbness should lessen in 24 hours, the weakness and soreness may last 72 hours or longer.

Depending on the severity of the strain and the exact muscles, ligaments, or tendons involved, the person will have edema, soreness, limitation of function, and bleeding into the tissue or joint. The person limits weight bearing, noted by a limp, or if the upper extremity is involved, will carry or hold the injured tissues.

*Groin Pull.* A groin pull is a strain of either the iliopsoas muscle or the adductor muscles of the leg. The iliopsoas is a muscle attached to the lumbar vertebrae posteriorly then coursing anteriorly to insert into the lesser trochanter of the femur. Its function is to flex the thigh and pull it forward.

The mechanism of injury is sudden bursts of speed—as during skiing, gymnastics, or skating—that pull on the muscle. A history of a sharp pain in the groin following a lunge or spreading of the legs is suggestive of a diagnosis of groin pull. On physical examination, edema is noted in the groin. Pain is produced when the patient is placed supine and the extended leg is lifted straight up in external rotation.

Treatment includes rest and wrapping a compression bandage around the groin and pelvis. Analgesics are given for pain. Ice may or may not be useful in reducing edema, because of the deep placement of the iliopsoas, but it may ease painful episodes. Return to usual activities may usually be resumed in 1–2 weeks.

*Hamstring Pull.* The hamstring muscle extends the thigh and bends the knee. It is attached proximally to the ischium and femur and distally to the posterior proximal tibia and fibula. Injury occurs in runners—especially sprinters and hurdlers. As with groin pull, sudden bursts of speed can cause hamstring pull.

Symptoms include immediate pain at the point of strain. Ice, rest, and compression are indicated. Stretching exercises should be performed following healing to promote return of function. Support of the hamstring muscles when activities are resumed is indicated.

The majority of strains heal without permanent sequelae, though a severe strain may require longer immobilization and, rarely, surgical repair if tendons are avulsed from their muscles or bone attachments. Rehabilitative exercises are also required following surgical repair. A brace may also be worn during the recovery and healing times.

*Sprain.* A sprain is a tear in or of a muscle, ligament, or tendon and is a more severe injury than a strain. Sprains are classified as first degree (some tearing of fibers with bleeding), second degree (moderate tearing with more extensive hemorrhage), and third degree (full tearing or avulsion of the tendon or ligament from its bony attachment, with or without some attached bone), accompanied by marked hemorrhage, edema, pain, and loss of function. Sprains require more intense treatments for longer periods and may include, along with ice, wrapping, elevation, and nonuse, application of a cast, and occasionally, surgical intervention to repair and reattach the detached ligaments or tendons if they are repairable. A third-degree sprain may require up to 6 or more weeks for full healing to occur. Rehabilitative exercises will be prescribed to aid the patient to regain full function. Because the ankle is the area most commonly sprained, this area will be the focus of the discussion on sprains.

*Ankle Sprain.* Inversion sprain is by far the most common type of ankle sprain; it occurs when the foot is twisted inward and the force of body weight stretches the lateral soft tissues and anterior talofibular ligament. This injury occurs most often in athletes who have high arches. Eversion sprain occurs when the foot is twisted outward and the force stretches the medial soft tissues. This sprain most often occurs in athletes who are flat-footed.

Classification of ankle sprains is:

Class I— (no ligament tear) minimal swelling, mild discomfort over the injured ligament, no abnormal motion;

Class II— swelling and hemorrhage, pain moderate to severe at rest and on motion;

Class III— egg-shaped injury within 2 hours of injury, marked swelling and pain (complete rupture may be pain-free), and loss of normal function.

Diagnosis involves a history of the above-described mechanisms for injury and physical examination, including stress tests for laxity of the ligaments, and arthroscopy.

Treatment for a Class I sprain is RICE. Class II sprains involving ligament tears require RICE with the use of an ankle support (see Fig. 4.2) or cast brace for 3 days to 3 weeks depending on the extent of the ligamentous injury. Class III sprains require use of a posterior splint for 3 weeks or RICE for 72 hours until soft tissue swelling decreases and surgery can be performed.

Complications include recurrent sprains and ankle instability. An ankle sprain can take up to 26 weeks to fully heal. Ankle strengthening exercises are the best prevention for ankle sprains.

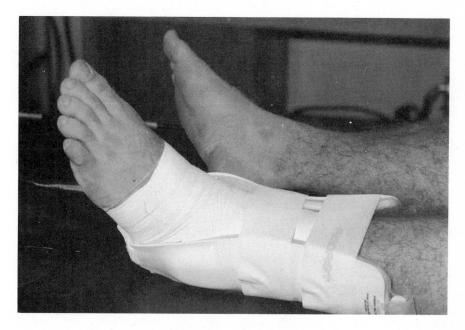

**Figure 4.2** *Aircast for support of a sprained ankle.*

## KNEE INJURIES

The knee is commonly affected by trauma, because of its anatomy, location, and the demands placed upon it (see Fig. 4.3 for anatomy). Knee injuries can be categorized into soft tissue injuries, including muscular, ligamentous, and cartilage injuries, and osseous injuries involving bones.

The bony structures of the knee include the patella, the proximal tibial condyles or plateaus, and the distal femoral condyles. Dislocations, fractures, or abnormal bone growth are the main problems associated with knee injuries.

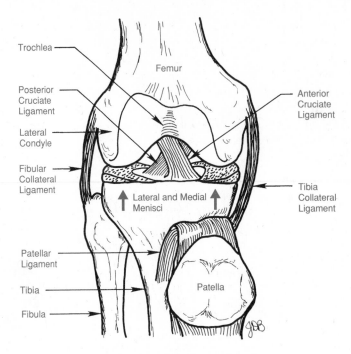

**Figure 4.3** Normal anatomy of the knee.

## Patella Dislocation

The mechanism for injury is a severe blow to the flexed knee while it is in external rotation. The most frequent dislocation is laterally. Dislocation and subluxations can recur due to laxity of the ligaments. Symptoms include a feeling of "the knee going out," presence of a knee deformity, and swelling. Diagnosis consists of assessing the mechanism of injury and x-rays, which reveal the dislocated patella.

Treatment includes ice, analgesics, elevation, and closed reduction. Reduction is obtained by flexing the hip and applying lateral pressure while extending the knee. Immobilization of the knee with a knee immobilizer or in a cast for 6 weeks in full extension is indicated following reduction. Crutches can be used for mobility. Recurrent dislocations may require surgery.

## Meniscal Injuries

The meniscus (knee cartilage) is comprised of the C-shaped medial meniscus and oval-shaped lateral meniscus. The medial meniscus is more fixed on the tibia and, therefore, can be injured more easily. The menisci are cartilage shock absorbers that protect the joint surfaces during loading; therefore, weight bearing and rotation at the time of knee injury increase the likelihood of meniscal injury. A bucket-handle tear of the medial meniscus is most common and aptly describes the appearance of the injury (see Figs. 4.4 and Fig. 4.5).

Diagnosis begins with a history of the mechanism of injury. Meniscal injuries occur with sudden rotary or extension-flexion injuries and are commonly found in conjunction with cruciate ligament tears. Symptoms of a meniscal injury include joint line pain, locking, and swelling. (Joint effusion immediately following an injury is a symptom of ligamentous rather than meniscal injury.)

The squat test consists of repeatedly squatting with legs and feet rotated internally and then externally. A meniscus tear will produce pain at the site and to the side of the tear.

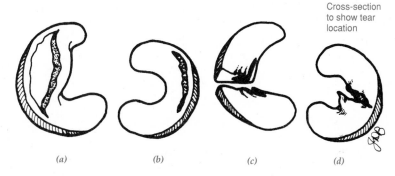

Cross-section to show tear location

(a)          (b)          (c)          (d)

**Figure 4.4** Meniscal tears of the cartilage of the knee: (a, b) bucket-handle tears; (c, d) transverse tears.

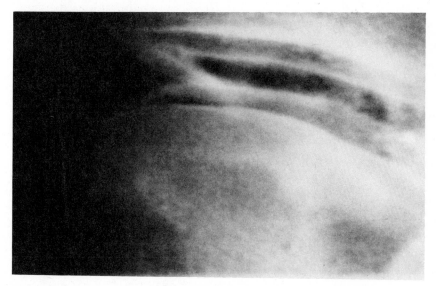

**Figure 4.5** Arthroscopic view of a bucket-handle meniscal tear.

McMurray's test helps to evaluate medial or lateral menisci. A positive medial meniscus tear will produce pain and crepitation when the patient is supine and the knee is flexed to 90° and gradually extended when the leg is rotated internally. A positive lateral meniscus tear produces the same symptoms of pain and crepitus when the knee is flexed to 90° and gradually extended when the leg is rotated internally.

A medial meniscus tear may be determined by a positive Bragard's sign. The patient's leg is placed in internal rotation and extension, which forces the medial meniscus anterior to the joint line. There is pain or tenderness along the anterior medial joint line if the medial meniscus is torn.

Payr's sign produces pain anterior-medially at the joint line when the patient sits cross-legged and pressure is placed on the flexed, externally rotated knee. A positive Payr's indicates a medial meniscus tear.

Patients with meniscal tears, but without ligament injury, may be treated conservatively with a splint, brace, or cast and nonweight bearing. Quadriceps exercises will be initiated early. Crutches will be used for 4 or more weeks. Surgical treatment might be required to remove a torn meniscus that causes a "locked knee" (see Fig. 4.5). A meniscectomy may be done by arthroscopic surgery or by arthrotomy.

Following surgery, the leg will be placed in a splint or cast for 1–2 weeks. Quadriceps exercises and "straight leg raises" will be initiated early in the postsurgical period. Application of ice to the knee and elevation of the leg to heart level will be used for 2 days postoperatively.

Complications following knee surgery include hemarthrosis and chronic synovitis. Postoperative care requires assessment of the dressings, neurovascular checks, patient education to perform quadriceps exercises and straight leg raises, and psychological support of the athlete, who will be nonactive in sports participation for a period of time.

The question of long-term effects of meniscectomy is still unanswered as to effects on the articular surfaces without complete menisci and the long-term effects of repeated loading activities—such as running—and load transmission across the joints.

## Knee Ligament Injuries

The knee ligaments provide stability to the knee joint and prevent nonphysiologic movement. Ligaments of concern include the anterior and posterior cruciate ligaments, medial collateral and lateral collateral ligaments (see Fig. 4.3). The anterior and posterior cruciate ligaments crisscross within the knee providing rotational stability and anterior-posterior stability to the knee. The medial and lateral collateral ligaments prevent varus and valgus instability. They run vertically from femur to tibia and fibula on the medial and lateral aspects of the joint.

Classification of ligament injuries are Class I mild—with only a few liga-ment fibers involved; Class II moderate—with more ligament fibers torn; and Class III severe—complete disruption of the ligament.

The "terrible triad" is an injury resulting in a tearing of the medial meniscus, anterior cruciate, and medial collateral ligaments. This injury usually requires surgical repair.

Common causes for ligamentous injury involve valgus stress with a flexed knee in rotation, as is common in football or skiing. Anterior stress on the tibia results in anterior cruciate tears, and posterior stress results in posterior cruciate injury.

Symptoms of ligamentous injury include Class I—slight pain, mild swell-ing; Class II—moderate pain, moderate swelling; and Class III—mild pain, varied swelling, mild-to-moderate joint instability, severe disability.

Diagnosis of ligament injury requires x-rays to rule out fractures and a thorough history and examination, including description of sensations or sounds during injury. A rupture of the anterior cruciate ligament may involve an audible pop at the time of injury followed by a hemarthrosis. The physical exam may include an anterior or posterior "drawer test" (see Table 2.6), although there is controversy as to the exact reliability of these tests, which assess the amount of laxity of the ligaments and should only be done after a knee x-ray yields "normal results." More than 1 cm of motion (more than normal) of the tibia forward or backward may indicate cruciate ligament damage.

Arthroscopy may be used to definitively determine the extent of injury. An arthrogram, if performed, may reveal no dye extravasation in Class I, minimal dye extravasation in Class II, and definite dye extravasation in Class III injuries.

Treatments for specific ligament injuries include:

Class I:   RICE followed by a progressive rehabilitation program.
Class II:  RICE followed by protected weight-bearing for 1-6 weeks. A protective brace may be used with range of motion exercise.
Class III: RICE followed by surgery to repair the ligaments. Brace protec-tion for up to 8 weeks is indicated.

Crutches and analgesics, anti-inflammatory drugs, or muscle relaxants may also be used in all classes of ligament injuries.

## SHOULDER INJURIES

The shoulder is a joint that relies on soft tissue support for stability (see Fig. 4.6a–d). The bony component consists of the humerus, scapula, and clavicle. The humerus articulates with the scapula at the glenohumeral joint. The acromial process—a posterior projection of the scapula—articulates with the

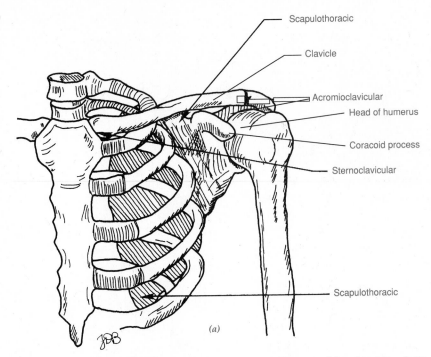

**Figure 4.6** (a) Anterior view of the bones and some ligaments of the shoulder girdle.

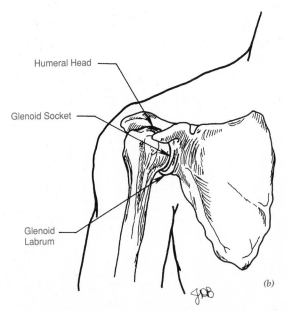

**Figure 4.6** (b) Posterior view of the bones of the shoulder girdle.

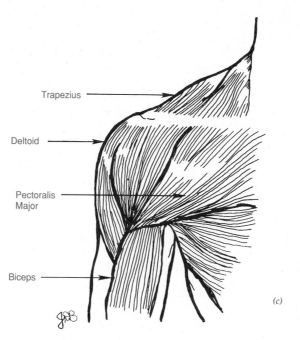

**Figure 4.6** (c) Muscles of the shoulder.

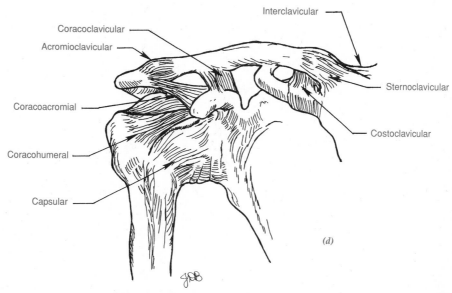

**Figure 4.6** (d) Ligaments of the shoulder.

clavicle at the acromioclavicular joint. The clavicle articulates with the sternum at the sternoclavicular joint. The supporting structure consists of the rotator cuff, which is composed of four muscles: the infraspinatus, supraspinatus, teres minor, and subscapularis and their tendons (see Fig. 4.6e).

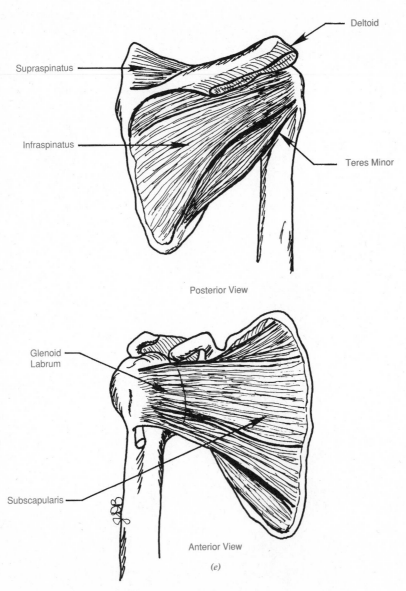

**Figure 4.6** (e) Rotator cuff muscles of the shoulder.

Four bursae lie in muscles around the shoulder (see Fig. 4.7). The subacromial or subdeltoid bursa lies between the deltoid muscle and the rotator cuff. The subcoracoid bursa lies under the coracoid process. The subscapularis bursa is in the tendonaris junction of the lesser tuberosity with the subscapularis. Located at the superior and inferior medial borders of the scapula is the scapular bursa.

Shoulder injuries include sprains, subluxations, dislocations, and fractures. The acromioclavicular, glenohumeral, and sternoclavicular joints are frequent sites for shoulder injuries. These injuries are classified by Class I—sprain; Class II—subluxation; and Class III—dislocation.

## Acromioclavicular Injury (Shoulder Separation)

The mechanism for this injury is usually caused by falling on the elbow, as when a football player holds on to the ball and, therefore, is unable to extend his arm to break his fall. The elbow receives the upward force, and the acromioclavicular joint is disrupted. Injuries to the acromioclavicular joint often includes sprains (ligament injury) of the acromioclavicular and coracoclavicular ligaments.

## Glenohumeral Injury (Shoulder Subluxation or Dislocation)

The mechanism for injury is abduction and external rotation, as in the case of the football arm tackle or the moving skier with a skipole entrapped behind. The

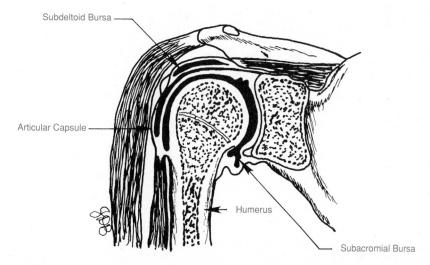

**Figure 4.7** Bursae of the shoulder.

injury usually occurs to the anterior portion of the capsule. The shoulder is the most frequent joint to dislocate, with fingers and elbows closely following.

## Sternoclavicular Injury

The mechanism for injury is a blow that forces the shoulder toward the midline. This force can disrupt the sternoclavicular joint. The major danger with this injury is the subsequent damage that may be done to underlying vascular structures; therefore, a thorough assessment must be made for possible vascular complications.

Diagnosis is made following a complete physical examination with attention to the mechanism of injury and site of the pain. A neurovascular assessment determines any circulatory or neurological impairment. X-rays are taken to rule out fractures or dislocations.

Treatments include closed reduction, followed by rest and immobility with a sling and swathe for 2 or more weeks to permit healing of the ligaments, and application of ice and compression dressing to minimize edema. Surgery may be indicated for Class II injuries.

Class III acromioclavicular injuries may require a resection of the clavicle with ligamentous repair or the use of oral anti-inflammatory agents.

Class III glenohumeral injuries may be surgically treated if dislocation occurs more than two or three times and if the person is unable to continue participation in sports because of repeated dislocations. Nonsurgical treatment may include exercises to improve strength in the adductors and internal and external rotators.

Rehabilitation includes motion as early as possible to prevent development of a stiff shoulder. The length of immobility will be determined by the physician and will depend on the extent of the injuries.

An isokinetic machine is recommended for testing and rehabilitating upper-extremity injuries. This machine provides data about the strength and endurance of muscle groups and, therefore, minimizes the possibility of an athlete's return to competition before complete motion and strength have returned.

Recurrent shoulder pain may necessitate the use of oral anti-inflammatory agents or steroids. The use of steroid injections is controversial, however, due to the risk of avascular necrosis, focal necrosis, and further tendon injury.

Return to active competition may be allowed 6 or more weeks after injury. The athlete must be fully healed before strenuous exercise is attempted.

## Rotator Cuff Injuries

Rotator cuff injuries are strains or tears of one or more rotator muscles or tendons. The most common site is the supraspinatus muscle. Severe rotator cuff tears involve two or more tendons, with retraction and scarring.

Acute tears result from trauma, such as falls on an outstretched hand or injuries from football throwing, baseball or softball pitching, racquetball serving, or manipulation of a frozen shoulder.

Symptoms include severe pain and loss of motion in forward flexion and abduction. Chronic tears originate from overuse or constant stress. Symptoms of chronic tears include pain on motion, weakness in elevation, and limited range of motion.

Diagnosis includes a history of the mechanism of injury, physical examination, x-rays to rule out fracture; an EMG (electromyogram) may help rule out nerve injury. Physical examination includes testing for a positive arc sign, which is indicative of cuff injury if pain is present at 70-100° range of abduction. The drop arm test is positive for a cuff tear if the patient is unable to maintain 90° of abduction against gravity. The patient may require an injection of lidocaine into the cuff to permit this test.

An arthrogram may be performed to diagnose the extent of the tear. Dye is injected into the space between the humeral head and the glenoid cavity. A rotator cuff tear is evident if the dye extravasates into the subacromial region; however, a negative arthrogram may not rule out a partial tear. Arthroscopy of the shoulder may be done to visualize the condition of the joint and its tissues (see discussion of arthroscopy, p. 101).

Conservative treatment with rest, a sling and swathe dressing, application of ice, anti-inflammatory agents, and analgesics is indicated for partial tears and for more severe tears without major disability or pain.

Surgical repair is indicated for persons with acute, complete rupture of the cuff or for persons with continued disability and pain (see Chapter 12 for surgical repairs).

Rehabilitation following conservative or surgical treatment is basically the same, including pain management using analgesics, ADL training for one-handedness, and physical therapy to regain muscle strength, endurance, and flexibility. Exercises begin with pendulum exercises.

The patient may not be able to participate in competition for several weeks following injury. Some persons find that they are unable to regain full strength and mobility and may need to substitute another sport that does not require so much shoulder stress. These are difficult decisions for an athlete and require full support and encouragement from the entire medical team.

## ELBOW INJURIES

Tennis elbow (lateral epicondylitis) or golfer's elbow (medial epicondylitis) are fully discussed in Chapter 5, pp. 178–181 (see Fig. 4.8).

### Dislocated Elbow

The elbow is the third most common joint to dislocate; the shoulder and fingers are the two most common, respectively. Although the elbow may

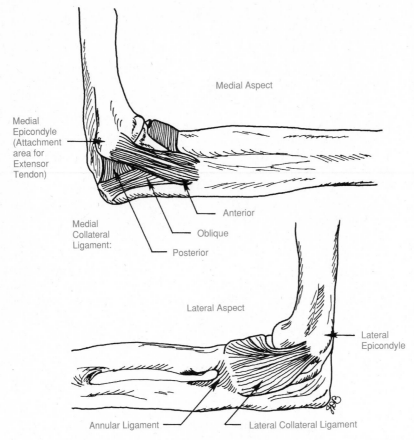

Medial Aspect

Medial Epicondyle (Attachment area for Extensor Tendon)

Medial Collateral Ligament:

Anterior

Oblique

Posterior

Lateral Aspect

Lateral Epicondyle

Annular Ligament

Lateral Collateral Ligament

**Figure 4.8** Medial and lateral epicondyles and collateral ligaments of the elbow (sites of golfer's and tennis elbow, respectively).

dislocate anteriorly, posteriorly, laterally, or medially, posterior dislocation is the most common.

The mechanism for a posterior dislocation injury is a fall with the arm in abduction and extension. The dislocated elbow shows moderate edema and a posteriorly protruding olecranon.

Diagnosis is made based on the results of a history of the mechanism of injury and a physical examination, including assessment of the neurovascular status. The brachial artery and median or ulnar nerves may be compromised with a posterior dislocation. X-rays confirm dislocation and rule out fractures of the coronoid process or medial epicondyle.

Treatments include stabilizing the elbow in flexion and adduction and applying ice to decrease edema. Closed reduction by the physician using gentle traction and pressure over the olecranon while lifting it distally and anteriorly is indicated as early as possible to avoid neurovascular compromise from soft tissue swelling and prevent articular cartilage damage.

## MISCELLANEOUS SOFT TISSUE CONDITIONS

### Osteochondritis Dissecans

Loose bodies in the knee can come from several sources, including disrupted menisci, fractured articular surfaces, or, more commonly, from osteochondritis dissecans. In this disease, subchondral bone and its covering cartilage develop avascular necrosis, and eventually the cartilage separates from adjacent bone to become a loose body. This may occur in the knee, shoulder, elbow, ankle, or hip, but it is most common in the knee.

Trauma is the suspected cause of the lesion, because it often occurs in persons who have participated in contact sports. Symptoms include dull, aching knee pain with "locking." Diagnosis involves a medical history that might reveal a momentary locking of the knee, observance of the person's gait (the tibia will appear externally rotated), and arthroscopy. If the bone has not yet separated from the cartilage, treatment will include rest and protected or nonweight bearing to allow the avascularized bone to heal. A cast might be applied for a few weeks. If the bone is separated from the cartilage, surgical treatment might be indicated for fixation or removal of the loose piece.

### Baker's Cyst

Baker's cyst is a popliteal cyst that can arise from fluid accumulation in the posterior bursa or from a collection of synovial fluid from the knee joint. The transmission of fluid into the bursa causes a cyst and reduces intra-articular pressure.

Symptoms include posterior knee swelling, chronic knee pain, and giving way of the knee. Symptoms of a ruptured cyst closely approximate those of thrombophlebitis; therefore, an accurate differential diagnosis must be made using ultrasonography and arthrography. Treatment includes aspiration of fluid, injection of steroids, and administration of anti-inflammatory drugs.

### Shin Splints

Shin splints are transient pain over one or both shins from running. Pain can be mild to severe and is evinced on palpation of the tibia.

This injury can be prevented by the runner's wearing shoes with better cushioning and having training in proper running techniques. Shin splints can happen to highly trained runners but are more prevalent in untrained runners. Treatment consists of stopping running for 6–10 days. If the pain continues following conservative treatment, an x-ray should be taken to rule out stress fractures.

## Blisters

Blisters are layers of skin that are separated by an abnormal amount of fluid, producing a noticeable lump. Pressure, friction, or a burn may cause a blister to develop.

Symptoms include a raised area that is filled with serum and is painful and very tender, and diagnosis is made by examination of the area, referred to as vesicle.

Treatments include covering the blister or vesicle with a small occlusive dressing and application of an antiseptic. There is controversy about puncturing blisters, because this breaks the skin integrity and allows possible infection. Puncturing the blister relieves the pressure pain and prevents further edema; however, the skin over the blistered area should not be removed, because it protects the area, which is considered a wound once the skin is punctured.

## FRACTURES

A fracture is a break in a bone (see Figs. 4.9, 4.10, 4.11, and 4.12). The break may be through only one cortex (greenstick) or through both cortices (transverse, oblique, or spiral), and may contain more than two pieces (comminuted) (see Fig. 4.13). Table 4.2 lists common types of fractures, descriptive features, and the force or power causing the fracture.

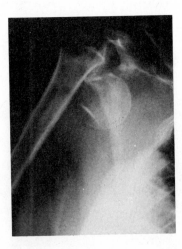

**Figure 4.9** Transverse fracture and dislocation of the head of the humerus.

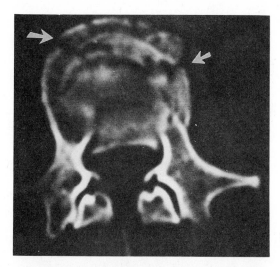

**Figure 4.10** Burst comminuted fracture of the vertebra (arrows).

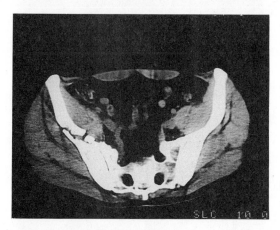

**Figure 4.11** Fracture and separation of ilium bone of the pelvis (left on picture).

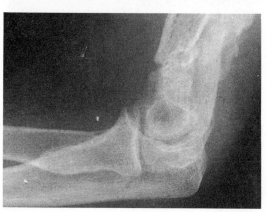

**Figure 4.12** Intra-articular comminuted fracture of the humerus and elbow.

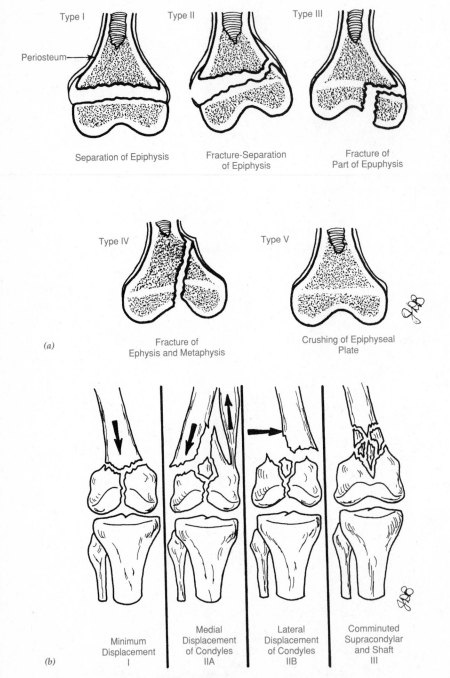

Type I · Type II · Type III

Periosteum→

Separation of Epiphysis · Fracture-Separation of Epiphysis · Fracture of Part of Epuphysis

Type IV · Type V

Fracture of Ephysis and Metaphysis · Crushing of Epiphyseal Plate

(a)

Minimum Displacement I · Medial Displacement of Condyles IIA · Lateral Displacement of Condyles IIB · Comminuted Supracondylar and Shaft III

(b)

**Figure 4.13** (a) Salter-Harris fractures involving the epiphysis. (b) Fractures and dislocations of the femur.

**Table 4.2** Descriptions of Types and Causes of Fractures

| Type of Fracture | Descriptive Factors | Force or Energy Causing Fracture and Injury |
|---|---|---|
| Closed | Skin is closed but bone is fractured. | Minor energy |
| Open | Skin is open, bone is fractured, and there may be trauma to soft tissues. | Moderate to severe energy that is continuous and exceeds tissue tolerances |
| Greenstick | Break in only one cortex of the bone. | Minor direct or indirect energy |
| Transverse | Horizontal break through the bone. | Direct or indirect energy toward the bone |
| Spiral | Fracture curves around both cortices and may become displaced by twist. | Direct or indirect twisting energy or force with the distal part held or unable to move |
| Oblique | Fracture at an oblique angle across both cortices. | Direct or indirect energy with angulation and some compression |
| Comminuted | Fracture with more than two pieces; may have much associated soft tissue trauma. | Direct crushing energy or force to tissues and bone |
| Compression | Fracture of bone which is squeezed or wedged together at one side. | Compressive, axial energy or force applied directly from above the fracture site |
| Avulsed | Fracture that pulls bone and other tissues from their usual attachments. | Direct energy or force with resisted extension of the bone and joint |
| Stress | Crack in one cortex of a bone. | Repetitive direct energy or force as from jogging, running, or striking a lever, or from osteoporosis |
| Pathologic | Transverse, oblique, or spiral fracture of a bone weakened by tumor presence. | Minor energy or force, which may be direct or indirect |
| Linear | As a line so can be transverse or oblique. | Minor or moderate energy or force directly to bone |
| Impacted | Fracture with one end wedged into the opposite or inside of the fractured fragment. | Compressive, axial energy or force directly to the distal fragment |

A fractured bone and its surrounding tissues cannot carry out their normal activities and functions. Bleeding may be pronounced, with a hematoma forming around the fracture fragments. Edema develops from the blood vessel disruption. Numbness is initially present, lasting for approximately 20 minutes, followed by pain, which can become progressively severe until it is relieved by medication and fracture treatments. Use of the body part containing the fractured bone will be limited by the pain and associated tissue trauma (see Fig. 4.14). The surrounding tissues may be cooler and paler than similar contralateral tissues.

Before any first aid or any other measures are performed, an accurate assessment of the extent of the injury must be made to avoid additional injury. The initial injury may precipitate a fainting episode or lead to increased bleeding, shock, and hypovolemia. The injured tissues should be immobilized in a splint or air cast, or the person may be placed on a backboard. Care must be taken to maintain the head and neck in a neutral position if head or neck trauma is suspected. Multiple trauma can involve the thorax, lungs, heart, pelvic bones, and other abdominal trauma. Pressure should be applied to open, bleeding wounds, and clean or sterile dressings should be applied to decrease the chance of contamination and aid hemostasis. Gentle handling, with support of joints above and below the fracture site, along with calm explanations and manner, increase the victim's confidence in the caregiver.

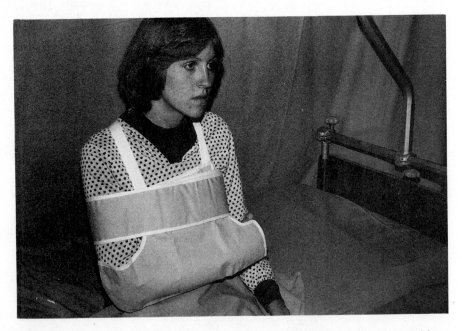

**Figure 4.14** Sling and swathe to support and immobilize the arm and shoulder.

## Stress Fractures

Stress fractures occur in runners and result in hairline cracks in bones of the lower extremities. Symptoms include pain at the fracture site, swelling, or limping. X-rays might appear normal, but a follow-up x-ray performed 2–3 weeks after injury reveals periosteal bone formation. Treatment includes rest for at least 3 weeks. Crutches may be used if extreme pain is present on ambulation.

Table 4.3 contains a listing of treatment usually used for each of the types of fractures. Use of a cast and the care involved is discussed in Chapter 10, and the use of various forms of traction is discussed in Chapter 11. Surgical repairs of fractures are discussed in Chapter 12.

## Processes of Bone Healing

Injured or traumatized bones heal themselves through the same process of inflammation as the soft tissues of the body. Because of the nature and function of the bony skeleton, however, the healing process appears more complex and takes longer. The exact nature of bone healing is still not completely understood; however, the use of the electron microscope has clarified more of the local cellular activities that aid or hinder bone healing.

A summary of the steps of bone healing may be given as follows:

*Development of a Hematoma at the Site of the Injury.* The presence of a hematoma may or may not be an absolute requirement for bone healing; it may be merely a consequence of the disruption of the blood vessels from the injury. It apparently promotes healing, however, by bringing clotting factors necessary for fibrin formation to the area and maintaining a "solid" area for fibrin strands to form. On the negative side, too large a hematoma could delay the entrance and exit of macrophages, platelets, oxygen, and other nutrients necessary to effect bone callus formation. Hematomas form from the bleeding of disrupted blood vessels, but they are also caused by increased capillary permeability, permitting extravasation of blood into the injured area. Redness, heat, and edema are evidence of this inflammatory healing step.

*Consolidation.* Fibroblasts invade the injured area and adhere to themselves and other tissue cells, forming a fibrin meshwork. White blood cells, such as lymphocytes, polymorphonuclear neutrophils, and monocytes, also migrate to the area, walling it off to keep the area of inflammation localized. Tissue chemotactic factors keep the fibroblasts and white cells adhered in the area, consolidating and continuing the inflammatory response, as noted by edema, heat, pain, and loss of function, because the tenuous fibrin meshwork is inadequate for carrying weight or moving without pain. Some mucopolysaccharides, which are either present in or are brought to the injured area, assist with the consolidation and adherence of fibrin meshwork. Osteoblasts congregate in the injured area.

**Table 4.3** Common Fractures, Their Usual Treatments, Weight-bearing Restrictions, and Common Complications

| Fracture Site | Type of Fracture or Injury | Usual Treatment | Weight Bearing/ Mobilization | Complications |
|---|---|---|---|---|
| | | Upper Extremities | | |
| Shoulder | Fracture/dislocation | Closed reduction Sling and swathe (see Fig. 4.14) ORIF* for repeated dislocation | Temporary immobility; early active motion. | Nonunion, dislocation |
| Head of Humerus | Comminuted (more than two pieces) | Total shoulder arthroplasty | Temporary immobility for 3–5 days; sling and swathe, then motion beginning with forward flexion and external rotation | Infection, loosening of prosthesis |
| Proximal Humerus | Avulsion fractures of tuberosities | ORIF using wire suture | Early motion | Infection, nonunion, delayed union |
| | Displaced fractures | Closed reduction | Immobility with sling and swathe, then movement encouraged | Stiff shoulder, nonunion, malunion |
| Shaft of Humerus | Fracture/dislocation | Closed reduction with hanging arm cast (dependent traction) | Cast for 10-21 days, then cast removed and movement encouraged | Nonunion, malunion, delayed union |
| | Pathological fracture | ORIF with plate and screws or intramedullary rod | Early movement of arm encouraged | Infection, stiff shoulder and elbow |

(continued)

| | | Treatment | Immobilization/Management | Complications |
|---|---|---|---|---|
| Distal Humerus | Supracondylar fracture | Hanging arm cast; ORIF if unable to reduce closed or if neurovascular compromise present | Immobility from cast presence | Nonunion, pain, limited motion, weakness, instability, loss of function, infection, radial nerve palsy |
| | Transcondylar fracture | ORIF | Splint for up to 7 days, then motion begun | |
| | Intracondylar fracture | Screws inserted | Immobility for varying periods | Degenerative joint problems |
| Olecranon | Articular fracture/dislocation | Plates/pins; If fragments separated: ORIF using wire, pin, or screw | As above; Immobilized in a splint for 7–10 days, then motion; Forceful extension to be avoided for up to 3 months | As above; Infection, nonunion, malunion, delayed union, degenerative joint problems |
| Radius Head and Neck | Nondisplaced fracture | Cast | Immobilized 2–6 weeks | Weakness, mild discomfort |
| | Comminuted fracture | ORIF; removal of free fragments; excision of radial head | Immobilization for 1 week, then motion encouraged | Infection, limited motion, weakness |
| Distal Radius (nonarticular) | Colles fracture with displacement of the radius | Cast, unless severely comminuted, then ORIF with Kirschner wires; application of external fixator | Immobilization in cast above the elbow with wrist and forearm in neutral position for 5–7 weeks. Finger exercises begun early | Median nerve compression, nonunion, malunion, stiff hand, infection, weakness, pain |

(continued)

**Table 4.3** (Continued)

| Fracture Site | Type of Fracture or Injury | Usual Treatment | Weight Bearing/ Mobilization | Complications |
|---|---|---|---|---|
| Ulna | Transverse or oblique fracture/dislocation | ORIF with intramedullary rod or plate or screws; application of external fixator. If fixator, may begin active movements earlier in recovery period. | Cast for 3–6 weeks, then removal, and gentle active motion begun. | Loss of motion, malunion, nonunion infection |
| Wrist Scaphoid or carpus | Transverse or oblique fracture/dislocation | Closed treatment in a cast from uppermost forearm to distal thumb. | Immobilization for 8–10 weeks in cast | Delayed union, nonunion, avascular necrosis |
| Phalanges and Metacarpals | Transverse or oblique | Reduction and splint or cast or ORIF if unstable fracture | Immobilization in cast or splint for 3 weeks | Malunion, nonunion, weakness, loss of function, infection |
| Base of thumb | Bennett's fracture, an intra-articular fracture through base of 1st metacarpal, the thumb | Closed pinning with Kirschner wire, or ORIF with insertion of Kirschner wire | Immobilization in cast for 3–7 weeks, or use of splint to maintain immobility | Nonunion, limited motion, pain, weakness of grip |
| Lower Extremities | | | | |
| Proximal Femur | Intertrochanteric fracture | ORIF with nails, compression screw, or plate | Mobility 1–2 days post-surgery, weight bearing as tolerated (WBAT) | Hemorrhage, nonunion, infection, avascular necrosis, deep vein |

| | | with a walker and then crutches | thrombosis, pneumonia |
|---|---|---|---|
| **Proximal Femur** (continued) | | | |
| Femoral neck or subcapital fracture | ORIF with screw or pins (Knowles), or sliding pin and blade plate, or prosthesis to replace head of the femur | Protected weight bearing 5–10 lbs. with walker or crutches | Avascular necrosis, nonunion, infection, hemorrhage |
| Subtrochanteric | ORIF with Zickel or other nail with screw into femoral head and neck | Protected weight bearing with increasing weight bearing over 6–8 weeks; full weight bearing at 8 weeks | Appliance failure, nonunion, infection |
| **Shaft of Femur** Transverse or oblique | Closed reduction with intramedullary fixation or external fixation device, or ORIF with intramedullary fixation with nails or rod | Touch down weight bearing (TDWB) for 4–6 weeks using walker or crutches | Nonunion, infection, rotation, malunion, delayed union, shortening, fat emboli |
| **Distal Femur** Condylar fracture (single condyle), displaced | ORIF using skeletal pins or cancellous screws; blade plate with screws | Quadriceps exercises begun immediately postoperatively, crutch walking; nonweight bearing (NWB) begun at 3–5 days and continued for 4–6 weeks until callus is well-formed | Nonunion, infection |

(continued)

**Table 4.3** (Continued)

| Fracture Site | Type of Fracture or Injury | Usual Treatment | Weight Bearing/ Mobilization | Complications |
|---|---|---|---|---|
| Distal Femur (continued) | Intercondylar fracture | ORIF with blade plate and screws and Kirschner wire (K-wire) for comminuted intercondylar or skeletal traction for 2–3 weeks or longer | Active, gentle, assisted exercises begun at 4–5 days; crutch walking at 2–3 weeks, NWB or partial WB for 10–12 weeks | Nonunion |
| | Supracondylar fracture | Skeletal traction with K-wire through the proximal tibia for several days followed by cast brace application | Bedrest while in traction; ambulation with NWB after fracture reduction for 8–10 weeks | Nonunion, refracture |
| | Epiphyseal fracture (Salter-Harris type) | ORIF with pins if soft tissue is caught between fragments, or closed reduction under anesthesia and spica or long leg-cast application | Pins removed at 4–6 weeks | Growth disturbance with shortening or angulation in children |
| | | | Immobilization in cast with knee at 45° flexion for 4–6 weeks, weight bearing at 8–10 weeks | |
| Knee | Fracture of the patella, nondisplaced | Knee immobilizer | Quadriceps exercises begun | Chronic bursitis, infection, malalignment resulting in loss of knee motion |

| | | | | |
|---|---|---|---|---|
| Knee (continued) | Comminuted | Fixation of fragments with wire loops; knee immobilizer | After removal of sutures, a cast-brace may be used; quadriceps exercises begun immediately postoperatively | |
| Tibia | Condylar fractures Nondisplaced with intact ligaments | Posterior splint | Immobility in traction or splint, weight bearing delayed for 8–10 weeks | Deep vein thrombosis, nonunion, loss of knee motion |
| | Comminuted | Skeletal traction with K-wire through calcaneus or distal tibia or ORIF with cancellous screws and buttress plates | Posterior plaster splint in 45° flexion for 3–4 days; quadriceps and active assisted exercises are then started, NWB for 12–16 weeks; begin use of crutches at 2 weeks | Loss of knee motion |
| Shaft of Tibia | Transverse | Varies: may be treated in a cast only or by ORIF | Cast for 8–10 weeks, then weight bearing begun or encouraged | All tibial fractures: Delayed union, malunion, nonunion, infection, potential shortening of leg |
| | Comminuted or open | ORIF with screws and plate or external fixation device | Cast worn for 3–6 weeks; pins removed at 3–4 weeks, and long leg | |

(continued)

**Table 4.3** (Continued)

| Fracture Site | Type of Fracture or Injury | Usual Treatment | Weight Bearing/ Mobilization | Complications |
|---|---|---|---|---|
| Comminuted or open (continued) | | | cast applied; NWB on crutches if able | |
| | Spiral or long oblique | ORIF with screws | Cast from midthigh to toes for 3–4 weeks, then partial weight bearing with crutches | |
| Ankle | Potts fracture (fracture of the lateral and medial malleoli) | ORIF with pins or screws | Cast from toes to tibial tuberosity for 4 weeks, then protected weight bearing with crutches | Infection, loss of motion, posttraumatic arthritis |
| | Cotton fracture (fracture of the lateral and medial malleoli and the posterior lip of the articular surface of the tibia) | ORIF with screws and compression plate with screws | As above | As above |
| Tarsal Bones Calcaneus | Transverse or oblique | Treatment options: ORIF with pin (Essex-Lopresti technique) or Closed reduction with pin or ORIF with staples | Cast; exercise toes and ankle; weight bearing in 8–10 weeks; cast and pin removed in 4–6 weeks | Infection |

| | | | | |
|---|---|---|---|---|
| Talus | Transverse or oblique | ORIF with screws | Foot in neutral position in a short leg cast, NWB for 6–8 weeks, then a walking cast | Avascular necrosis, posttraumatic arthritis, loss of motion, residual pain |
| Metatarsal bones | Transverse or oblique | Closed reduction or | Foot padded and placed in wooden shoe for 4–8 weeks, then protected weight bearing with cane or crutches | Nonunion, pain |
| | | ORIF with wire or plate | Cast or padded dressing with wire exposed; wire removed at 3 weeks, wooden shoe in 4–6 weeks | Nonunion, pain |
| Clavicle | | Closed reduction | Arm in sling and swathe for 8 weeks, then movement encouraged | Nonunion, malunion with protrusion of fragments |
| | | ORIF with intramedullary pin | Ambulatory with arm in sling for 1–2 weeks | Nonunion |
| Pelvis Ring of Pelvis | Comminuted or Oblique and lateral | ORIF or | Early ambulation if other injuries permit | Hemorrhage, disruption of vessel and nerves, injuries to intestines, bladder, and urethra |
| | | Closed treatment with external fixation | Bedrest and immobility 3–5 days or longer, then up with a walker | Deep vein thrombosis, pneumonia, paralytic ileus |

*ORIF = Open Reduction with Internal Fixation.

*Granulation.* Osteoblasts continue to cross in and through the fibrin bridge to help firm it; capillary buds gradually develop into new blood vessels and bring nutrients to the area to form collagen, the tough scar tissue. Again, these collagen fibers are held together with more mucopolysaccharides, gradually becoming longer and longer collagen strands, incorporating calcium deposits throughout to form bone or callus. *Bone is the only tissue that heals itself with new bone, not scar tissue.*

*Callus formation.* *Osteoblasts* continue in this step as they did in granulation, laying the network for bone buildup. *Osteoclasts* destroy dead bone and help in the synthesis of new bone. This stage is critical to bone formation and healing for several vital reasons: (1) the environmental nutrients must be present and in sufficient quantity—particularly the proper amount and tension of oxygen, as well as the above-mentioned vitamins, minerals, carbohydrates, proteins, insulin, and water; (2) bone healing is enhanced by just the right amount of compression on the immature bone. Too little compression may result in pseudobone, and too much compression may decrease oxygen tension too greatly, causing too much bone-end absorption, ultimately creating too great a space for collagen fibers to form strong callus. The mucopolysaccharides gradually decrease in this stage as the collagen strengthens and is impregnated with calcium forming the healed bone.

*Remodeling.* During this stage, excess callus is resorbed, and trabecular (fibrous) bone is laid down along the lines of stress and according to Wolff's law of stress lines. Wolff's law states that bone will respond to stress by becoming thicker and stronger. Osteoclasts resorb excess or poorly placed trabecular bone until it is strong and has been remodeled according to its usual structure and function. Osteoblasts help in forming new haversian canals to complete the remodeling stage.

Bone formation and healing are thought to be controlled by electrical charges of the various cells involved. The electropositive osteoblasts act on the convex side of the bone, whereas the electronegative osteoblasts build up new bone on the concave side.

## Local Factors in Bone Healing

- *Severity of Trauma.* Too much trauma in the contiguous soft tissues contributes to increased edema formation, decreasing or blocking the passage of substances such as blood with vital nutrients to the area, causing dissipation of the "bonogenic" (bone forming) cells to too large an area of bone and soft tissue. The cells appear confused; too much healing (bone and soft tissue) is required; thus, the entire healing process is delayed (see Figs. 4.12 and 4.13b).

- *Insufficient Bridge of Bone.* If the osteoblasts cannot build a sufficient bridge on the concave side of the traumatized bone—because of a lack of either nutrients or oxygen—healing is delayed and retarded; it may ultimately proceed only to the point of cartilage formation (cartilage is bone without calcium) and not continue to form solid bone.
- *Too Much Bone Loss.* If too much bone was lost in the original injury, the distance to be bridged may either be too great or may be unbridgeable for a long time, thus delaying or prohibiting healing.
- *Type of Bone Injured.* Cancellous (spongy) bone heals fairly quickly because of the presence of cells and blood in this type of bone. Cortical bone, being more solid and relatively low in cells and blood, must heal with end-to-end contact and have more rigid immobilization to prevent disruption of the fragile blood supply and nutrients.
- *Degree of Immobilization.* If immobilization is inadequate, healing is delayed, because motion or movement of the parts disrupts the hematoma and/or the fibrin bridge; this could eventually result in formation of only cartilage, a condition known as pseudoarthrosis (false joint formation) (see Fig. 4.15).
- *Infection.* Local tissue defenses would have to mobilize to fight and wall off the infection, possibly retarding or, at times, preventing healing.
- *Local Malignancy.* As with infection, the presence of malignant cells depletes local resources, delaying or preventing healing. Usually the primary malignancy must be treated before healing can proceed.

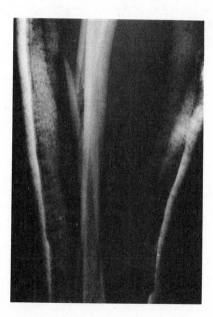

**Figure 4.15** Inadequate immobilization of a comminuted fracture of the tibia. (Cast is too loose; reduction has been lost.)

- *Necrosis of Bone* (for example, radiation necrosis). Such scarring (necrosis) prevents blood from getting in, resulting in nonunion or markedly prolonged healing time.
- *Intra-articular Fractures (through the joint).* Such fractures free synovial joint fluid containing fibrinolysins, which destroy the initial clot or hematoma, delaying the first-stage process of healing as shown in Fig. 4.12, which is an intra-articular fracture.
- *Use of Bone Growth Stimulators.* Use of low-voltage electric impulses enhances bone healing.

## Systemic Factors in Bone Healing

- *Age.* Young children heal rapidly because of their more-rapid cell differentiation, whereas older persons experience a longer healing time. Though there is no "average" time for fracture healing, children show beginning callus formation as early as 7–10 days after injury; whereas older persons have evidence in 10–14 days. In children, fractures may be totally healed in 4–6 weeks; it might take 6–8 weeks or longer in older adults.
- *Hormones.* Growth hormone promotes bone healing, whereas corticosteroids inhibit bone healing because of their anti-inflammatory nature. Thyroid hormone, insulin, and vitamins A and D are anabolic (tissue building).
- *Debilitating Diseases.* Diabetes, cancer, or other cachectic diseases hinder bone healing.
- *Local Stress Around a Fracture.* Healing is retarded or slowed by stress at the site.
- *Exercise, Including Quadriceps ("Quad") Setting and Some Weight Bearing.* Exercises enhance healing by promoting calcium retention in bone. Weight bearing of a limited degree aids bone healing.

## NURSING PROCESS IN THE CARE OF PERSONS WITH FRACTURES

## NURSING DIAGNOSIS

*IMPAIRED PHYSICAL MOBILITY RELATED TO FRACTURE OF BONE(S) AND SOFT TISSUE TRAUMA*

### Assessment

1. Assess for presence of deformity, edema, tenderness or pain, and condition of contiguous soft tissues.

2. Assess for open areas of skin, bleeding, dirt or foreign substances in fracture area.

3. Assess for ability to use part or protective measures to prevent further injury.

## Expected Outcomes

The patient will:

- regain physical mobility following treatments.
- regain intact skin tissues with healing and recovery.

## Nursing Interventions

1. Gently assist patient to a position of comfort; support injured tissues at joints above and below fracture site to prevent additional injury.

2. Elevate injured limb or part on pillows to aid venous return.

3. Apply ice bag(s) to injured area to lessen edema and bleeding.

4. Perform neurovascular checks q 1–2 hrs as ordered (see p. 255 for steps of neurovascular checks.)

5. When ordered, assist patient to be up in chair; elevate injured limb on pillows or stool to decrease edema formation. Observe patient for amount of weight bearing permitted.

6. Teach patient use of crutches or walker to aid ambulation; monitor ambulation to note any unsafe practices.

7. Apply sling to maintain upper extremity nonweight bearing; teach patient self-application of sling to increase independence.

8. Teach patient how to use trapeze and shift positions in bed; teach "post" position by having patient bend knee of uninjured leg and place foot firmly on bed, then grasp trapeze and lift self with all weight on arms and uninjured leg and foot.

9. Monitor traction setup (if used; see Chapter 11 for care of patients in traction) for proper functioning.

10. Explain upcoming surgical procedure, if surgical correction is to be done. See Chapter 12 for surgical care.

## Evaluation

The patient:

- gradually regained physical mobility after treatments.
- regained intact skin tissues with healing and recovery.

# NURSING DIAGNOSIS

## PAIN RELATED TO FRACTURE(S) AND SOFT TISSUE TRAUMA

### Assessment

1. Assess amount of pain, severity, sites, and characteristics of pain.
2. Assess efforts of pain relief and results.

### Expected Outcomes

The patient will:

- regain freedom from pain with treatments and recovery.
- have no lingering or recurring pain episodes.

### Nursing Interventions

1. Assist patient to reposition self to ease pain and relieve sore or painful muscles and tissues.
2. Monitor patient's complaints of pain; have patient describe pain using 1–10 pain scale; have patient describe pain in own words.
3. Apply ice to injured site to lessen edema and pain.
4. Elevate injured area to increase venous return to decrease edema.
5. Administer narcotic and non-narcotic analgesics q 3 to 4 hours as ordered; monitor effects and side effects of medications or PCA (patient controlled analgesia), if present. Around-the-clock administration of analgesics helps maintain therapeutic blood levels to control pain.
6. Administer muscle relaxant or nonsteroidal anti-inflammatory medications between narcotics to help resolve soft tissue reactions and ease inflammatory response.

### Evaluation

The patient:

- gradually experienced pain relief over time and with medications. Was able to control pain with intermittent medications at home.
- had no lingering or recurring pain episodes after healing of fracture and soft tissue trauma.

# NURSING DIAGNOSIS

## ALTERED PERIPHERAL (PULMONARY) TISSUE PERFUSION AND IMPAIRED GAS EXCHANGE RELATED TO FAT EMBOLISM

### Assessment

1.  Assess for signs of fat embolism: disorientation, shortness of breath, petechiae over chest, neck, and in conjunctivae, tachypnea, sense of danger or doom, anxiety.

2.  Assess vital signs and temperature.

### Expected Outcomes

The patient will:

- regain normal peripheral tissue perfusion with no pulmonary sequelae.

- regain satisfactory gas exchange with blood gases within normal ranges.

### Nursing Interventions

1.  Monitor physical status q 1–2 hrs for initial 72 hours or longer after long bone fracture. Majority of fat emboli become manifested in first 72 hours after long bone fractures.

2.  Monitor vital signs carefully: tachycardia and elevated temperatures are early signs; tachypnea and shock symptoms may follow quickly.

3.  Check for petechial rash over chest, neck, and conjunctivae—sites different from those associated with allergic or hypersensitivity reactions.

4.  Monitor orientation or changes in sensorium carefully. Disorientation is an early sign of fat embolism.

5.  Listen for breath sounds in all lobes. Breath sounds may be decreased in affected areas.

6.  Administer oxygen therapy by mask or respirator, if needed. $PaO_2$ may be as low as 50 to 60 mm Hg in fat embolism syndrome because of impaired alveolar exchange from obstruction and lung inflammation. $PaCO_2$ levels may be elevated above 45 mm Hg if obstruction from fat embolization is present.

7.  Initiate intravenous fluid therapy as ordered; monitor infusion rates carefully to avoid pulmonary edema.

8. Assist with blood gas determination and chest x-ray as ordered.
9. Administer steroids as ordered. Steroids aid pulmonary microcirculation and are anti-inflammatory.
10. Administer volume expanders (albumin) or whole blood as ordered to restore or maintain blood volume to counteract shock. Albumin also binds free fatty acids in vascular tree.
11. Administer antipyretic drugs as ordered for hyperpyrexia (elevated temperatures); if temperature markedly elevated, external cooling via hypothermia blanket may be needed.
12. Monitor patient closely for progression or relief of symptoms; patient may need to be transferred to intensive care unit for mechanical ventilatory assistance.

## Evaluation

The patient:
- regained normal peripheral tissue perfusion with no pulmonary sequelae after treatments.
- regained satisfactory gas exchange with $Pa\,O_2$ and $Pa\,CO_2$ levels within normal ranges after treatments.

## NURSING DIAGNOSIS

### ANXIETY RELATED TO SUDDEN INJURY AND LOSS OF MOBILITY.

## Assessment
1. Assess presence of or degree of anxiety.
2. Assess effects of anxiety on patient's coping behavior.

## Expected Outcomes
The patient will:
- experience only mild anxiety following injury
- regain emotional stability over time and with care.

## Nursing Interventions
1. Monitor responses to sudden injury, loss of mobility, and hospitalization: may be hyperactive, restless, angry, hostile, fearful, anxious, or quiet and withdrawn.
2. Explain all upcoming events and care; reexplain as needed. Anxiety may prevent patient from completely hearing or understanding initial explanations.

3. Explain use of surgery, casts, or traction, and purpose of each treatment.
4. Discuss healing processes related to fracture and inflammation; use pictures as needed.
5. Administer analgesics, muscle relaxants, and anti-inflammatory medications as ordered to ease pain, muscle spasms, and anxiety. Pain and muscle spasms may increase patient's anxiety that healing is not progressing normally.
6. Assist patient with diversionary activities as desired to distract patient from self-absorption.
7. Teach relaxation techniques to lessen anxiety.
8. Assist with ambulation as ordered, with proper ambulatory aid and amount of weight bearing as ordered.
9. Prepare for discharge by teaching self-care and long-term healing as appropriate.

## Evaluation

The patient

- experienced only mild anxiety controlled with patient's coping mechanisms and medications (analgesics, muscle relaxants, and anti-inflammatories).
- regained emotional stability over time with explanations, knowledge, relaxation techniques, and positive stress response behaviors.

## BIBLIOGRAPHY

Galli, R.L., Spaite, D.W., & Simon, R.R. (1989). *Emergency orthopedics: The spine.* Norwalk, CT: Appleton & Lange.

Ghelman, B. (1985). Meniscal tears of the knee: Evaluation by high resolution CT combined with arthrography. *Radiology, 157,* 23–27.

Goss, T.P. (1986). Rotator cuff injuries. *Orthopaedic Review, 15*(8), 496–503.

Hall, A.J., & Stenner, R.W. (1985). *Manual of fracture bracing.* New York. Churchill Livingstone.

Kaplan, P.E., & Tanner, E.D. (1989). *Musculoskeletal pain and disability.* Norwalk, CT: Appleton & Lange.

Kim, M.J., McFarland, G.K., & McLane, A.M. (1991). *Pocket guide to nursing diagnoses* (4th ed.). St Louis: Mosby-Yearbook.

Leach, R.E. (1986). Lower extremity injuries sustained while playing tennis. *Journal of Musculoskeletal Medicine, 3*(6), 44–54.

McMaster, W.C. (1986). Painful shoulder in swimmers: A diagnostic challenge. *The Physician and Sports Medicine, 14*(12), 108–122.

Mears, D.C., & Rubash, H.E. (1986). *Pelvic and acetabular fractures.* Thorofare, NJ: Slack.

Mourad, L. (1991). *Orthopedic disorders.* St. Louis: Mosby-Yearbook.

Rand, J. (1984). The role of arthroscopy in the management of knee injuries in the athlete. *Mayo Clinic Proceedings, 59,* 77–82.

Reicher, M. A., Hartzman, S., Duckwiler, G. R., Bassett, L. W., Anderson, L. J. & Gold, R. H. (1986). Meniscal injuries: Detection using MR imaging. *Radiology, 159,* 753–758.

Simon, R.R., & Koenigsknecht, S.J. (1987). *Emergency orthopedics: The extremities* (2nd ed.). Norwalk, CT: Appleton & Lange.

Spiegel, P.C. (1984). *Topics in orthopaedic trauma.* Baltimore: University Park Press.

Tucker, C. (1990). *The mechanics of sports injuries.* London: Blackwell.

Turek, S.L. (1984). *Orthopaedic principles and their application* (Vols. 1, 2) (4th ed.). Philadelphia: Lippincott.

Wilkerson, C.B. (1985). Treatment of ankle sprains with external compression and early mobilization. *The Physician and Sports Medicine, 13*(6), 83–90.

# 5

# NURSING PROCESS IN INFLAMMATORY CONDITIONS OF MUSCULOSKELETAL TISSUES

Inflammatory conditions are those that result in local or systemic inflammatory reactions. Some of these conditions are caused by autoimmune responses to some antigen. Rheumatoid arthritis (R.A.), systemic lupus erythematosis (SLE), and progressive systemic sclerosis (PSS) are three autoimmune conditions that affect musculoskeletal tissues, primarily due to arthritis involving one or more joints, joint tissues, and muscles and their functions. Other inflammatory conditions, such as bursitis and epicondylitis or tenosynovitis, are usually secondary to trauma or overuse, yet they also affect the muscles and joints. These two types of inflammatory conditions are the topics of this chapter (see Table 5.1).

## RHEUMATOID ARTHRITIS (R.A.)

R.A. is a chronic, systemic, autoimmune inflammatory condition affecting many tissues in the body. It usually causes severe illness in the affected person, and its course is unpredictable.

R.A. has been estimated to affect 1 to 3% of the population in the United States, with up to 200,000 new cases per year. Onset of symptoms of R.A. can occur at any age and females have a steady progression of onset with increasing age, with females being affected 3:1 over males. In males, R.A. symptoms have two peak incidences, one between ages 24 to 34 and the second after age 65. It appears to affect blacks and whites in the Unites States at equal rates. It may have a genetic or familial basis, although no definite studies have validated those bases. The disease has been shown to shorten life expectancies from 3 to 18 years.

**Table 5.1** Local, Regional, and Systemic Signs of Inflammation

| Sign | Tissue Response | Local Evidence | Regional Evidence | Systemic Evidence |
|------|-----------------|----------------|-------------------|-------------------|
| Redness (rubor) | Vasodilation from histamine liberation or other irritants, increased red blood cells (RBCs) in capillaries | Area redder than surrounding tissues | Extended area of redness in extremity, conjunctiva, or other tissues (cellulitis) | Flushed face, rash over body or parts of body |
| Heat (calor) | Increased metabolism in area and increased arterial blood supply | Area hotter than surrounding tissues | Large area of hotter-than-normal tissues (e.g., the entire finger, hand, leg) | Low-grade or spiking temperatures |
| Edema (tumor) | Slowing of blood flow, lymphatic compression, cellular debris, irritation, increased venous congestion, increased capillary permeability, increased WBCs and RBCs in area | Swelling, wheal, papule, blister (vesicle), and so on | Edema of area surrounding inflamed cells, enlarged lymph nodes | Generalized edema over body with edema of eyelids, sacral area, and legs |
| Pain (dolor) | Pressure on nerve endings or from chemical irritants in area | With movement; wincing or avoidance behavior, limping, guarding; verbal evidence of pain, tenderness, numbness, tingling | Pain in area of cellulitis or inflammation from increased pressure of edematous tissues; headache; nuchal rigidity; low back pain; abdominal pain | Generalized malaise, soreness, aching throughout body possibly localizing to the back, joints, appendix, or other areas |

| | | | | |
|---|---|---|---|---|
| Loss of function (functio laesa) | Triggered reflexly to decrease use to prevent more injury; use prevented by edema and degree of injury | Lack of movement, lack of use of part, or protective behaviors; holding, supporting to part where applicable; possible stiffness or decreased flexion or extension | Joint weakness, stiffness, tightness or flaccidity of muscles | Inability to carry on activities of daily life, such as walking, moving, lifting |
| Metastasis (spread) | Cells from capillaries into area of inflammation to wall off area and phagocytize if needed | Not externally observable initially (possible eventual abscess or pustule) | Regional lymph node enlargement, edema of entire finger or extremity | Generalized edema, rash, toxemia |
| Metaplasia (hypo- or hyperplasia) | Cell size decreased to adapt to decreased nutrients or increased due to permeability, compared with normal tissues | Not externally observable initially | Swollen or indented area in inflamed site | Systemic weight loss |

## Pathophysiology

The onset of R.A. can be acute or insidious, and, most commonly, the sites involved are the fingers and wrists (50%), feet and ankles (20%), and 10% each in the knee, shoulder, and other joints. Pain and stiffness in the affected joints usually are two of the first symptoms. The joints become swollen and painful, and a common finding is that symmetric joints are affected bilaterally. The joints become red, warm, and are very tender as the disease progresses through the synovial lining. The lining becomes markedly inflamed, thickened, and overgrown, extending outside the joint, and is referred to as pannus formation. Joint swelling increases and the joint feels "doughy." Deformity may be noted as tendons around the affected joint become inflamed and decrease joint range of motion. Ligaments also can become inflamed and tender. As the disease progresses, the joint cartilage becomes frayed and fibrillated, causing more limitation of movement and increased pain. Cartilage loose bodies and tendon nodules may cause clicking with joint motion.

Signs of inflammation may be noted in other body tissues, especially the heart, lungs, kidneys, and skin. Subcutaneous nodules appear near joints but outside the joints in the soft tissues. Cardiac arrhythmias may be noted, and respiratory and renal functions may show gradual decreases.

Many of the following symptoms must be present for the diagnosis of R.A. to be made: morning stiffness in one or more joints for 6 or more weeks; symmetric involvement bilaterally; pain and tenderness on movement in at least one joint, swelling in two or more joints; subcutaneous nodules over bony prominences; elevated erythrocyte sedimentation rate; positive serum rheumatoid factor (an immunoglobulin). Radiologic studies usually show characteristic bony decalcification localized to or around the affected joint. Physical examination gives evidence of the above symptoms, limitation of joint functions and deformities of the metacarpophalangeal (MCP) joints, with or without ulnar deviation at wrist (see Fig. 5.1). The proximal interphalangeal (PIP) joints also are affected in R.A. Synovial fluid examination may rule out infection, but does not help for making the diagnosis of R.A. Anemia is usually present in the majority of patients. Approximately 80 to 90% of patients with R.A. have a positive rheumatoid factor test, although other conditions can cause a positive test, also.

A childhood variant of R.A. affects children between 5 and 15 years of age. It is referred to as Still's disease as it was first described by Dr. Still. In juvenile R.A., the joint symptoms may be less prominent initially, with fever, red rash, and lymphadenopathy noted.

Treatments for R.A. are multiple, as might be expected, and not one is useful for all patients affected. Patients are usually started on nonsteroid, anti-inflammatory medications, such as aspirin (see Table 5.2 for commonly used medications); education of the family and patient is done and is discussed at each visit; use of hot or cold applications may be initiated (see pp. 442 and pp. 445

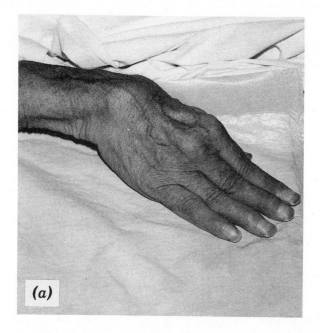

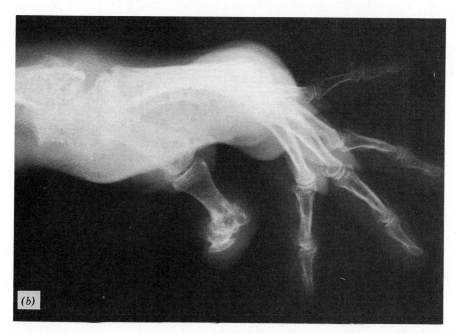

**Figure 5.1** Deformities of the fingers and metacarpal bones from rheumatoid arthritis.

**Table 5.2** Medications Commonly Used for Musculoskeletal Conditions

| Name of Medications | Adult Dosage (Orally) | Side Effects/ Adverse Reactions | Conditions Used |
|---|---|---|---|
| Salicylates | | | |
| Aspirin, plain or buffered | 600–3000mg/d | Anorexia, nausea, vomiting, gastric distress, gastro-intestinal bleeding, decrease in clotting, ringing in ears (tinnitus) | Arthritis—all types; sports injuries (sprains, tennis elbow) |
| Choline magnesium trisalicylate (Trilisate) | 250–1000 mg b.i.d. or t.i.d | Anorexia, nausea, headache, gastric distress | Low back pain; arthritis— all types |
| Choline salicylate (Arthropan) | 2000–3000 mg t.i.d. | Same as for choline magnesium trisalicylate | Arthritis—all types |
| Salsalate (Disalcid) | 1000–3000 mg/d | Same as for choline magnesium trisalicylate | Arthritis—all types |
| Nonsteroidal Anti-inflammatory Drugs | | | |
| Ibuprofen (Motrin) | 400 mg q.i.d | Anorexia, nausea, vomiting, gastric distress, gastro-intestinal bleeding, headache, dizziness, edema, fluid retention, skin rash, diarrhea or constipation, blurred vision, anemia | Arthritis—all types; low back pain |
| Fenoprofen (Nalfon) | 600–3200 mg/d | Same as for Ibuprofen plus dysuria, cystitis, hematuria, proteinuria | Rheumatoid arthritis |

| | | | |
|---|---|---|---|
| Naproxen (Naprosyn) | 250–750 mg/d | Same as for Ibuprofen plus dysuria, cystitis, hematuria, proteinuria | Rheumatoid arthritis |
| Sulindac (Clinoril) | 150–400 mg/d | Same as for Ibuprofen plus dysuria, cystitis, hematuria, proteinuria | Arthritis—all types; ankylosing spondylitis |
| Tolmetin (Tolectin) | 400–2000 mg/d | Same as for Ibuprofen plus dysuria, cystitis, hematuria, proteinuria | Rheumatoid arthritis |
| Meclofenamate (Meclomen) | 50–100 mg | Same as with Ibuprofen | Arthritis—all types |
| Piroxicam (Feldene) | 20 mg/d | Same as with Ibuprofen, but peptic ulceration and bleeding can be severe | Arthritis—all types |
| Indomethacin (Indocin) | 25–75 mg/d to 150–200 mg/d for some clients | Same as with Ibuprofen | Arthritis—all types |
| Phenylbutazone (Butazolidin) | 300–400 mg/d | Same as with Ibuprofen plus aplastic anemia | Rheumatoid arthritis |
| Oxyphenbutazone (Tandearil) | 300–400 mg/d | Same as for Phenylbutazone | Rheumatoid arthritis |
| Diflunisal (Dolobid) | 500–1000 mg/d | Same as with Ibuprofen plus eyesight changes (patients should see an ophthalmologist frequently | Osteoarthrosis |
| Diclofenac (Voltaren) | 25–75 mg, 2 to 4 times daily | Same as with Ibuprofen | Rheumatoid arthritis; osteoarthritis; ankylosing spondylitis |

(continued)

**Table 5.2** (Continued)

| Name of Medications | Adult Dosage (Orally) | Side Effects/ Adverse Reactions | Conditions Used |
|---|---|---|---|
| Steroids | | | |
| Prednisone (Deltasone, Meticorten, Fernisone) | 5–60 (or more) mg/d | Anemia; edema, hypertension; sodium retention; potassium excretion; alteration in carbohydrate, protein, and fat metabolism, osteoporosis, bruising, moon facies, cataracts, hirsutism | Rheumatoid arthritis |
| Antigout | | | |
| Colchicine (Colsalide) | 1–1.2 mg. followed by 0.5–0.6 mg/hr until pain is relieved or diarrhea occurs | Nausea, vomiting, diarrhea, abdominal cramping, and with long-term administration: bone marrow depression, aplastic anemia | Acute attack of gout |
| Probenecid (Benemid) | 250 mg–500 mg/d | Headache, anorexia, nausea, vomiting, diarrhea, constipation, rash, fever | Gout—long-term therapy |
| Sulfinpyrazone (Anturane) | 200–400 mg/d | As with Probenecid | Gout—long-term therapy |
| Allopurinol (Zyloprim) | 200–600 mg/d | Skin rash, fever, malaise, cataracts, nausea, vomiting, diarrhea, drowsiness | Gout—long-term therapy |

for types and purposes of applications); physical therapy exercises are begun to increase joint mobility. Other treatments include steroid medications, cytotoxic drugs such as methotrexate; injection or oral administration of gold; application of resting or dynamic splints; occupational therapy to help with ADL and home management; immunosuppressive medications may be given; and surgical procedures, such as arthroplasty, silicone implants after synovectomy, arthrodesis, and total joint replacements may be done. Some of the above treatments may be given or used simultaneously, and which treatments are used varies with the patient's specific condition.

Nursing aspects for R.A. are given on pp. 160–170.

## SYSTEMIC LUPUS ERYTHEMATOSUS (SLE)

SLE is another autoimmune disease which affects connective tissues in the body that contain collagen fibers; thus it affects collagen-containing tissues in and around joints, blood vessels, heart, lung, kidneys, and skin. A mild form of lupus erythematosus, called discoid lupus, primarily affects the skin tissues, noted by patchy areas of red rash. Systemic lupus erythematosus, however, is a life-shortening chronic disease that requires thorough patient-family education and compliance for best results.

Symptoms of SLE include presence of a reddish rash over the bridge of the nose and cheeks, referred to as a butterfly rash as it resembles the shape of a butterfly, fever, arthritis of many joints, alopecia, Raynaud's phenomenon (see p. 00), photosensitivity, and signs of heart, lung, or renal involvement, such as infections, edema, extreme tiredness, and blood vessel changes. As with R.A., women are affected over men by a ratio of 9:1, with an age range from about 15 to 50 years.

The diagnosis of SLE is made from the patient's history, physical examination, serologic studies, and radiographs. Serologic studies include complete blood count, hemoglobin, hematocrit, albumin/globulin ratio, total protein, creatinine, antinuclear antibodies, immunofluorescence studies, immunoglobulin assay, electrocardiogram, renal scan, and erythrocyte sedimentation rate. Urinalysis is also done to determine renal involvement. In SLE, the arthritis does not erode the cartilage, affecting the capsule and supporting structure causing joint instability and subluxations (partial dislocations).

Treatments for SLE include joint protective measures including use of orthoses and splints, heat and cold applications, rest periods during the day, education in joint and muscle sparing techniques, use of active and passive ROM exercises, relaxation exercises, low to high doses of corticosteroid medications, and other medications specific for particular organ involvement, such as antimalarial drugs, immunosuppressives, and others.

The nursing aspects are given on pp. 160–170.

## PROGRESSIVE SYSTEMIC SCLEROSIS (PSS)

PSS was formerly called scleroderma, but PSS is a more inclusive name. PSS is a disease of the small blood vessels and connective tissues with the development of ischemic, fibrotic (scars), and degenerative changes in the skin, joints, and internal organs. Frequently, PSS involves the alimentary tract, lungs, heart, kidneys, and synovium of joints.

PSS involves excess deposition of fibrous (scar) tissue of unknown cause. Causes may be immunological or secondary to vascular trauma or inflammation. The disease is most common in women (3 of 4 patients are women), from ages 20 to 50 years of age.

Symptoms of PSS are clustered in the CREST syndrome consisting of C = calcinosis, R = Raynaud's phenomenon, E = esophageal dysfunction, S = sclerodactyly, and T = telangiectasis. Other symptoms include tightened, tough skin of the fingers and face, edema eventually replaced with scarring (fibrosis) of facial tissues, hyperpigmentation, and limitations of ROM of joints. Thickening of subcutaneous tissues, muscles, tendons, and joint capsules also cause stiffness and decreased ROM, and skin ulcerations.

Diagnosis is made from the presence of CREST syndrome, and the characteristic tightening of the skin.

Treatments include active ROM exercises, dynamic orthoses, mild heat applications, wrapping of affected joint, and massage, discontinuing use of tobacco products as nicotine causes vasoconstriction, avoidance of cold by wearing mittens or gloves, wearing warm clothing, and eating in moderation (large meals reduce peripheral circulation). Medications include nonsteroid anti-inflammatory and steroidal medications (only for patients with polymyositis), cardiotonic and antihypertensive medications.

The nursing aspects for PSS are given on pp. 160–170.

## NURSING PROCESS FOR RHEUMATOID ARTHRITIS, SYSTEMIC LUPUS ERYTHEMATOSUS, AND PROGRESSIVE SYSTEMIC SCLEROSIS

## NURSING DIAGNOSIS

### IMPAIRED PHYSICAL MOBILITY RELATED TO JOINT INFLAMMATION, TIGHTENED TISSUES, OR DEFORMITIES

### Assessment

1. Assess all joints for signs of inflammation, deformity, taut or tightened tissues around joints, deviation from midline and symmetry.

2. Assess ROM of joints bilaterally.

3. Assess for Raynaud's phenomenon (color changes of blanching, redness, and cyanosis).

4. Assess for ulcerations or calcium deposits.

5. Assess for sensory changes: numbness, tingling, pins and needles.

6. Assess for systemic organic involvement: cardiac arrhythmias, shortness of breath, bowel sounds.

## Expected Outcomes

The patient will:

- maintain full ROM of unaffected joints.
- regain satisfactory ROM in affected joints.
- regain some ROM in affected joints with treatments.
- regain satisfactory physical mobility with treatments.

## Nursing Interventions

1. Explain purposes of frequent assessments of joint functions and physical mobility as bases for care; explanations ease concerns.

2. Clarify planned treatment regimen to ease joint problems: exercises, heat/cold applications, use of orthoses and splints.

3. Secure consultation with physical and occupational therapists for active and passive exercises and for assistance with ADL and home management.

4. Apply ordered hot or cold applications q 4 hours; monitor effects of applications. Patients use the type of application that provides most relief of inflammation and discomfort.

5. Encourage exercise program between physical therapy sessions.

6. Apply orthoses, splints, or other joint supports as ordered to allow rest to joints and to maintain proper joint positions.

7. Reposition patient q 3 to 4 hours; use only small pillows under back, head, and knees to prevent contractures.

8. Assist with ambulation as needed; monitor use of ambulatory aid if used.

## Evaluation

The patient:

- maintained full ROM in unaffected joints for long periods and years.
- retained satisfactory ROM in affected joints by doing own ADL and self-care.

- regained some ROM in affected joints as shown by 5 degrees more ROM after exercises.
- regained satisfactory physical mobility after treatments by walking greater distances.

## NURSING DIAGNOSIS

### ACTIVITY INTOLERANCE RELATED TO TIGHTENED SKIN TISSUES, FATIGUE, ANEMIA, AND RAYNAUD'S PHENOMENON

#### Assessment

1. Assess degree or amount of activity tolerated per 24 hours.
2. Assess sites of tightened skin tissues.
3. Assess laboratory data for evidence of anemia.
4. Assess for Raynaud's phenomenon in fingers and toes.
5. Assess for memory losses.

#### Expected Outcomes

The patient will:
- have more activity tolerance after treatments.
- have fewer periods of fatigue per 24 hours.
- regain normal hematocrit and hemoglobin levels.
- have fewer episodes of Raynaud's phenomenon after treatments.
- have no memory lapses or losses after treatments.

#### Nursing Interventions

1. Assess skin of fingers and toes for color changes of Raynaud's phenomenon: color changes from blanching to redness to cyanosis; assess color of conjunctivae and nail beds—paleness is associated with anemia.
2. Assess lab data for signs of anemia: hematocrit below 30% and hemoglobin below 12 gms.
3. Assist patient with ADL and self-care to conserve available energy.
4. Provide time for a.m. and p.m. nap or rest times to lessen fatigue.
5. Provide rest periods after exercise or activity periods to help patient regain physical strength.

6. Straighten bed linens and provide back massage to promote nighttime rest. Patient should have 8–10 hours sleep if possible.

7. Consult with dietitian for diet of iron-rich foods after assessing patient's likes and dislikes; monitor amount of food intake.

8. Administer ordered iron replacement medication; discuss taking medication with orange juice to aid absorption; discuss side effects of iron tablets, such as constipation, blackish stools, and gastric irritation (lessened by administering iron with food and not on an empty stomach). Iron tablets help restore iron stores in conjunction with iron-rich foods.

9. Encourage patient to wear mittens or gloves when handling hot or cold containers or when in cold temperatures; encourage to wear gloves at night to lessen vascular responses to temperature changes.

10. Administer vasodilator medication, if ordered, to lessen vasoconstriction; explain to patient to change positions slowly to avoid hypotensive episodes or fainting.

11. Explain memory lapses or losses related to anemia and decreased oxygenation; as anemia lessens, lapses should be reversed.

## Evaluation

The patient:

- gradually increased physical activities as anemia lessened and skin tissues were more pliant after exercises.

- had more energy and less fatigue as anemia lessened.

- gradually regained low normal ranges of hematocrit and hemoglobin levels.

- had no recent memory lapses or losses as anemia lessened.

- had fewer Raynaud's reactions while wearing mittens or gloves and while taking vasodilator medications.

## NURSING DIAGNOSIS

### PAIN RELATED TO JOINT TISSUE INFLAMMATION, DEFORMITIES, AND MUSCLE/TENDON INVOLVEMENT

## Assessment

1. Assess type, amount, duration, and characteristics of pain; relief efforts and effects.

2. Assess effects of medications on pain episodes.

## Expected Outcomes

The patient will:

- experience much pain relief with treatments.
- have pain controllable with medications.

## Nursing Interventions

1. Discuss types of treatments for pain relief: use of exercises, heat and cold, and medications.

2. Have patient describe and monitor pain episodes and monitor effects of treatments.

3. Administer nonsteroidal anti-inflammatory or analgesic medications as ordered (see Table 5.2).

4. Monitor effects of medications for relief of pain; note side effects of medications.

5. Assist with exercises, use of hot or cold applications for relief of pain; monitor effects of treatments. Caution: Use hot applications cautiously if peripheral circulation is already compromised with Raynaud's phenomenon.

6. Provide time for patient to express feelings about having R.A., SLE, or PSS; clarify any misunderstood information if feasible.

7. Encourage use of relaxation techniques, diversionary activities, biofeedback, or other techniques to help control pain experiences.

## Evaluation

The patient:

- experienced marked decrease in pain episodes with treatments.
- had pain controlled with medications.

## NURSING DIAGNOSIS

### IMPAIRED GAS EXCHANGE RELATED TO PNEUMONITIS, PULMONARY EDEMA, AND ANEMIA

## Assessment

1. Assess breath sounds in all lobes.
2. Assess vital signs and weight.
3. Assess lab data for signs of anemia.

## Expected Outcomes

The patient will:

- regain satisfactory gas exchange following treatments.
- regain normal ranges of hematocrit and hemoglobin.
- not develop congestive heart failure.

## Nursing Interventions

1. Assess vital signs, paying special attention to respiratory rates and depth; listen to breath sounds in all lobes.
2. Check for orthopnea and color of lips and extremities to note progression or relief of pulmonary edema.
3. Position patient in high Fowler's position to ease dyspnea.
4. Administer diuretics, antibiotics, and bronchodilator drugs as ordered to decrease pulmonary inflammation and edema.
5. Encourage deep breathing exercises q 2 hours; note any sputum expectorated, checking amount and color.
6. Have patient use respiratory aid q 2 hours to increase respiratory reserve.
7. Monitor hematocrit and hemoglobin to note effects of medications and diet to lessen anemia.
8. Monitor breath sounds in all lobes q 4 hours to note changes in response to treatments.

## Evaluation

The patient:

- regained satisfactory gas exchange following treatments.
- did not develop pneumonia or congestive heart failure.
- regained low normal ranges of hematocrit and hemoglobin.

## NURSING DIAGNOSIS

### SELF-CARE DEFICIT RELATED TO JOINT DEFORMITIES, INFLAMMATION, AND PRESENCE OF R.A., SLE, OR PSS

## Assessment

1. Assess ability to do own self-care or ADL.
2. Assess stage of disease in body.

## Expected Outcomes

The patient will:

- be able to do own self-care and ADL.
- have disease controlled with treatments and medications.

## Nursing Interventions

1. Clarify patient's abilities to do self-care and ADL.
2. Monitor patient's current state of disease activity through patient's comments, chart data, and physician's comments.
3. Assist patient with self-care and ADL as needed.
4. Assess effects of increasing self-care activities; suggest rest periods as appropriate.
5. Encourage participation in treatment regimen to ease disease activity.
6. Provide modified utensils to ease muscle and joint strain—may use long-handled grabbers, rubber-handled utensils, cords on zippers, and such.
7. Consult with occupational therapist for self-care assistance, if needed.

## Evaluation

The patient:

- gradually participated in own self-care and ADL.
- had remission of acute symptoms of R.A., SLE, and PSS with treatments and medications.

## NURSING DIAGNOSIS

### POTENTIAL FOR INJURY RELATED TO GI DISTENTION, OBSTRUCTION, OR BLEEDING.

## Assessment

1. Assess for bowel sounds, abdominal girth, and bowel movements.
2. Assess for occult blood in stools or vomitus.

## Expected Outcomes

The patient will:

- have no bowel obstruction or abdominal distention.
- have regular, soft bowel movements.

- have no detectable GI bleeding.
- have active peristalsis and bowel sounds.

### Nursing Interventions

1. Assess abdominal distention, abdominal girth, and bowel sounds in all four quadrants.
2. Assess bowel movements for characteristics of stool and occult blood.
3. Discuss dietary intake and fiber to increase bowel output and prevent constipation.
4. Assist patient to ambulate to increase circulation to abdominal tissues.
5. Note patient's complaints of abdominal pain, if present. Pain may be related to inflammatory condition or to iron tablets for anemia.
6. If patient with PSS has a bowel obstruction with surgical resection, provide postop care as needed.

### Evaluation

The patient:

- had mild abdominal distention only without bowel obstruction.
- had soft, formed bowel movements with dietary changes.
- had no positive occult bleeding signs.
- had peristaltic rushes every 30 to 40 seconds (normal is 30 seconds) and active bowel sounds in all quadrants.

## NURSING DIAGNOSIS

### BODY IMAGE DISTURBANCE RELATED TO "PINCHED" FACIAL APPEARANCE IN PSS, RASH WITH SLE, AND DEFORMITIES RELATED TO R.A.

### Assessment

1. Assess all skin tissues for tightness, presence of deformities, rash, nodules, or deviations from midline.
2. Assess for effects on body image.

### Expected Outcomes

The patient will have:

- a positive body image in regard to visible body changes.
- no increases in deformities, rash, nodules, or deviations from midline.

## Nursing Interventions

1.  Monitor feelings about changes in facial characteristics and pinched expression, butterfly rash on face, and rash in other places over body, about deformities of hands and wrists, and presence of subcutaneous nodules.

2.  Encourage participation in facial exercise program to "loosen" tight skin tissues.

3.  Administer ordered medications to treat specific disease, such as vasodilators, steroids, nonsteroidal anti-inflammatory medications, and others.

4.  Consult with mental health personnel, if necessary, to help patient clarify feelings about appearance.

5.  Encourage patient to verbalize concerns about specific disease, its effects on body image, and presence of deformities or rash.

6.  Provide reading materials that offer guidance to develop positive attitudes and positive body image.

## Evaluation

The patient had:

-   a more positive body image after counseling and reading materials.
-   no marked increases in deformities, rash, nodules, or deviations because of surgical resections, medications, and other treatments.

## NURSING DIAGNOSIS

### SLEEP PATTERN DISTURBANCE RELATED TO PAIN, MUSCLE, AND JOINT STIFFNESS

## Assessment

1.  Assess sleep patterns.
2.  Assess effects of pain on restful sleep, wake periods.
3.  Assess muscle and joint mobility.

## Expected Outcomes

The patient will have:

-   long periods (6–7 hours) of uninterrupted sleep.
-   restful sleep after brief wake periods.
-   proper positioning to lessen muscle/joint pressures.

## Nursing Interventions

1. Discuss sleep patterns since disease onset.
2. Discuss methods to lessen muscle/joint stiffness such as a warm bath or shower, massage, heat application to joints, medications.
3. Position patient with pillows to back and between legs; bed should be flat to lessen development of contractures.
4. Tighten bed linens and change damp linens to lessen pressure on tender skin areas.
5. Administer medications for sedation and pain relief.
6. If desired, provide a snack or warm milk at bedtime. Milk contains l-tryptophan, which induces sleep.
7. Reduce noise and noisy activities so environment is quiet to promote sleep.

## Evaluation

The patient had:

- long periods (7–8) hours of uninterrupted sleep.
- return of sleep after brief wake periods.
- nonpainful muscle/joint pressure through proper positioning.

## NURSING DIAGNOSIS

### ALTERED ROLE PERFORMANCE RELATED TO DEFORMITIES AND FATIGUE

## Assessment

1. Assess usual roles and responsibilities.
2. Assess changes in roles and responsibilities due to present conditions and fatigue.

## Expected Outcomes

The patient will:

- be able to resume usual roles and responsibilities after treatments.
- be stronger and less fatigued with treatments.

## Nursing Interventions

1. Discuss effects of deformities and fatigue on usual roles and responsibilities.
2. Monitor progress in healing after synovectomies, if done, or after bowel resection if needed in PSS; provide needed care after corrective surgery. See Chapter 12 for surgical techniques.
3. Discuss patient's responses to various therapies in health care conferences.
4. Encourage open communications with family and patient.
5. Encourage patient to participate as able in usual roles and responsibilities.
6. Encourage patient to verbalize feelings related to deformities and fatigue (see p. 169 for nursing care for fatigue).

## Evaluation

The patient:

- was gradually able to resume some of usual roles and responsibilities.
- regained strength and was markedly less fatigued after treatments.

## BURSITIS

Bursitis is inflammation of a bursa, a small sac located between muscles and tendons, containing synovial fluid that helps lubricate muscles and tendons. It can become inflamed from trauma or overuse. Surrounding tissues can also become inflamed around the bursa, and more than one bursa can become inflamed. Bursae that are commonly inflamed are the anserine bursa located near the knee (see Fig. 5.2a), the olecranon or elbow bursa, the greater trochanteric bursa lateral to the hip (see Fig. 5.2b), and the subdeltoid and subacromial bursae of the shoulder (see Fig. 5.2c). Bursae that are chronically inflamed may develop calcifications.

### Pathophysiology

Bursitis can develop from continuous friction between the bursa and its surrounding tissues. The friction causes irritation, edema, and, later, inflammation. The bursal sac becomes swollen and engorged, and the area around the bursa becomes very tender and painful. Movement of the tissues enclosing the bursa causes more pain and pressure. Joint movements become affected and are limited by the pain. The area may be red, hot, and edematous with pain radiating to surrounding tissues. At times, the patient can point to the area of greatest tenderness, referred to as "point tenderness."

Bursitis can also develop from repeated microtrauma which leads to thickening of the bursal sac and possibly some leaking (effusion) of the bursal fluid. Such repetitive irritation and inflammation can lead to calcifications in

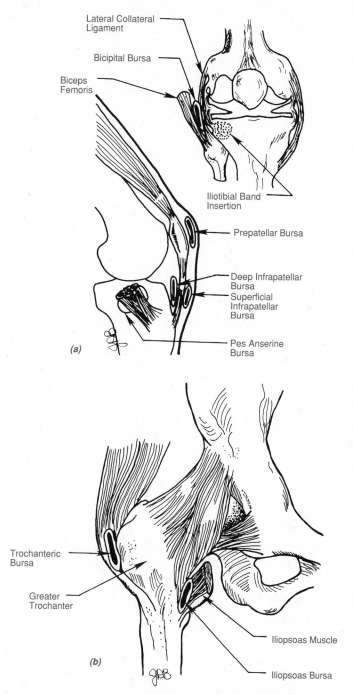

**Figure 5.2** Bursae of the (a) knee; (b) hip.

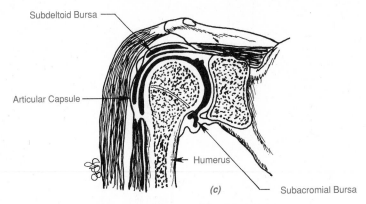

**Figure 5.2** Bursae of the (c) shoulder.

the bursa and adhesions around the bursa which limit movements of the associated tendons.

Symptoms include localized, point tenderness, and pain; heat and swelling around bursal site with limitation of movements. The person may hold the joint close to the body to lessen strain or pain.

Diagnosis is made from the patient's history, physical examination, and roentgenograms which may show enlarged bursa with or without calcified deposits.

Treatments include avoiding activities that can cause constant irritation, such as throwing a ball, kneeling, or raising arms above shoulders. Moist heat applications can be placed over the involved site, and, rarely, the arm may be placed in a sling for elbow or shoulder bursitis. Non-narcotic analgesics may be given for pain, and nonsteroidal anti-inflammatory medications may be given for the treatment of the inflammation. Corticosteroids may be injected into the bursal area in individualized doses. If infection of the bursa is present, an antibiotic may be prescribed. Rarely, excision of the calcified deposits and bursal wall may be necessary.

## NURSING PROCESS

## NURSING DIAGNOSIS

### IMPAIRED PHYSICAL MOBILITY RELATED TO BURSAL INFLAMMATION

Assessment

1. Assess area for presence of edema, heat, redness, tenderness and point tenderness, and limitation of motion.

2. Assess ROM of contiguous joints.

## Expected Outcomes

The patient will:

- regain usual physical mobility after treatments.
- regain full ROM of affected joints.

## Nursing Interventions

1. Assess bursa and surrounding area to determine present condition.
2. Monitor amount of limitation of motion and ROM of surrounding joints.
3. Apply moist warm compresses to area every 4 hours to aid resolution of inflammation.
4. Apply sling or elastic bandage to area as ordered to lessen strain and provide external support.
5. Discuss activities that could lead to chronic irritation and inflammation to decrease recurrence.
6. Monitor resolution of inflammation with treatments.

## Evaluation

The patient:

- regained usual physical mobility after treatment.
- regained full ROM after resolution of inflammation.

## NURSING DIAGNOSIS

### PAIN RELATED TO INFLAMED BURSA

## Assessment

1. Assess type, amount, duration, and severity of pain.
2. Assess relief measures undertaken and their results.

## Expected Outcomes

The patient will:

- experience relief of pain.
- have no recurrence of bursitis and pain.

## Nursing Interventions

1. Assist patient to position of comfort using pillows or sling (if upper extremity affected); handle affected tissues gently.

2. Monitor results of warm, moist applications.

3. Administer ordered analgesics and anti-inflammatory medications every 4 hours to maintain therapeutic blood levels.

4. Assist with injection of corticosteroids into bursal sites; clarify temporary increase of pain after injection, followed by relief of pain and tenderness.

5. Encourage use of extremity to retain joint and muscle functions.

## Evaluation

The patient:

- experienced relief of pain with treatments.
- had no recurrence of bursitis or pain to date.

## ANKYLOSING SPONDYLITIS

Ankylosing spondylitis (AS) is an inflammatory disease affecting the vertebral column, the sacroiliac joints, and later, the joints of the shoulders, hips, and knees. The affected bones and joints become deformed and ankylosed (stiff and immovable).

AS usually develops in late adolescence or early adulthood. Males are affected over females in an 8:1 ratio, between ages 20 to 40 as peak incidence, and it is rare over age 50. The antigen HLA-B27 is present in 90% of persons with AS, but is normally present in about 8 percent of the population. Blacks have a lower incidence of AS than other racial groups.

AS is also known as Marie-Strumpell arthritis and Bechterew disease, but AS is the preferred name as it is descriptive of its pathologic lesions (see Fig. 5.3).

### Pathophysiology

The process initiating the inflammation in AS is unknown. It begins insidiously in an adolescent or young adult, noted initially by morning lumbar-area backache, pain and stiffness in the sacroiliac joints. As the disease progresses, fibrosis (scarring) and ankylosis are common. Activity eases the pain and stiffness, which return with sitting in the same position over long periods. The pain and stiffness worsen over several months with involvement of more spinal components, muscles, and ligaments. Severe muscle spasms pull the vertebral column into forward flexion, increasing the thoracic rounding producing marked kyphotic curvature and obliteration of the lordotic curves of

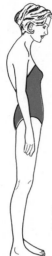

**Figure 5.3** Posture of person with ankylosing spondylitis.

the cervical and lumbar areas. The entire vertebral column becomes flexed forward and ankylosed. Inflammatory changes in the intervertebral discs cause scarring and calcification along the entire vertebral column, giving rise to the name "bamboo spine," as the spinal column looks like bamboo stalks on x-rays. Other joints also are inflamed and calcify as the disease progresses. Eventually patients cannot raise and extend their heads and necks upward. The neck becomes ankylosed with the head pointed nearly horizontally.

Symptoms include loss of normal spinal curves, calcification and ankylosis of the vertebrae, back pain and pain in hips and shoulders; the head and neck are flexed forward with marked increase in thoracic kyphosis. The hip joints become ankylosed in advanced AS.

Diagnosis is made from the patient's history, physical examination, presence of HLA-B27 antigen, and elevated erythrocyte sedimentation rate. X-rays show the characteristic "bamboo spine" and ankylosis of vertebral, sacroiliac, hip, and shoulder joints.

Treatments include active exercises to back, hips, and other affected joints; deep breathing exercises to main respiratory reserve; application of warm, moist compresses to lessen muscle spasms, use of firm mattress and flat bed position to help maintain a straighter spinal column; application of a molded plastic jacket to help maintain spinal curvatures; use of head halter traction to lessen muscle spasms. Surgical treatments include total hip or shoulder replacements; cervical spinal fusion to help maintain an upright position, and osteotomy to correct severe curvatures. Medications include analgesics such as aspirin, nonsteroidal anti-inflammatories, cortisone, and indomethacin in individualized doses. Phenylbutazone (Butazolidin) may be used for short-term therapy, but because of its toxicity cannot be used for long-term therapy.

**NURSING PROCESS**

## NURSING DIAGNOSIS

### IMPAIRED PHYSICAL MOBILITY RELATED TO INFLAMMATION OF VERTEBRAE AND MAJOR JOINTS

Assessment

1. Assess posture, gait, and ROM of joints.
2. Assess areas for signs of inflammation.

Expected Outcomes

The patient will:

- maintain as much physical mobility as possible for long periods.
- regain some ROM of affected joints for long periods.

Nursing Interventions

1. Observe patient's posture and gait, noting limitations when standing, walking, sitting, or lying down.
2. Assist to a position of comfort; keep bed flat to maintain extension of vertebral column.
3. Teach patient proper bed positions and to avoid lying prone.
4. Massage back several times daily.
5. Encourage maintaining exercise regimen to maintain joint functions; assist with ROM exercises as needed.
6. Teach deep breathing exercises to maintain respiratory capacity.

Evaluation

The patient:

- maintained satisfactory physical mobility as long as possible.
- regained moderate ROM of affected joints for long periods.

## NURSING DIAGNOSIS

### PAIN RELATED TO INFLAMMATION OF SPINAL COMPONENTS AND MAJOR JOINTS

Assessment

1. Assess amount, type, severity, and characteristics of pain.
2. Assess results of efforts to relieve pain.

## Expected Outcomes

The patient will have:

- relief of pain with treatments.
- have only controllable pain episodes.

## Nursing Interventions

1. Assess pain experiences: have patient describe and chart pain severity, duration, sites, and results of pain relief efforts.
2. Monitor the results of warm, moist compresses for relief of pain.
3. Reposition patient to relieve aching or tired muscles and joints; massage areas as needed.
4. Administer medications as ordered: analgesics, anti-inflammatories, steroids, and others; monitor for effects of pain relief, and for side effects.
5. Have patient keep a pain relief chart with effects of all therapies.
6. Encourage active participation in usual activities as able.

## Evaluation

The patient:

- had relief of pain with treatments.
- had only controllable pain after treatments.

## NURSING DIAGNOSIS

### ALTERATION IN BODY IMAGE AND USUAL ROLES RELATED TO INFLAMMATORY CHANGES AND PRESENCE OF ABNORMAL, NONFUNCTIONAL CURVATURES

## Assessment

1. Assess effects of AS on body image.
2. Assess usual daily roles and activities.

## Expected Outcomes

The patient will:

- regain a positive body image over time.
- return to usual roles and activities after treatments.

## Nursing Interventions

1. Discuss patient's statements of effects of abnormal curvatures on body image and activities.
2. Encourage participation in desired activities as condition permits.
3. Apply soft collar to neck if ordered.
4. Discuss surgical options, as feasible.
5. Consult or secure guidance from mental health consultant if patient is depressed.
6. Encourage patient to maintain usual roles and responsibilities as able.
7. Secure consultation with occupational therapists for home management activities as necessary.

## Evaluation

The patient:

- gradually regained a positive body image over time.
- returned to usual roles and activities after treatments.

## EPICONDYLITIS AND TENDINITIS (TENOSYNOVITIS)

Epicondylitis is inflammation of the tendons at the condyles where the tendons attach to bones. Tendinitis is inflammation of the sheath covering a tendon or group of tendons. Tendinitis or tenosynovitis are interchangeable terms.

Epicondylitis and tendinitis frequently occur together because of their closeness to each other. These conditions may be related to sports injuries or to overuse syndromes. Half of persons with epicondylitis are younger persons with usually a sports-related injury, while the other half are older persons with overuse injuries from repetitive motions, such as in offices or work areas with activities that require repetitive turning, twisting, or striking motions. Epicondylitis is called *tennis elbow* when it affects the lateral epicondylar area, and is *golfer's elbow* when the medial epicondylar area is involved (see Fig. 5.4).

Tendinitis affects the same populations as above but it can also be diagnosed in persons with chronic diseases such as diabetes and rheumatoid arthritis. Athletes also have tendinitis of particular tendons such as the Achilles tendon and patellar tendon. Adolescents to older adults can develop tendinitis.

### Pathophysiology

Repetitive motions or overuse activities appear to cause microtraumatic changes leading to partial tears, edema, bleeding, and pain in and around the affected tendons. Often patients can point to the area of greatest tenderness or

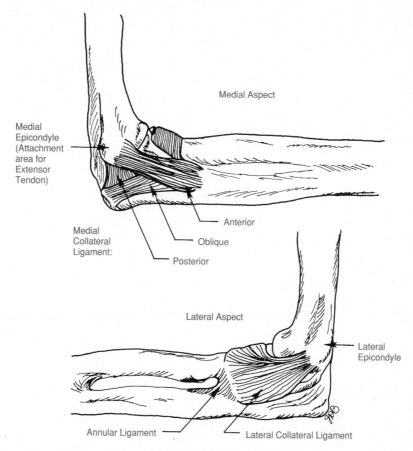

**Figure 5.4** *Medial and lateral epicondyles and collateral ligaments of the elbow (sites of golfer's and tennis elbow, respectively).*

soreness in the epicondylar area. The condition occurs most commonly in the dominant extremity; however, it can occur bilaterally if repetitive pronation and supination motions of both extremities are done. Pathologic signs also include avascularity of the tendon and, at times, calcification at the tendon attachment. Scar tissue may form due to the repetitive trauma and avascularity. At times, the tendon ruptures from these degenerative changes. Pain associated with epicondylitis may be from the bleeding, avascularity, and ischemia.

Tendinitis involves inflammation of the tendon sheath which is lined with synovium. The sheath thickens from the inflammatory changes leading to limitations of motion and pain as the trapped tendon tries to move within the thickened, tight sheath.

Common sites for tendinitis include bicipital tendinitis of the shoulder, patellar tendinitis of the knee, Achilles tendinitis of the heel, and de Quervain's tenosynovitis of the radial area of the wrist.

Symptoms of each condition differ somewhat according to the severity of the condition. Inflammatory signs such as pain, edema, tenderness (point tenderness often), pain reproducible with pronation or supination, redness, and heat in the affected area are common in both conditions. The pain of tendinitis is more poorly localized than in epicondylitis. Also, numbness or muscle weakness may more often accompany tendinitis. Finkelstein's test (see p. 63) is positive in de Quervain's tendinitis.

Diagnosis is made from the patent's history and a physical examination during which motions can reproduce the symptoms. X-rays may show calcifications and an MRI may show partial or full tears of the tendon.

Treatments include rest and avoiding the motions that cause an increase in symptoms. A forearm band may be used for lateral epicondylitis or tennis elbow. Ice applications may be used for 24 to 48 hours, and moist heat applications may be used after ice use is discontinued. Range of motion exercises are done after the initial inflammation is resolved. A knee splint may be used for patellar tendinitis and heel pads or orthotic inserts may be used for Achilles tendinitis. Corticosteroids may be injected into the inflamed area but extreme care must be taken to be certain the injection is not intratendinous as it could cause tendon rupture. Medications much as nonsteroidal anti-inflammatory and non-narcotic analgesics are given to ease pain and inflammation. If surgery is required after conservative measures have not resolved the condition, surgical removal of calcified deposits may be done, or removal of exostoses (bony outgrowths) around the lateral epicondyle and repair of tears of the specific tendon. The tendon sheath may be released and repaired to permit more movement of the tendon.

## NURSING DIAGNOSIS

### IMPAIRED PHYSICAL MOBILITY RELATED TO INJURY TO SPECIFIC TENDON AREA (MEDIAL OR LATERAL EPICONDYLE) OR TENDINITIS

#### Assessment

1. Assess lateral epicondylar area for signs of inflammation and pain for tennis elbow.
2. Assess medial epicondylar area for signs of inflammation and pain for golfer's elbow.
3. Assess areas for tenderness, often point tenderness.
4. Assess movements that reproduce symptoms.

## Expected Outcomes

The patient will:

- experience relief of inflammation and pain.
- regain full ROM in affected joints.

## Nursing Interventions

1. Determine amount and site of inflammation by noting amount of edema, pain or tenderness, color, temperature in area.
2. Explain or clarify rationale for rest to affected part and avoidance of activities that reproduce symptoms.
3. Explain purposes and steps for use of hot or cold applications.
4. Teach patient how to apply wrap, splint, placement of pads or orthosis as needed.
5. Administer ordered anti-inflammatory medications to aid resolution of inflammation.
6. Assist with injection of corticosteroid medications as needed; explain temporary postinjection increase in pain followed by marked decrease in pain and tenderness.
7. Secure physical therapy consultation for prescribed exercises.

## Evaluation

The patient:

- experienced relief of inflammation and pain following treatments.
- regained full ROM in affected joints after treatments and recovery.

*Note:* Another nursing diagnosis for epicondylitis and tendinitis is: Pain related to the inflammation. Outcomes and interventions are the same as those given above for impaired physical mobility, thus they will not be repeated.

## LYME DISEASE

This is a newly discovered disease first diagnosed in 1975 in Lyme, CT, from which it received its name. It is an infectious disease caused by the spirochete *Borrelia burgdorferi*. It has become the most common vector-transmitted disease in the United States, being transmitted by the deer tick, which may be carried by raccoons, mice, deer, and other vectors. It has been diagnosed in 43 states and 5 continents. In the U.S., the majority of cases have occurred in the northeast, upper midwest, and far west. All persons are vulnerable.

## Pathophysiology

The vector carries the tick and transmits it to its human host through the bite of the tick. The hallmark diagnostic finding is a pinkish-red rash called erythema migrans, which develops in about half the infected patients. This rash may be missed, however, as it occurs only in the first week of the infection along with flulike symptoms. If medical attention is not sought, the diagnosis may be delayed until other symptoms become more prominent. About 60% of patients develop arthritis, 15% neurologic complications, and 5% cardiac problems. The rash has a characteristic red circle, referred to as a target lesion, resembling a bull's-eye target. The rash covers the area of the tick bite, with the axillae and groin frequent sites. If untreated, the rash fades in 1 to 4 weeks.

Along with the rash, flulike symptoms, and arthritis, other symptoms include fever, headache, and fatigue. Neurologic symptoms may simulate meningitis, but rarely persist over time. Myocarditis may be a sign of cardiac involvement. Most patients recover completely if treated.

Diagnosis is by the ELIZA test (enzyme-linked immunoassay), which is positive for antibodies of IGM or IGG after 2 to 4 weeks, the history of tick exposure, and possible bite sites and/or ticks found on body or clothes. The specific rash is also diagnostic with its target lesion.

Treatment is to remove the tick and take to physician for identification; bed rest or activity restriction is used for neurologic or cardiac complications. Medications include use of ceftriaxone (Rocephin), given intravenously for 14 to 21 days for patients with meningeal symptoms; doxycycline for 10 to 21 days or erythromycin orally for 10 to 21 days.

Prevention involves wearing shirts tucked into pants and pants tucked into boots when person goes into wooded areas. Bug repellent should be applied prior to entering wooded areas or fields with long grasses. The clothing and body should be carefully checked after emerging from wooded areas or fields.

## NURSING PROCESS

## NURSING DIAGNOSIS

### IMPAIRED PHYSICAL MOBILITY RELATED TO SYSTEMIC AND LOCAL INFECTION IN JOINT OR JOINTS

Assessment

1. Assess all joints for ROM.
2. Assess joints for signs of inflammation.

## Expected Outcomes

The patient will:

- recover from acute illness and arthritis.
- regain physical mobility after recovery.

## Nursing Interventions

1. Monitor amount of inflammation by checking redness, pain, soreness, warmth, and edema of all joints affected to note progression or regression.
2. Check ROM of joints daily to note any losses.
3. Encourage active ROM to unaffected joints to help maintain strength.
4. Assist with self-care and ADL, if needed, because of joint pain.
5. Encourage ambulation as permitted; assist if needed.

## Evaluation

The patient:

- recovered from illness and arthritis with treatments.
- regained physical mobility without limitations.

## NURSING DIAGNOSIS

### HYPERTHERMIA RELATED TO SYSTEMIC INFECTION

## Assessment

1. Assess vital signs and temperature q 1 to 2 hours initially.
2. Assess skin surfaces for rash and perspiration.

## Expected Outcomes

The patient will:

- regain normal body temperatures after treatments.
- regain healthy skin tissues.

## Nursing Interventions

1. Monitor vital signs and temperature every 1 to 2 hours as needed; report elevations over 101°F (38.3°C).
2. Administer antibiotic and antipyretic medications as ordered; note changes in temperature after administration.

3. Check skin surfaces for presence of or fading of rash to note resolution of symptoms.

4. Change bed linens when damp from perspiration or diaphoresis as fever drops.

5. Encourage intake of fluids as tolerated to 3000 ml per 24 hours to help maintain proper hydration.

## Evaluation

The patient:

- regained normal body temperatures after treatments.

- regained healthy skin tissues with no rash.

## NURSING DIAGNOSIS

### PAIN RELATED TO SYSTEMIC INFECTION, ARTHRITIS, OR NEUROLOGIC SIGNS.

## Assessment

1. Assess type and sites of pain, its severity, and duration.
2. Assess for headache, its location and severity or associated symptoms.

## Expected Outcomes

The patient will:
- regain a pain-free existence after treatments.
- have no lingering complications.

## Nursing Interventions

1. Monitor pain episodes, the sites, duration, and efforts for pain relief with results.

2. Monitor headache site, severity, duration, and relief efforts.

3. Monitor relief of joint pain after administration of anti-inflammatory medications.

4. Monitor symptoms associated with headache, such as nausea, nuchal rigidity, and vomiting as signs of neurologic complications; record and report such signs promptly.

5. Maintain a darkened room if patient has photophobia; monitor relief of photophobia over time.

6. Administer non-narcotic analgesics q 4 hours as ordered for relief of systemic pain; monitor results of medications for pain relief.

7. Assist patient to reposition self every 2 hours to help relieve sore or painful joint or headache pain.

8. If headache or neurologic signs lead to confusion or disorientation, maintain a safe environment by raising the siderails and staying with patient, or have relatives with patient.

## Evaluation

The patient had:
- complete relief of pain related to systemic and local (joint) disease following treatments.
- no remaining or lingering sequelae after recovery.

## BIBLIOGRAPHY

Abelson, R. (1991). The autoimmune gold rush. *Forbes, 148*(12),198–200.

Ball, G.V. & Koopman, W.J. (1986). *Clinical rheumatolgy.* Philadelphia: Saunders.

Bynum, T.E. (1989). NSAID-induced gastropathy: A gastroenterologist's point of view. *Journal of Musculoskeletal Medicine, 4*(3)(suppl.),S18–20.

Grimes, D.E. (1991). *Infectious diseases.* St. Louis: Mosby-Yearbook.

Gulanick, M., Klopp, A., & Galanes, S. (eds.) (1991). *Nursing care plans, nursing diagnosis, and interventions.* St. Louis: Mosby-Yearbook.

Hicks, J.E. (1989). Exercise for patients with inflammatory arthritis. *Journal of Musculoskeletal Medicine, 6*(10),40–56.

Kaplan, P.E., & Tanner, E.D. (1989). *Musculoskeletal pain and disability.* Norwalk, CT: Appleton & Lange.

Kim, M.J., McFarland, G.K., & McLane, A.M. (1991). *Pocket guide to nursing diagnoses* (4th ed.). St Louis: Mosby-Yearbook.

Lawson, J.P., & Steere, A.C. (1985). Lyme disease: Radiographic findings. *Radiology, 154,*37–43.

Legwold, G. (1989). Lyme disease: Diagnosis by observation. *Cleveland Clinic Journal of Medicine, 56*(3),230–231.

Legwold, G. (1984). Tennis elbow: Joint resolution by conservative treatment and improved technique. *The Physician and Sports Medicine, 12*(8),168–182.

LeNoir, J.L. (1986). Subacromial-subdeltoid bursitis of the shoulder. *Orthopaedic Review, 15*(11),730–732.

McCance, K.L., & Heuther, S.E.(1989). *Pathophysiology.* St. Louis: Mosby-Yearbook.

Melvin, J.L. (1989). *Rheumatic disease in the adult and child: Occupational therapy and rehabilitation* (3rd ed.). Philadelphia: Davis.

Mourad, L. (1991). *Orthopedic disorders.* St. Louis: Mosby-Yearbook.

Paulus, H.E., Furst, D.E., & Dromgoole, S.H. (1987). *Drugs for rheumatic disease.* New York: Churchill Livingstone.

Riggs, G.K., & Gall, E.P. (1984). *Rheumatic diseases: Rehabilitation and management.* London: Butterworth.

Scherr, L. (Reporter). (June 30, 1989). *Lyme disease* [Television broadcast].

Schumacher, H.R., & Gall, E.P. (1988). *Rheumatoid arthritis.* Philadelphia: Lippincott.

Taylor, D.L. (1983). Inflammation: physiology, signs and symptoms. *Nursing '83, 13*(1),52–53.

Walker, L.G., & Meals, R.A. (1989). Tendinitis: a practical approach to diagnosis and management. *Journal of Musculoskeletal Medicine, 6*(5),24–54.

Wong, A.L., & Weesbart, R.H. (1989) Rheumatoid arthritis: A review of current medical therapies. *Journal of Musculoskeletal Medicine, 6*(11),39–58.

Zwolski, K. (1990). Lyme disease. *Journal of Orthopaedic Nursing, 9*(1),10–17.

# 6

# NURSING PROCESS IN THE CARE OF PATIENTS WITH DEGENERATIVE CONDITIONS OF MUSCULOSKELETAL TISSUES

Degenerative musculoskeletal conditions affect many areas in the body, with muscles and joints being the primary tissues affected. Degenerative conditions are associated with trauma, abuse, wear and tear over time, and developmental and other influences. Even with treatment, degenerative conditions frequently worsen over time and limit one's mobility and socialization.

## OSTEOARTHRITIS

Osteoarthritis (OA) is a degenerative condition of articular (joint) cartilage, primarily in the major weight-bearing joints, although other joints can also be affected. In this disease, the joint cartilage becomes thinner, frayed, split, and eroded over the bone ends (see Fig. 6.1).

Osteoarthritis is referred to as an older person's disease, and, indeed, the incidence increases with each decade of aging. Persons as young as 40 years can have some symptoms of OA but the predominant ages are 60 years and up. It has been estimated that up to 50 million Americans have OA, with a slightly higher female incidence. It is found in all regions of the world and in all climates. Some osteoarthritis is found in all persons over age 75.

OA was thought to be a disease of aging; however, the recent discovery of a gene related to defective cartilage growth and regeneration indicates that OA may have a genetic basis in many cases. The gene appears to involve the proteoglycan complexes that provide the matrix for cartilage growth, strength, and regeneration. Obesity has also been implicated in OA due to the greater weight-bearing stresses on joint cartilage. Mechanical alterations in joints secondary to injury, fractures, or other trauma may and do contribute to the development of OA.

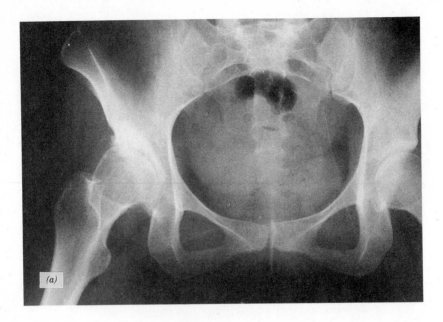

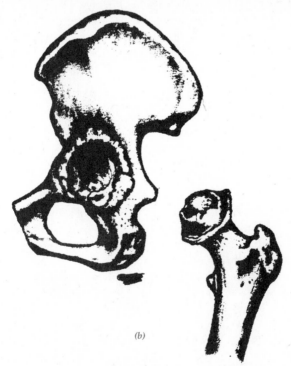

**Figure 6.1**     (a, b) Degeneration of cartilage in osteoarthritis of hip.

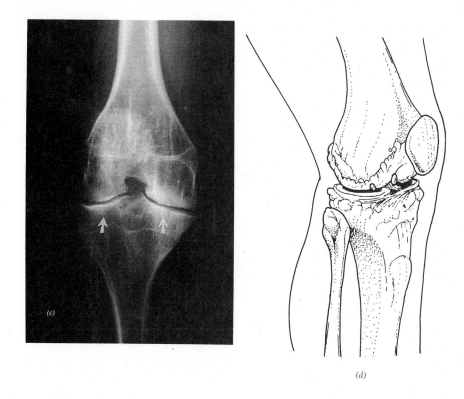

**Figure 6.1** (c, d) Degenerative changes in cartilage of the knee.

## Pathophysiology

In OA, the joint cartilage becomes progressively deteriorated, noted by eburnation (wearing away), fraying, splitting, and fibrillation. The area of cartilage nearest the joint surface wears away first, then deeper layers become involved. There may be variations in wear from area to area within a joint and from joint to joint. Water content of the cartilage may become less than normal, and the cartilage becomes thinner and less able to bear the shock and weight during weight-bearing activities. Fragments of cartilage may loosen or become unattached, setting up irritation and low-grade focal inflammatory areas in the affected joint. Over time, the loosened, eroded, frayed cartilage is worn away, exposing the underlying bone. Exposed bone develops spurs of new bone, called osteophytes, which gradually increase in size to try to fill the empty spaces, but they eventually affect mobility and cause painful movement. Bone cysts may also develop in the subchondral bone due to infiltration of synovial fluid through the eroded joint cartilage. Attempts of the body to repair the joint cartilage fail as the areas enlarge and more cartilage is involved.

Eventually all the layers of joint cartilage are involved and much of the cartilage is lost over the bone ends, as shown in Fig. 6.1a–d.

The destruction of cartilage can proceed over relatively long periods without the patient having symptoms beyond mild soreness until large portions are eroded. Once inflammation develops, pain becomes more noticeable with joint use and weight bearing. The range of motion of the affected joint becomes affected as the bone cysts and osteophytes enlarge, and pain episodes increase in severity and duration. The patient becomes hesitant to use the joint(s) and soon muscle atrophy secondary to disuse develops. Bone enlargements in the distal interphalangeal joints become noticeable and are referred to as Heberden's nodes. Bouchard's nodes are in the proximal interphalangeal nodes in OA. Bone spurs may also limit movement in the vertebral column, producing irritation, limitation of motion, and numbness and tingling with nerve root impingement (see Fig. 6.2).

The major weight-bearing joints of the hips, knees, and vertebral column are the most commonly affected in OA, along with the distal finger joints. Less commonly affected is the shoulder, elbow, wrist, or ankle, unless secondarily following trauma. Secondary OA can also occur in hemophilia from repeated hemorrhaging into joint areas.

Symptoms of OA vary from individual to individual, related to the joint involved and the severity of the condition. Dull, aching pain, which gradually becomes sharper, more frequent, and accompanied by joint stiffness, and soreness are the commonest symptoms. Later, joint swelling and deformity

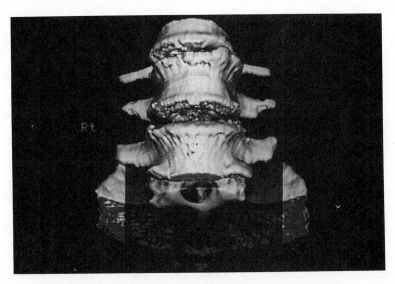

**Figure 6.2**   Degerative change in vertebral osteoarthritis.

become noticeable, accompanied by limitation of motion, tenderness, and joint instability. Increasingly, pain on weight bearing and at rest are common experiences in persons with OA.

The diagnosis of OA is made from the patient's history, physical examination, deformity of joint(s), and radiologic studies. Plain x-rays may show narrowing of joint space, presence of osteophytes, bone spurs, and cysts, "lipping" of osteophytes and, at times, calcification of ligaments, especially along the spinal column. A CT scan may show impingement of the spinal canal or narrowing of nerve pathways. Gait analysis may show abnormal weight-bearing patterns and a positive Trendelenburg sign. Muscle testing will show muscle weakness. If a bone scan is done, it will show increased uptake in the area of OA.

Treatments vary with the joint involvement and the severity of the condition. Ambulatory aids such as a cane, walker, or crutches may be used for relieving pain with weight bearing; rest is prescribed for inflamed and tender joints; a splint or other orthotic device may be applied to maintain joint strength and shape. Range of motion exercises and physical therapy may help maintain joint functions. Medications such as anti-inflammatory analgesics, nonsteroidal anti-inflammatory medications, and muscle relaxants are commonly prescribed (see Table 5.2). Surgical procedures include varus or valgus osteotomy, arthrodesis (joint fusion), or total joint replacement as treatments for OA.

## NURSING PROCESS

## NURSING DIAGNOSIS

### IMPAIRED PHYSICAL MOBILITY RELATED TO OA AND LIMITED RANGE OF MOTION

#### Assessment

1. Assess posture and gait: note "hunched" shoulders, increased kyphosis, decreased lordosis, limp, length of step.
2. Assess all joints for shape, deformity, signs of inflammation, ROM, and pain.

#### Expected Outcomes

The patient will:

- have increased ROM of affected joints.
- have increased physical mobility with ambulatory aid.

## Nursing Interventions

1. Teach patient use of ordered ambulatory aid; observe use of aid and distance traveled to note progress and if changes are needed.
2. Consult with physical therapist for specific exercises according to physician's orders and patient condition to increase functions.
3. Encourage rest periods to lessen inflammation.

## Evaluation

The patient:

- had increased range of motion of affected joints.
- had increased physical mobility using ambulatory aid, walking up to 2 miles daily.

## NURSING DIAGNOSIS

### PAIN (ACUTE) RELATED TO DEGENERATIVE JOINT CHANGES AND MUSCLE SPASMS

## Assessment

1. Assess type, amount, degree and severity, duration, and occurrence of pain.
2. Assess muscle strength, joint ROM, and presence of muscle spasms.

## Expected Outcomes

The patient will:

- experience relief of pain with medications.
- experience freedom from muscle spasms.

## Nursing Interventions

1. Monitor pain episodes: have patient describe type, amount, duration, and occurrence of pain.
2. Discuss when pain is better or worse with rest or activity.
3. Administer ordered analgesic, anti-inflammatory medication (see Table 5.2); monitor results of medications.
4. Administer ordered muscle relaxant medication; monitor results.

## Evaluation

The patient had:
- relief of pain with medications.
- relief of muscle spasms with medications.

## NURSING DIAGNOSIS

### SELF-CARE DEFICIT RELATED TO OSTEOARTHRITIS

## Assessment

1. Assess ability to do own ADL (activities of daily living).
2. Assess usual roles in relation to OA.

## Expected Outcomes

The patient will:
- increase ability to do own ADL following treatments.
- resume usual roles following treatments.

## Nursing Interventions

1. Explain proposed surgical procedure for patient's specific condition (see pp. 368–372 for surgical treatments and care).
2. Provide appropriate postoperative care as given on pp. 377–393.
3. Assist patient to do ADL as needed, such as assisting with bath or shower, dressing, grooming, preparing foods for eating, and such.
4. Observe patient's progress toward total self-care as appropriate.
5. Discuss usual roles and care needed to resume usual roles: consult with occupational therapist if appropriate.

## Evaluation

The patient:
- gradually was able to do own ADL as healing progressed.
- gradually resumed usual roles over time as recovery progressed.

## HALLUX VALGUS

Hallux valgus is a degenerative deformity in which the great toe (hallux) angulates away from the midline (valgus angulation) toward the second and other toes. At times the great toe may deviate over or under one or more toes.

Hallux valgus may become progressively worse and more painful or aggravated by wearing shoes that fit improperly or do not properly support the foot. Wearing high-heeled shoes over extended periods may contribute to the progression of hallux valgus.

Hallux valgus is more common in women than men and there is a familial tendency for the condition. Adolescent females also develop hallux valgus. It can also be associated with rheumatoid arthritis as well as osteoarthritis. Additionally, in nearly all cases of hallux valgus, a bunion develops at the first metatarsophalangeal (MTP) joint which can become inflamed and then is very painful (Fig. 6.3).

Pathophysiology. Hallux valgus (HV) develops secondary to OA of the first metatarsophalangeal (MTP) joint, or to medial angulation of the first metatarsal bone. A "flat" foot also contributes to HV because a fallen or dropped longitudinal arch causes dorsiflexion of the first cuneiform-metatarsal joint, with the distal end of the first metatarsal bone becoming displaced dorsally and medially, causing the adductor hallucis tendons to draw the big toe laterally or in a valgus direction (see Fig. 6.4). The great toe may ride over or under the second toe, and the other toes are crowded, leading, at times, to the development of hammer toe, claw toe, or mallet toe. The angulation and degeneration of the first MTP joint may lead to development of a bunion on the medial side of the first MTP. A bunion is an inflamed bursa which forms adventitiously at the first MTP because of pressure and inflammation. There may also be valgus deviation of the heel.

Hallux valgus can progress to become hallux rigidus which is narrowing and rigidity of the MTP joint making flexing the joint extremely painful and subsequently lost from bone spurs in the MTP joint. Hallux rigidus is more common in men.

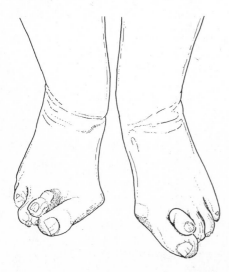

**Figure 6.3** Hallux valgus with bilateral bunions and elevation of second toe over great toe due to deviation of great toe.

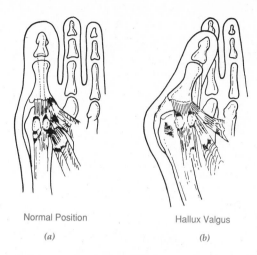

Normal Position

Hallux Valgus

(a)

(b)

**Figure 6.4** Pathomechanics of bunion deformity with the metatarsal heads slipping out of the sesamoid complex and deformity of the large toe.

Symptoms of hallux valgus include the development of the deformity and deviation and, at times, a bunion. Pain is another common symptom and centers around the MTP joint. Painful standing, sitting, and walking are other symptoms.

Diagnosis is made from the patient's history and physical examination. Radiological evidence shows the degenerative changes in the MTP joint and valgus displacement of the great toe; bone spurs may be noted.

Treatments include changing shoes to those with larger toe areas and lower heels. Using a felt ring around a bunion may relieve pressure and pain. Using metatarsal pads taped under metatarsal heads change weight-bearing surfaces. Medications such as analgesics and intra-articular injections of steroids relieve pain and inflammation. Surgical treatments include various osteotomies, arthrodesis, arthroplasty, and bunionectomy (see Table 6.1). The fact that there are over 100 different operative techniques indicates that this condition is a perplexing one for surgeons.

**Table 6.1** Operative Procedures for Hallux Valgus

Proximal metatarsal osteotomy
Distal metatarsal osteotomy
Shaft osteotomy
Metatarsal cuneiform fusion
Arthroplasty
Combinations of these operations

## NURSING PROCESS

## NURSING DIAGNOSIS

### IMPAIRED PHYSICAL MOBILITY RELATED TO PAIN AND DEFORMITY

#### Assessment

1. Assess gait and mobility.
2. Assess for presence of osteoarthritis in MTP and other joints.
3. Assess feet bilaterally.

#### Expected Outcomes

The patient will:
- have relief of impaired mobility following treatments.
- have no recurrence of hallux valgus or bunion.

#### Nursing Interventions

1. Teach patient about use of pads and other orthotic devices to improve mobility.
2. Refer patient to podiatrist or orthotist for measurement and shoe fitting or for orthotic devices.
3. Refer patient to medical physician, if desired, for surgical correction if orthoses insufficient to relieve pain.
4. Refer patient to physician or podiatrist for correction of hallux valgus, bunion, and bursitis.

#### Evaluation

The patient
- experienced relief of pain and easing of bursitis.
- had improved mobility after treatments.

## NURSING DIAGNOSIS

### BODY IMAGE DISTURBANCE RELATED TO DEFORMITIES OF FOOT OR FEET

#### Assessment

1. Assess amount of and sites of pedal deformities.
2. Assess concerns related to body image and deformities.

## Expected Outcomes

The patient will:

- have removal of deformities from foot or feet.
- develop a more positive body image.

## Nursing Interventions

1. Provide time for patient to verbalize concerns related to deformities.
2. Encourage patient's decision to have corrective procedures to remove deformities.
3. Encourage postoperative compliance with care to prevent recurrence.

## Evaluation

The patient:

- developed a more positive body image following removal of hallux valgus and bunion.
- had improved mobility with treatments.

## NURSING DIAGNOSIS

### PAIN RELATED TO BUNION AND BURSITIS

## Assessment

1. Assess type, amount, duration, and events related to pain, such as when pain occurs.
2. Assess relief measures taken and results of each measure.
3. Assess bunion and hallux valgus sites for signs of inflammation: redness, heat, and edema.

## Expected Outcomes

The patient will:

- have relief of pain with treatments.
- have no further bunion or bursitis.

## Nursing Interventions

1. Discuss etiology of bunions and bursitis.
2. Discuss use of low-heeled shoes and orthotic devices to ease muscle strain, pressure, and pain.

3. . Discuss use of mild analgesics to relieve pain as feasible.

4. Discuss application of ice bag to lessen edema and pain.

## Evaluation

The patient:

- had corrective removal of pedal deformities without recurrence.
- had relief of pain after treatments.

## LOW BACK PAIN RELATED TO DEGENERATIVE DISC DISEASE OR SPINAL STENOSIS

The incidence of low back and related leg pain has increased in the last 40 years, most commonly in the 30- to 40-year-old person. This age of incidence is vital because it accounts for 30–50% of work absences, and directly impacts the work force. The cause is often chronic musculoskeletal strain, and is often not diagnosed because the majority of persons affected return to work in one month. Persons not returning to work require exploration of the etiology of the pain and possibly treatment for the pain. Exploration of the full etiology of the low back pain is often not done until conservative treatment measures have failed to relieve the pain.

Conservative treatment of initial acute low back pain is empirical, with 1–2 or more days of bed rest as the first treatment choice. Bed rest for low back pain requires that the person lie in a "lawn chair" type position, being allowed up for bathroom privileges. This treatment is difficult for people to comply with because, as previously stated, the pain occurs during the peak earning years, when people have families and many other responsibilities and activities.

Along with bed rest, conservative treatment also includes use of anti-inflammatory medications, muscle relaxants, and at times, narcotic medications. Anti-inflammatory medications may cause gastric irritation and ulcerations, drowsiness, weight gain, or edema. The patient should be instructed to take the medication with food to prevent gastric problems. The patient must also take the medications as prescribed to maintain a therapeutic blood level. A decrease in inflammation brings a subsequent relief of pain, which may not be seen for 5–7 days after initiation of medications. Narcotic use is usually confined to the initial 3–6 weeks, as continued use may lead to dependency and decreased effectiveness of the medication over time, possibly causing the patient to increase the dose or frequency.

Conservative treatment also may include physical therapy for strengthening the lower back, increasing flexibility, for aerobic exercises, and for proper body mechanics. Strengthening exercises lessen the weakness of back or abdominal muscles to provide more support to the vertebral column. Abdominal strengthening exercises consist of abdominal curls with the knees flexed and the feet flat on the floor. Strengthening of paraspinal muscles (muscles on either side of the spine) is accomplished by lying flat with knees bent and pushing the lower lumbar area into the floor, then relaxing the muscles. Flexibility exercises assist the person to bend and change position with less possibility of injury. Men are generally less flexible than women, which may be due to larger muscle masses in men.

Aerobic exercises assist the person to attain and maintain an ideal weight, increase general conditioning, and promote a sense of well-being.

Physical therapy also teaches the person to perform daily and work-related tasks in non-injury-producing positions. Correct body mechanics are taught, and modifications in job and household tasks are made to avoid additional injury. These "back regimes" usually assist the person to return to productive life activities again. If acute pain persists beyond 6 weeks, it then becomes chronic pain. At this point, the physician may proceed with a full diagnostic evaluation, or the patient may be referred to a back school.

Back schools were developed to provide comprehensive programs to assist the patient and family to deal with the disability of back pain without use of narcotics. The program is multifaceted, with physical therapy, counseling, and work hardening as some of the programs provided.

Evaluation of low back pain after the pain has persisted for longer than 6–8 weeks, or when there is progression to radicular pain or sciatica, is thorough. Determination of etiology of the pain begins with a comprehensive history, including a description of which positions aggravate the pain, distances the patient can walk, pattern of weakness or numbness of the back or extremity, and a thorough discussion of the pain, its type, duration, extent, and characteristics. Defining the severity of pain in a scale of 1–10 is very useful for comparison following one or more treatments.

The physical examination begins with a spinal examination. With the patient standing, the physician observes the posture of the person from the front, back, and each side. The spinal column is examined for straightness and normal or exaggerated curves. The patient bends forward and the shoulders are examined for asymmetry in height or size. During various position changes, the patient is observed for indications of pain, which are compared to the patient's verbal history of when the pain occurs, to establish whether or not there may be a psychological component to this patient's expression of low back pain. Evidence of a psychological component may be when the patient displays signs of pain during standing/forward flexion, but not during straight leg raising checks, which may indicate that the pain is non-physiologic. If indications of a psychologic component are detected, the physician may order an MMPI (Minnesota Multi-Phasic Inventory) or other psychologic evaluation to determine what extent of the patient's pain is non-physiological and to ascertain if secondary gain is involved.

The physical examination also entails assessment of the presence or absence of paraspinal muscle spasms, presence or absence of deep tendon reflexes, pulsations and palpation of peripheral pulses to help rule out peripheral vascular diseases, an abdominal assessment to rule out abdominal aneurysm, and assessment of individual muscle groups which may demonstrate weakness in one or more muscles if there is any nerve entrapment. Testing of sensory functions may be evaluated through Semmes Weinstein monofilaments, which are synthetic filaments of varying diameters. As the filaments are touched to the skin, the patient reports when and where they are felt. The smaller the filament felt, the higher the degree of sensation. Decreased sensation is evident when a large monofilament must be used before the patient can feel the touch.

Muscle and reflex grading are somewhat subjective, but the most commonly used parameters are listed in Tables 2.4 and 2.5.

Diagnosis of low back pain etiology involves putting together pieces of information from the history, physical examination, and diagnostic examinations such as x-rays, CT scan, MRI, or other examinations. Table 6.2 delineates differences in symptoms of two common causes of low back pain, spinal stenosis and herniated (ruptured) disk.

Spinal stenosis is the result of an inadequate size of the spinal canal and causes compression of the neural elements (dural sac and nerve pathways and nerve roots). The symptoms differ from herniated disk as described in Table 6.2. Other differences between spinal stenosis and herniated disk include a gradual increase in walking difficulty. Patients often relate that pushing a lawn mower or grocery cart helps relieve pain when walking because forward flexion of the spine provides more space in the spinal canal, thereby lessening symptoms.

Conservative treatment of spinal stenosis may include use of nonsteroidal anti-inflammatory drugs, physical therapy, pain blocking electrical units (TENS), and epidural steroid injections.

**Table 6.2** Differences Between Symptoms of Spinal Stenosis and Herniated Nucleus Pulposus

| Spinal Stenosis | Herniated Nucleus Pulposus |
| --- | --- |
| Gradual onset of pain | Abrupt onset of pain |
| Pain increased with walking | Pain increased with sitting |
| Bilateral pain relieved with sitting or lying down with hips flexed | Unilateral pain distribution |
| Bowel or bladder problems | Positive sciatic stretch test on straight leg raises |

Herniated nucleus pulposus or ruptured disk is related to degeneration of the cartilaginous intervertebral annulus, which allows the semigelatinous nucleus pulposus to herniate through the cracked or frayed cartilage. Herniations cause low back pain and sciatic neuropathy that require the conservative treatments discussed above. Surgical treatments for low back pain are discussed in Chapter 12.

## BIBLIOGRAPHY

Altman, R.D. (1984). Osteoarthritis: Pathogenesis, differential diagnosis, treatment. *Orthopaedic Review, 13*(5), 53–63.

Bordelon, R.L. (1987). Evaluation and operative procedures for hallux valgus deformity. *Orthopedics, 10*(1), 38–44.

Buchanan, W.W. (1989). Managing arthritis in elderly patients. *Journal of Musculoskeletal Medicine 4*(3) (Suppl.), 516–17.

Cooke, T.D.V. (1988). Pathogenesis of osteoarthritis. *Orthopaedic Review, 17*(5), 527.

Frymoyer, J.W. (Ed.) (1991). *The Adult Spine Principles and Practice* (Vols. 1–2), New York: Raven Press.

Gulanick, M., Klopp, A., & Galanes, S. (Eds.). (1986). *Nursing care plans, nursing diagnosis, and interventions.* St. Louis: Mosby-Yearbook.

Hoaglund, F.T. (1984). Confirming the diagnosis of osteoarthritis. *Journal of Musculoskeletal Medicine, 1*(5), 66–81.

Karpman, R.R., & Baum, J. (Eds.). (1988). *Aging and clinical practice: Musculoskeletal disorders.* Tokyo: Igaku-Shoin.

Kengora, J.E. (1988). A rationale for the surgical treatment of bunions. *Orthopedics, 11*(5), 777–789.

Kim, M.J., McFarland, G.K., & McLane, A.M. (1991). *Pocket guide to nursing diagnoses* (4th ed.). St Louis: Mosby-Yearbook.

Mann, R.A. (1987). Treatment of the bunion deformity. *Orthopedics 10*(1), 49–56.

Moskowitz, R.W. & Haug, M.R. (Eds.). (1986). *Arthritis and the elderly.* New York: Springer.

Mourad, L. (1991). *Orthopedic disorders.* St. Louis: Mosby-Yearbook.

Phillips, R.H. (1989). *Coping with osteoarthritis.* Garden City Park, NY: Avery.

Weinstein, J.N., & Wiesel, S.W. (1990). *The lumbar spine.* Philadelphia: Saunders.

# 7

## NURSING PROCESS IN
## THE CARE OF PERSONS
## WITH BONE TUMORS

Tumors of the musculoskeletal tissues may affect cartilage, muscle, or synovium, but most frequently they affect bones. Many tumors are benign, but those that are malignant are usually aggressive and of great concern. Musculoskeletal tumors make up only about 3% of all malignant tumors, and about 6,000 new primary bone and soft tissue sarcomas are diagnosed yearly in the United States. Secondary tumors, or metastatic ones, occur in bones more often than primary tumors but the incidence is very difficult to determine with accuracy.

Benign musculoskeletal tumors (see Table 7.1) are not life-threatening, but malignant tumors are always life-threatening because of their uncontrolled growth. Musculoskeletal malignant tumors are graded according to their malignancy as shown in Table 7.2. They are also identified as being intracompartmental (entirely within a compartment) or extracompartmental (growing both inside and outside compartmental boundaries), and according to whether or not there is evidence of metastasis. Careful, accurate grading and staging are necessary for the best treatment to be devised. Many malignant bone tumors occur in young people and radical resection and even amputation may be necessary, making it extremely vital that accurate diagnosis precedes such surgical procedures. Treatments for malignant bone tumors must take into consideration the patient's age, life style, life goals, and quality of life when decisions on radical excision or amputation are made. Other surgical procedures may also be done for specific tumors, as will be discussed later. Table 7.3 lists common bone, cartilage, and muscle tumors, whether they are benign or malignant, common diagnostic procedures, and usual treatments.

**Table 7.1** Classification of Benign & Malignant Tumors with Tissue of Origin

| Tissue of Origin | Benign | Malignant |
|---|---|---|
| Bone | Osteoma | Primary osteosarcoma |
| | | Central osteosarcoma |
| | | Low-grade medullary osteosarcoma |
| | | Telangiectatic osteosarcoma |
| | | Multicentric osteosarcoma |
| | | Paget's disease |
| | | Juxtacortical osteosarcoma |
| | | Parosteal osteosarcoma |
| Cartilage | Osteochondroma | Chondrosarcoma |
| | Endochondroma | |
| | Periosteal chondroma | |
| | Chondroblastoma | |
| Muscle | Leiomyoma | Leiomyosarcoma |
| | Rhabdomyoma | Rhabdomyosarcoma |
| Fibrous tissue | Fibroma | Fibrosarcoma |
| | | Malignant fibrous histiocytoma |
| Adipose connective tissue | Lipoma | Liposarcoma |
| Bone marrow | | Ewing's sarcoma |
| | | Plasma cell myeloma (multiple myeloma) |
| Uncertain cell | Giant cell | Malignant giant cell |
| | Unicameral bone cyst | |
| | Aneurysmal bone cyst | |
| Vascular tissue | Hemangioma | Hemangioendothelioma |
| Neural | Neurofibroma | |

# BONE AND CARTILAGE TUMORS

## Benign Tumors of Bone and Cartilage

Osteoma. An osteoma is a benign tumor of children and young adults between ages 10 and 20. It is found in the bones of the face or skull, and makes up about 20% of benign bone tumors. It is commonly an external tumor, but may also be located within sinuses, nasal passages, ocular orbit, and inside the skull. It forms a hard, immovable, nontender swelling over the involved soft tissues. Internally growing osteomas may produce symptoms referable to their

**Table 7.2** Surgical Staging System for Bone Tumors

| Stage | Grade (G)* | Site (T)** | Metastasis (M)*** |
|---|---|---|---|
| 1A | Low ($G_1$) | Intracompartmental ($T_1$) | None ($M_0$) |
| 1B | Low ($G_1$) | Extracompartmental ($T_2$) | None ($M_0$) |
| 11A | High ($G_2$) | Intracompartmental ($T_1$) | None ($M_0$) |
| 11B | High ($G_2$) | Extracompartmental ($T_2$) | None ($M_0$) |
| 111A | Low ($G_1$) | Intracompartmental or extracompartmental ($T_1$ or $T_2$) | Regional or distant ($M_1$) |
| 111B | High ($G_2$) | Intracompartmental or extracompartmental ($T_1$ or $T_2$) | Regional or distant ($M_1$) |

* *Grade (G)*
  $G_0$ = Benign; well-differentiated cells.
  $G_1$ = Low-grade malignant; moderate cell differentiation; occasional distant metastasis.
  $G_2$ = High-grade malignant; poorly or undifferentiated cells; frequent distant metastasis.
** *Site (Tumor)*
  $T_1$ = Localized, encapsulated; intracompartmental (entirely confined in anatomical boundaries of tissues of origin).
  $T_2$ = Extracompartmental (spread outside of tissues of origin).
*** *Metastasis (M)*
  $M_0$ = Has no lymph node or distant metastasis.
  $M_1$ = Has lymph node and/or distant metastasis.

**Table 7.3** Common Bone, Cartilage, and Muscle Tumors, Their Specific Characteristics, Diagnostic Procedures, and Usual Treatments

| Tumor | Characteristics | Diagnostic Procedures* | Usual Treatments |
|---|---|---|---|
| | | Tumors of Bone and Cartilage | |
| Osteoma | Benign | Bone scan: may show increased uptake. | Left untouched or may be resected to relieve symptoms. |
| Osteochondroma | Benign | X-ray, CT scan, or MRI: shows outpouching of trabecular bone in metaphyseal area of bone. | Excision of tumor and resection of tendon above its point of attachment to remove all precartilaginous tissues to prevent recurrence. |
| Chondroma, chondromyxoma, or enchondroma | Benign; about 25% are malignant | X-ray, CT scan, or MRI: may show thinned cortex of bone. | Wide, en bloc excision or amputation, if malignant and in a long bone. |
| Chondroblastoma | Benign | X-ray, CT scan, or MRI: may show osteolytic tumor with points of calcification. | Excision, curettage of tumor bed and placement of bone chips; about one-third of these tumors recur. |
| Giant cell tumor (osteoclastoma) | Benign | X-ray, CT scan, or MRI: show bone-destroying, osteolytic with large cells; bone scan shows increased uptake. | Thorough excision to prevent recurrence; if recurs, wide excision with bone grafts to fill defect. |
| Aneurysmal bone cyst | Benign | X-rays show cyst-shape; arteriogram should show aneurysmal nature of cyst; MRI shows outline of cyst. | Curettage to remove cyst; cryo-surgery with liquid nitrogen. |
| Unicameral bone cyst | Benign | X-rays show multiloculated cyst. | Excision with bone grafts to fill defect; steroid injection into cyst. |

(continued)

**Table 7.3** (Continued)

| Tumor | Characteristics | Diagnostic Procedures* | Usual Treatments |
|---|---|---|---|
| Osteosarcoma | Malignant | X-rays, CT scan, or MRI: show "sunburst" appearance characteristic of this tumor; bone scan: helps determine tumor size and possible metastases; chest x-ray: shows metastases, if present; serum alkaline phosphatase is elevated. | Wide excision with limb salvage; may need joint replacement if joint involved with tumor or excision; chemotherapy and radiation therapy will be done both pre- and postoperatively; amputation may be required (less done recently with improved surgical techniques). |
| Parosteal Sarcoma | Malignant, low-grade | X-ray, CT scan, and MRI: show metaphyseal tumor attached to cortex of bone but outside periosteum of bone; bone scan shows increased uptake. | Wide excision of tumor. |
| Chondrosarcoma | Malignant | X-ray, CT scan, MRI to aid diagnosis. | Wide excision; possible limb amputation; radiation and chemotherapy if of high-grade malignancy. |
| Ewing's Sarcoma | Malignant | X-ray, CT scan, or MRI aid diagnosis. | Radiation therapy, as tumor is radiosensitive; chemotherapy also used. |
| Fibrosarcoma | Malignant | X-ray, CT scan, or MRI outline tumor. | En bloc wide excision. |

### Tumors of Muscles

| | | | |
|---|---|---|---|
| Leiomyoma | Benign | Ultrasound: shows tumor mass. | Surgical removal. |
| Rhabdomyoma | Benign | Noted by physical examination of muscle mass. | Surgical removal. |
| | | | |
| Leiomyosarcoma | Malignant | Ultrasound. | Removal with wide resection. |
| Rhabdomyosarcoma | Malignant | Arteriogram outlines tumor. | Removal with wide resection; radiation therapy (tumor is radiosensitive); chemotherapy may also be given. |

*Securing a thorough health history and doing a physical examination are routine diagnostic procedures for each tumor.

specific site, as, for example, headache, seizures, or pain. The tumor grows slowly, and stops growing when it reaches a certain size. It is diagnosed by its site and size through x-rays or CT scans. Table 7.3 discusses its medical management. Recurrences are rare.

*Osteochondroma.* These tumors make up the largest group of benign bone tumors. They are composed of spongy bone covered with a cap of cartilage. They develop during growth periods, growing in the metaphysical area of the bone, near the knee. They may also grow in tendons, and are firm, hard growths fixed to the bone, where they may hinder or limit joint motions. Table 7.3 lists their diagnostic tests and treatments.

*Chondroma, also called Chondromyxoma and Enchondroma.* This benign tumor is most often noted in a finger or humerus of a young adult, where its growth destroys the cancellous areas of the affected bone. It can undergo malignant transformation if in the pelvis or a large long bone. It grows slowly and remains stationary unless it becomes malignant. Chondromas cause few symptoms unless complicated by a pathologic fracture which causes severe pain. Table 7.3 lists diagnostic and treatment parameters.

*Chondroblastoma.* This is a rare benign cartilage tumor, growing usually in a long bone near the epiphyseal area and metaphysis. It occurs most often in males between the ages of 5 and 25 years. Symptoms are mild, intermittent pain for long periods—sometimes as long as 2 years—with mild edema and tenderness. If a joint is involved, there may be some limitation of motion. Diagnostic and treatment parameters are found in Table 7.3.

*Giant Cell Tumor, also called Osteoclastoma.* This benign tumor occurs in young adults between the ages of 20 to 40 with an almost equal male-female distribution. It accounts for 4 to 5% of benign bone tumors in the United States. It grows in the epiphyseal area of bones, growing eccentrically and destroying the bone matrix as it grows. It is most often found in the femur after the epiphyseal growth plates are closed. This tumor is composed of large, giant cells which can grow into contiguous soft tissues. It grows slowly with no characteristic symptoms, except for dull, aching pain that is worse at night. Table 7.3 contains diagnostic and treatment options (see Fig. 7.1).

*Aneurysmal Bone Cyst.* This is a benign tumor consisting of a mass of vascular spaces enclosed in a shell of new bone growing out from the affected bone into the soft tissues. Males are most often affected between the ages of 10 and 30 years. It grows most commonly in the metaphyseal area of long bones. Symptoms may include a history of trauma, limitation of joint motion, edema, and pain increased with movement. If the bone cyst is in a vertebra, there may

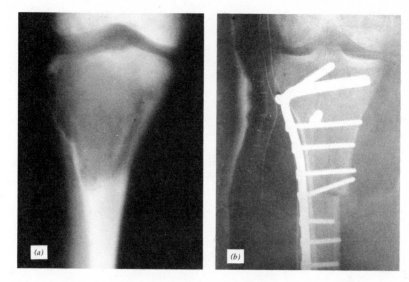

**Figure 7.1** (a) Osteoclastoma (giant cell tumor) of the proximal tibia. (b) Cadaver bone with plate and screws to replace the proximal tibia in (a). (Courtesy of Dr. Lawrence Weis, Ohio State University Bone and Extremity Tumor Unit.)

be nerve impingement symptoms of numbness or weakness. Again, Table 7.3 has diagnostic and treatment factors.

*Unicameral Bone Cyst.* This is a rare, benign growth in the metaphysis of a long bone near the epiphysis. It has a thin walled cavity filled with yellow fluid. It affects persons between 5 and 15 years of age. Over 50% of these bone cysts occur in the humerus. It has no symptoms and is discovered on x-ray after a fracture at the site. See Table 7.3 for diagnosis and treatment factors.

## Malignant Tumors of Bone and Cartilage

*Osteosarcoma.* This tumor is the most common tumor of bone, making up about 35% of malignant bone tumors. It grows rapidly and is highly malignant. Its peak incidence is between 10 and 20 years with slightly more males than females affected. Older persons between the ages 50 and 60 with Paget's disease also have osteosarcoma with that disease.

As listed in Table 7.1, there are several varieties of osteosarcomas. The majority occur around the knee area in the distal femur and proximal tibia. Others may be found in the mandible and humerus.

Its rapid growth pattern causes it to quickly destroy the inner cortex of the bone as it expands into contiguous soft tissues (see Fig. 7.2). Symptoms include dull, aching, almost constant pain, often worse at night. The patient

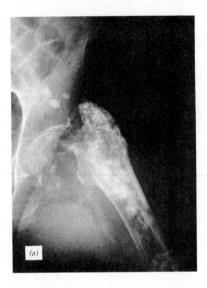

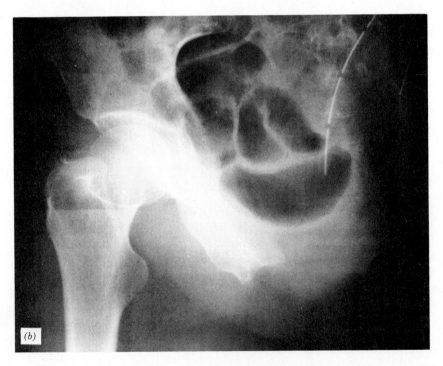

**Figure 7.2** Osteosarcoma of the left proximal femur.

avoids using the part because of discomfort. Other symptoms may include weight loss, malaise, and nausea. Table 7.3 contains diagnostic and treatment parameters.

*Parosteal Sarcoma.* This tumor grows outside the periosteum of bone; the name means abnormal site or disease. It is a tumor of low grade malignancy, and often recurs even with radical resection. Parosteal osteosarcomas occur in persons between 14 and 40 years of age, growing in the metaphyseal area of long bones, primarily the distal femur. The tumor is a hard mass that may encircle the bone. The major symptom is local pain and there may be some limitation of motion. Table 7.3 has the diagnostic and treatment patterns.

*Chondrosarcoma.* Chondrosarcoma is a malignant tumor of cartilage that affects males slightly more commonly than females. It most frequently occurs in the upper end of the humerus or femur. In contrast to malignant bone tumors, which occur most frequently in persons under 25 years of age, chondrosarcomas affect persons between 30 and 50. The tumor is slow growing and may not manifest itself for several years. As it grows, it erodes outward from the site and may have some bone cells in its matrix (see Fig. 7.3).

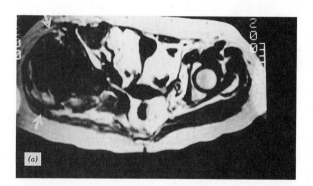

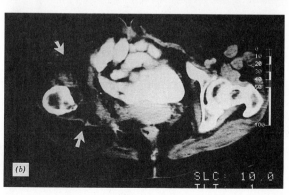

**Figure 7.3** (a) Chondrosarcoma of the pelvis and ilium (arrows). (b) Chondrosarcoma of the proximal femur (arrows) of a different patient.

Symptoms associated with chondrosarcoma depend on the area affected and the size of the tumor. The major symptom is pain, which is persistent and eventually severe. Eventually a mass may be palpated. Symptoms may persist for 5–10 years before a diagnosis is made because of the slow growth of the tumor.

Diagnosis is made from the medical history, physical examination of the tumor site, if possible, x-rays, CT scan, or MRI examinations. Biopsy is performed at the time of the definitive surgery selected from all the data. Surgical excision must be wide and thorough to make certain all tumor has been removed. Recurrence can occur at the site. Amputation may be required to be certain of complete tumor removal. When the tumor is not totally removed, it will metastasize to the lungs and may also recur locally at the site of the original tumor.

*Ewing's Sarcoma.* This tumor has an uncertain cell origin, as it may start in the marrow of bone, from the stem or reticulum cells, or from the supportive bone marrow. Persons ages 5 to 25 years are most commonly affected. This tumor grows in the diaphysis of bone, not the metaphysis. Pain that is worse at night is the major symptom. The tumor is a hard, tender mass that is fixed to the bone. The overlying skin is red and edematous. Systemic symptoms may be anemia, weight loss, and fever. See Table 7.3 for diagnosis and treatments.

*Fibrosarcoma.* This tumor is made of fibroblasts. It is identical with a fibrosarcoma that grows in soft tissues, although this is a tumor of bone fibrous tissues. It occurs mainly in the femur, but can also be found in the vertebrae, skull, or mandible. It grows in the metaphysis or diaphysis of bones, in persons over 30 years of age. Symptoms include onset of continuous pain that is worse at night, and as the tumor enlarges, there is gradual swelling with a firm, smooth mass firmly fixed to bone. See Table 7.3 for diagnosis and treatments.

*Metastatic Tumors of Bone.* These are tumors that spread to bones from their primary sites, such as the breast, lung, prostate, kidneys, bladder, and others. Sites of metastatic spread include the pelvis, vertebrae, ribs, hip, humerus, and femur other than the hip. The metastatic cells grow and weaken the affected bone. Frequently the patient has a pathologic fracture as the first indication of metastasis. There may also be some limitation of motion. A radionuclide bone scan may show several areas of metastasis. A biopsy of the metastatic site may lead to the primary tumor. Appropriate treatments may include radiation therapy, chemotherapy, and surgery to repair the pathologic fracture, if present. Hormone therapies may be used for hormonal-dependent tumors.

## MUSCLE TUMORS

### Benign Tumors of Muscle

*Leiomyoma.* This is a benign tumor of smooth muscle. It develops most often in the smooth muscles of the uterus, where it may remain symptom-free for long periods. Eventually, there may be soreness, abdominal or pelvic tenderness, and a mass may be palpable. The tumor may be removed if it leads to excessive bleeding or pronounced discomfort. If a leiomyoma occurs in other muscle tissues, it may be removed if it affects muscle actions. Biopsy confirms its benignity.

*Rhabdomyoma.* This is a tumor of striated muscles. It is a rare tumor, with tenderness and pain its only symptoms. It should be biopsied to confirm its benignity.

### Malignant Tumors of Muscle

*Leiomyosarcoma.* This is a malignant counterpart of a leiomyoma, with similar sites and symptoms. It can also be found in stomach muscles, prostate, small bowel, and esophagus. It grows in bizarre cell patterns, with radical growth and areas of necrosis. Surgical removal with wide excision is used, plus radiation therapy and chemotherapy to be certain all cells are killed.

*Rhabdomyosarcoma.* This is the malignant counterpart of rhabdomyoma. It grows in persons of all ages, with a slight male predominance. It is found in the inguinal, gluteal, popliteal, and interscapular areas. Symptoms include having a mass that is soft and enlarging slowly. There may be some tenderness and pain from pressure and use. The tumor frequently is shaped like the muscle in which it is located. An arteriogram aids in the diagnosis, showing large vessels that run in different directions, with arteriovenous shunts likely. These tumors are radiosensitive and radioresponsive. Surgical removal may also be used.

Nursing care of patients with bone or muscle tumors is intense because of the uncertain nature of these tumors. Before definitive treatments can be devised, the physician must attempt to make the most accurate diagnosis possible. Frequently, consultation with an orthopaedic oncologist is sought for the optimal treatment protocol or plan. All treatment options should be discussed with the patient and family, as often as needed, to be as certain as possible that all options are understood. Radical surgical excision with limb salvage may be opted by the patient and family, rather than amputation. All must agree that the suggested treatments are best for the patient's specific tumor.

## NURSING PROCESS

## NURSING DIAGNOSIS

### IMPAIRED PHYSICAL MOBILITY RELATED TO TUMOR MASS, PRESSURE, AND PAIN

#### Assessment

1. Assess for observable or palpable mass; may be subcutaneous or intramuscular and may or may not be easily palpable.
2. Assess for changes in skin tissues, such as thinning from stretching, shininess, edema, or redness from increased blood vessels.
3. Assess for effects of mass on mobility; presence of limp or hesitation; use of ambulatory aid; limitation of weight bearing.
4. Assess for pain: see next nursing diagnosis.

#### Expected Outcomes

The patient will:
- regain satisfactory mobility after treatments.
- experience relief of pressure and pain.

#### Nursing Interventions

1. Explain all upcoming diagnostic examinations to ease patient's concerns if physician has mentioned possible diagnosis of malignant tumor.
2. Prepare patient for diagnostic tests such as x-ray, CT scan, bone scan, MRI (magnetic resonance imaging; see p. 102), or other test.
3. Monitor results of serologic studies, such as complete blood count, alkaline phosphatase, acid phosphatase, and others.
4. Assist patient to ambulate with aid, if ordered.
5. Assist with ROM exercises, with caution for joints near tumor site.
6. Assist to positions of comfort if surgery performed.
7. Assist therapist in transfer of patient to chair if hemipelvectomy or above-knee amputation done.
8. Maintain desired position of operative limb, if limb salvage surgery done: position may be neutral, abduction, adduction, or internally or externally rotated. Foot of bed may be elevated.

9. Assist prosthetist when measuring patient for postoperative prosthesis, if necessary (see Chapter 12 for care after amputation).
10. Teach patient and assist in adduction, extension, or other exercises if limb amputated to prevent contractures.

## Evaluation

The patient:

- regained satisfactory mobility after surgical removal of tumor; is learning to walk with limited weight-bearing using crutches temporarily (had resection of muscle to remove tumor).
- had relief of pressure and pain with removal of tumor.

## NURSING DIAGNOSIS

### *PAIN RELATED TO PRESSURE OF ENLARGING MASS ON NERVE(S), BONE, OR OTHER TISSUES*

## Assessment

1. Assess for presence of pain, its type, amount, duration, when present, what relief measures used, and with what results.
2. Assess site or sites of pain related to tumor site or metastasis.
3. Assess medications used for pain relief and with what results.

## Expected Outcomes

The patient will:

- be relieved of pain following treatments.
- have no recurrence of pain after recovery.

## Nursing Interventions

1. Assist to positions of comfort; adjust position q 2–3 hours.
2. Monitor for anxiety or restlessness; restlessness may be related to metastatic disease to pelvis, vertebrae, or ribs; anxiety may be related to potential diagnosis.
3. Monitor for possible pathologic fracture: deformity, inability to bear weight; dull, aching, or sharp pain in specific area of bone; place limb in position of comfort; if in traction, monitor function of traction setup and position of limb.

4. Administer ordered analgesic and/or anti-inflammatory medications q 3 to 4 hours; monitor results of medications to relieve pain; patient may use PCA (patient-controlled analgesia) pump after surgery to administer own analgesics.

5. Use splint, pillows, or joint immobilizer to help position affected limb more comfortably.

6. Do neurovascular checks (see p. 255) to determine severity of pain or current condition.

7. Massage back and tired muscles q 6 hours; assist with ROM exercises to ease soreness and pain.

8. Teach relaxation exercises to lessen anxiety and pain.

9. Provide privacy and time for patient to verbalize concerns about diagnosis; secure consultation with therapists as needed.

## Evaluation

The patient:

- was gradually becoming pain free after treatments; was still taking non-narcotic analgesics intermittently.

- hopefully, will have no recurrence after recovery and tissue healing.

## NURSING DIAGNOSIS

### AFTER SURGERY: IMPAIRED GAS EXCHANGE RELATED TO ANESTHESIA, BED REST, AND OPERATIVE PROCEDURE (THORACOTOMY OR FOREQUARTER AMPUTATION)

## Assessment

1. Assess for respiratory rate, depth, splinting of respiratory muscles.
2. Assess breath sounds for rales, rhonchi, or breath sounds.
3. Assess for cough, sputum amount or color.

## Expected Outcomes

The patient will:

- regain satisfactory gas exchange during recovery.

- have no lingering cough or sputum production.

- have clear lung sounds.

## Nursing Interventions

1. Assess respiratory rates and depth with other vital signs.

2. Listen to breath sounds in all lobes; percuss lung areas as needed if breath sounds decreased or noisy.

3. Encourage to deep-breathe and cough to clear respiratory passages.

4. Have patient use incentive spirometer q 2 hours to expand lungs and clear respiratory passageways.

5. Check color and amount of sputum, if any coughed up; report yellow or green sputum to physician.

## Evaluation

The patient had:

- satisfactory gas exchange while recovering from surgery.

- no lingering cough or sputum production.

## NURSING DIAGNOSIS

### IMPAIRED SKIN INTEGRITY RELATED TO SURGICAL WOUNDS OR SKIN GRAFT

## Assessment

1. Assess incisional areas for signs of inflammation and healing: initially will have redness, edema, heat in incisional area, and pain (which should lessen over time).

2. Assess for presence of drainage from wound; check color of drainage if any present.

3. Assess skin graft, if present, for color, edema, raising off skin surface, dehiscence, and drainage.

## Expected Outcomes

The patient will:

- regain skin integrity and healing over time.

- have well-adhered skin graft, if present.

## Nursing Interventions

1. Monitor healing of incision by checking amount of redness, edema, heat in incisional area, pain, or tenderness when assisting or doing dressing changes. Redness, edema, heat, and tenderness should be markedly lessened in 5–6 days depending on length of incision, site, and closure of incision.

2. Monitor presence, amount, and color of drainage from incision: may be initially serosanguineous, then serous; it should not increase and become yellow or green, which could indicate infection; yellow or green drainage may need to be cultured to determine presence and type of pathogens.

3. Monitor skin graft site for adherence to recipient site; if ordered, roll graft with applicators to remove edema fluid to aid adherence of graft.

4. Use aseptic technique for wound and graft care to decrease chance of wound or graft infection.

5. If graft is split thickness, check donor site for type and amount of drainage, amount of pain, and signs of granulation or infection. Donor site may be covered with transparent sterile dressing or medicated gauze; change as ordered.

6. Monitor sutures for security of closure, and for signs of irritation or drainage; sutures should be cleaned during dressing changes.

7. Teach stump wrapping techniques if patient has amputation; see p. 423 for wrapping techniques.

8. Assist patient to positions of comfort as needed.

## Evaluation

The patient

- regained skin integrity and wound healing by first intention over time.
- had 100% adherence of split-thickness skin graft to operative wound site.

## BIBLIOGRAPHY

Beltran, J. (1990). *MRI musculoskeletal system.* Philadelphia: Lippincott.

Coombs, R., & Friedlaender, G. (1987). *Bone tumour management.* London: Butterworth.

Darr, K.F., Acker, J. Pesson, C. & D'Ambrosia, R.D. (1988). Giant cell tumor of bone. *Orthopedics, 11*(1), 209–221.

Enneking, W.F., (Ed.). (1987). *Limb salvage in musculoskeletal oncology.* New York: Churchill Livingstone.

Enneking, W.F. (1986). A system of staging musculoskeletal neoplasms. *Clinical Orthopedics & Related Research, 204,* 9–24.

Gebhardt, M.C., & Mankin, H.J. (1988). Osteosarcomas: The treatment controversy. *Surgical Rounds for Orthopaedics, 2*(7), 25–42.

Lane, J.M., Hurson, B., Boland, P., & Glasser, D. (1986). Osteogenic sarcoma. *Clinical Orthopedics & Related Research, 204,* 93–110.

Mourad, L. (1991). *Orthopedic disorders.* St. Louis: Mosby-Yearbook.

# 8

# NURSING PROCESS FOR PATIENTS WITH INFECTIONS OF BONES

Infection is an inflammatory response of the body to the invasion of pathogenic microorganisms. The pathogens multiply, set up local cellular responses, and—depending on the specific pathogen—liberate toxins. Toxins affect capillary blood flow, leading to fluctuations in blood volume and blood pressure, and may precipitate sepsis, systemic infection, and shock. Bacterial infections may either be contained locally by the white blood cells and lymph nodes or become systemic, resulting in severe, life-threatening sepsis. In orthopaedics, infections can be and sometimes are life threatening when associated with osteomyelitis.

## OSTEOMYELITIS

Osteomyelitis is infection of the bone and bone marrow. It can occur as a result of orthopaedic trauma or secondary to other infections. Osteomyelitis commonly develops when the host's resistance is low or when the focal site has impaired resistance or decreased blood flow, allowing the pathogenic organisms to implant and reproduce. Hematogenic (blood borne) osteomyelitis is more common in children and is usually secondary to throat infections; at times it results from the lowered oxygen tension in sickle cell disease. Older persons develop osteomyelitis secondary to open traumatic wounds, armed services, or war-related injuries, following joint replacements and secondary to instrumentation procedures in various organs, joints, or tissues. Osteomyelitis may develop along pin tracks from external fixators, related to inadequate management of an open fracture, not to the presence of the external fixator.

The incidence of osteomyelitis is difficult to determine with certainty because of the many sites or tissues that may become infected. Pin track

**220**

infections after removal of external fixators affect approximately 2% to 8% of patients. Of patients having total joint replacements, 0.5% to 1.0% may develop osteomyelitis, a very low percentage considering there are over 200,000 total hip replacements yearly, 150,000 total knee replacements yearly, and lesser numbers of replacements of the shoulder, elbow, wrist, and ankle.

## Pathophysiology

Osteomyelitis commonly develops in the metaphyseal area of the bone where the blood supply is decreased compared to other areas of the bone. The pathogenic organisms implant and reproduce until a mass of organisms is present. Exudates, such as pus and cellular debris, build up, and, along with the growing mass, can cause a feeling of tightness and pressure. The exudate (pus) may spread away along tissue planes to other areas of the bone, and can spread upward or outward from the site until it breaks through the skin, becoming a draining fistula. The area of osteomyelitic infection becomes hot, tender or painful, with redness around the site. The person may resist using the area (frequently an extremity) as the infection progresses. Pieces of infected bone die if the infection is unchecked and become surrounded by the purulent exudate. Such dead bone pieces are called sequestrum, and, if they are large, they must be removed or they become sources of continued infection. New bone sections, called involucrum, may surround the sequestra in an attempt to heal the area, but full healing is prevented because of the dead bone at the site (see Fig. 8.1). Occasionally the infection may become walled off and form a fibrous tissue capsule around the site. Such a walled-off capsule is called a Brodie's abscess. The organisms within a Brodie's capsule remain virulent and can cause a reinfection or flare-up at any time.

The major organisms that cause osteomyelitis include staphylococci, which account for approximately 90% of purulent osteomyelitis. Other causative organisms are streptococci, *Escherichia coli, Salmonella typhi,* and *Neisseria gonorrhoeae.* The bones most frequently infected are the femur, tibia, humerus, and radius, in the order named. The areas around the knee, lower end of the femur, upper tibia, and upper shaft of the humerus and radius are common sites for osteomyelitis to develop.

The diagnosis of osteomyelitis is made from the patient's history of open trauma, surgery, or an antecedent infection. Physical examination will usually reveal a tender, warm or hot, reddened, and edematous area, which may be open and exude purulent drainage. A mass may be felt. The patient is reluctant to use the affected part and may hold it in a flexed position. The patient may have a fever ranging from 101 to 104°F (38.3–40°C), and may feel tired, weak, and complain of headache and nausea.

Laboratory tests may show markedly elevated white blood cell counts up to 30,000 or more (normal range is 5,000–9,000/cmm), with counts of 80%

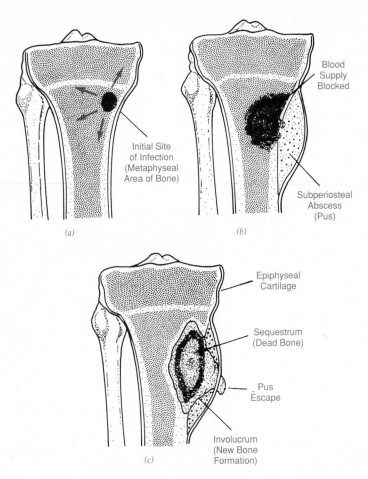

**Figure 8.1** Sites of osteomyelitis. (a) Metaphyseal area of bone; (b) development of pus and abscess of osteomyelitis; (c) fistula to skin.

polymorphonuclear neutrophils (normal is 50–70% of total WBC's). A culture of the drainage should grow the infecting pathogen. A blood culture may reveal a bacteremia or even a septicemia. The teichoic acid antibody test may show antibodies as soon as two weeks after infection (teichoic acid is a cell-wall component of *S. aureus*). The erythrocyte sedimentation test will be elevated above normal. The tuberculin skin test will be positive if the osteomyelitis is caused by tubercle bacilli.

Radiologic studies may be initially negative for the first 7–10 days after infection, but thereafter may show the localized destruction of bone with or without sequestrum and involucrum. The infected bone may appear moth eaten and eroded. A CT scan may show spread into contiguous tissues. A bone scan will show increased uptake in the infected area.

Treatments must be vigorous, intense, and long-term to effect total eradication of the infection. Initially, appropriate antibiotics are administered intravenously for 6 weeks, followed by oral administration of antibiotics for 3–6 months. Aspirin for adults and acetaminophen for children are given for temperature elevations above 102°F (39°C). Bed rest may be required initially during the acute infection to keep the infection localized and to lessen systemic stress.

Surgical debridement may be done after the intravenous antibiotic therapy has been concluded. The infected bone should be sterile (no actively growing pathogens) and the remaining debris will be scraped away. Tubes may be placed in the site for irrigation with antibiotic solutions until wound cultures are negative and the area is satisfactory for bone grafts to be placed, if needed. If the involved bone is markedly weakened, it may be placed in an external fixator to help prevent a fracture (see Fig. 8.2). Free muscle transfers may be placed in the site to obliterate dead space. Hyperbaric oxygen treatments with 100% oxygen for 2 hours daily for 30 treatments may be needed for refractory osteomyelitis. Rarely is amputation required in recent years because of more vigorous initial treatments (see Fig. 8.3).

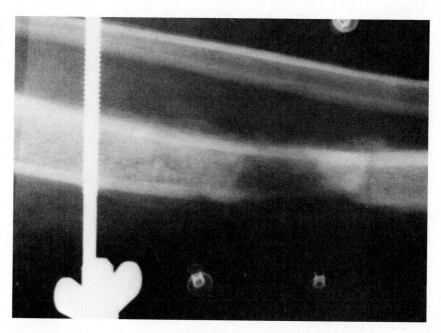

**Figure 8.2** Osteomyelitis of the tibia with transfixing pins.

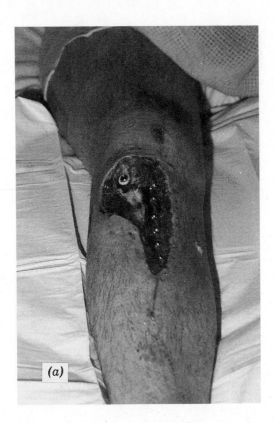

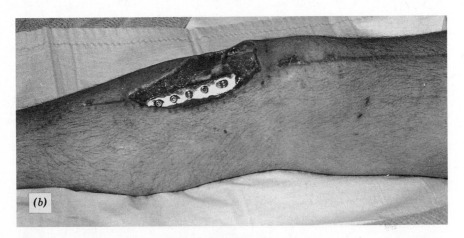

**Figure 8.3** (a) Infection, skin loss, and osteomyelitis in a fractured tibia treated with a compression plate and screws; (b) Lateral view of wound area in same patient.

## NURSING PROCESS

## NURSING DIAGNOSIS

### IMPAIRED PHYSICAL MOBILITY RELATED TO PRESENCE OF OSTEOMYELITIS

#### Assessment

1. Assess for presence of painful, sore, or tender area, with or without palpable mass.
2. Assess for presence of drainage; drainage may be blood-streaked and purulent.
3. Assess for fever.
4. Assess how person holds limb—may be in flexion.
5. Assess for presence of systemic disease, e.g., tuberculosis.

#### Expected Outcomes

The patient will:
- regain painless mobility with healed area.
- regain solid bone integrity.
- regain normal body temperatures.

#### Nursing Interventions

1. Place patient on bed rest, if ordered; arrange affected limb on pillows for comfort.
2. Demonstrate use of ambulatory aid (crutches) in anticipation of being allowed out of bed.
3. Administer ordered antibiotics intravenously.
4. Assist with transfer to hyperbaric chamber, if such treatments are ordered.
5. Administer antipyretic medication for temperature elevations.

#### Evaluation

The patient:
- was regaining painless mobility after treatments.
- was experiencing bone healing as shown by x-rays; eroded area was "filling in" due to presence of bone grafts (see later nursing diagnosis).
- regained normal ranges of body temperatures after treatments.

## NURSING DIAGNOSIS

*IMPAIRED SKIN INTEGRITY RELATED TO PRESENCE OF PURULENT DRAINAGE OR INSERTION OF IRRIGATION TUBES AT SITE OF OSTEOMYELITIS*

### Assessment

1. Assess site for drainage on dressings or from irrigating tubes.
2. Assess site for skin irritation, redness, edema, and hot areas.

### Expected Outcomes

The patient will:
- have resolution of infection; and no further drainage.
- regain skin integrity.

### Nursing Interventions

1. Do wound irrigations with ordered solutions (usually organism-sensitive antibiotics) at proper times.
2. Change wound dressings using aseptic technique.
3. Reposition patient q 2-3 hours.
4. Assess all skin tissues for signs of pressure.

### Evaluation

The patient:
- was regaining skin integrity without purulent drainage from site.
- was experiencing resolution of infection in bone with irrigations and antibiotics.

## NURSING DIAGNOSIS

*PAIN RELATED TO BONE INFECTION AND ALTERED TISSUE PERFUSION*

### Assessment

1. Assess type, amount, duration, and characteristics of pain.
2. Assess motor and sensory functions of involved and opposite limb.

## Expected Outcomes

The patient will:

- experience pain relief following treatments.
- regain normal peripheral tissue perfusion.

## Nursing Interventions

1. Administer analgesic medications as ordered; monitor effects of medications.
2. Assist patient to adjust positions as needed; handle affected tissues gently.
3. Encourage diversionary activities to help pass time; offer games, puzzles, cards, or other diversions, as needed.
4. Perform neurovascular checks to monitor peripheral perfusion; compare affected and normal limbs (see p. 255 for neurovascular checks).

## Evaluation

The patient:

- experienced pain relief with treatments and analgesics.
- regained normal peripheral perfusion without edema or tenderness.

## NURSING DIAGNOSIS

### *KNOWLEDGE DEFICIT RELATED TO OSTEOMYELITIS, ITS TREATMENTS, AND PROGNOSIS*

## Assessment

1. Assess patient's understanding of infectious process.
2. Assess patient's understanding of treatment plan and options.

## Expected Outcomes

The patient will:

- develop understanding of the nature of osteomyelitis.
- develop understanding of the treatments and prognosis of his/her osteomyelitis.
- comply with proposed treatment regime.

## Nursing Interventions

1.  Explain osteomyelitis, its causes, diagnostic tests, and treatments; use pictures or diagrams as appropriate.
2.  Explain the treatment time frame and progression of treatments over time.
3.  Explain the expected and side effects of antibiotics.
4.  Explain aseptic technique and its purposes.
5.  Explain proposed surgical care (saucerization, insertion of irrigating tubes, or placement of bone grafts).
6.  Explain symptoms the patient should report to physician following discharge: recurrence of pain, soreness, edema, and fever.

## Evaluation

The patient:

*   could explain osteomyelitis in his/her situation.
*   verbalized acceptance of treatment regimen and purposes of each treatment.
*   complied with each treatment protocol until completed.
*   verbalized methods to prevent recurrence and symptoms to report to physician.

## WOUND INFECTIONS

Superficial or deep wound infections are complications which may or may not be related to the orthopaedic patient's injuries or overall condition. They may be secondary to the treatments, e.g., surgical incision and/or joint replacements, for the primary condition. Wound infections may also result from a nosocomial infection acquired in the health care facility.

*Superficial wound infections* include abscesses, cellulitis, and carbuncles. This type of infection (superficial) is a localized infection. An *abscess* is a localized collection of purulent material which may be on the exterior of the skin, such as in a surgical wound, or may develop internally in visceral tissues, such as a brain, lung, or subdiaphragmatic abscess. A *carbuncle* is a localized abscess around a hair follicle or sweat gland, usually caused by staphylococci. *Cellulitis* is inflammation of the epidermal interstitial cells around an open area. The inflamed tissues may then become infected, such as in gas gangrene.

Treatments for superficial wound infections include application of warm soaks or compresses, incision, and drainage of the purulent material, irrigation and packing of the wound to permit second-degree healing, and administration of oral antibiotics at times.

Deep wound infections are very severe complications for orthopaedic patients as they may extend into the joint and its bones and other structures. Deep infections may result from the surgical exposure or from another undiagnosed infection, such as urinary tract infection, abscessed tooth, or pneumonia. Persons with diabetes, arteriosclerosis, and compromised immune systems are especially susceptible to deep infections.

Signs or symptoms of deep infections include pain in the affected area with or without pain referred to another distant area, elevated temperatures locally and systemically, drainage from the wound which may be serous or purulent, elevated WBC counts, cultures revealing the pathogens, and altered cerebral functions, if a brain infection is present. If the deep infection involves a joint, the patient would complain of pain on use or weight bearing, if allowed, and the wound may dehisce. Diagnosis of a deep infection may be made with a sinogram, which involves injection of a radiopaque solution into the involved area followed by x-rays to show the presence of purulent material at the site.

Treatments for deep infections are more intense and prolonged than for superficial infections. Antibiotic administration, frequently a cephalosporin-type of antibiotic, will be intravenous initially, followed by oral antibiotics for 6–9 months or longer, if a joint infection. Internal fixation devices, such as nails, prostheses, and rods are usually removed, since they are foreign bodies that resist antibiotics. Prostheses may be replaced into the joint after all infection is cleared.

## BIBLIOGRAPHY

Crenshaw, A.H., (Ed.). (1987). *Campbell's operative orthopaedics.* St. Louis: Mosby-Yearbook.

Epps, C.H., (Ed.). (1986). *Complications in orthopaedic surgery,* (2nd ed.). Philadelphia: Lippincott.

Esterhai, J.L., Pisarello, J., Brighton, C. T., Heppenstall, R. B., Gelman, H., & Goldstein, G. (1988). Treatment of chronic refractory osteomyelitis with adjunctive hyperbaric oxygen. *Orthop Rev, 17*(8), 809–815.

Gentry, L.O. (1987). Overview of osteomyelitis. *Orthop Rev, 16*(4), 91–106.

Green, N.E., & Edwards, K. (1987). Bone and joint infections in children. *Orthop Clin North Am.,* 18:1–22.

Hoare, K., & Donahue, K.M. (1990). Alterations in musculoskeletal function. In McCance, K.L. & Heuther, S.E. *Pathophysiology.* St. Louis: Mosby-Yearbook.

Mader, J.T., Hicks, C.A., & Calhoun, J. (1989). Bacterial osteomyelitis adjunctive hyperbaric oxygen therapy. *Orthop Rev, 18*(5), 581–585.

McGuire, M.H. (1989). The pathogenesis of adult osteomyelitis. *Orthop Rev, 18*(5), 564–570.

Perry, C.R., Pearson, R.L., Davenport, K., & Kippler, L. (1988). Local antibiotic treatment of orthopaedic infections. *Surg Rds for Orthop, 2*(4), 32–42.

Totty, W.G. (1989). Radiographic evaluation of osteomyelitis using magnetic resonance imaging. *Orthop Rev, 18*(5), 587–590.

Zaroukian, M.J., & Pera, A. (1988). Diagnosing osteomyelitis. *Surg Rds for Orthop, 2*(11), 17–26.

Zinberg, E.M. (1989). Free-muscle transfer for chronic osteomyelitis. *Surg Rds for Orthop, 3*(3), 26–32.

# 9

# NURSING PROCESS FOR PATIENTS WITH METABOLIC BONE DISEASES

Metabolic bone diseases are those that are related to inadequate bone synthesis or accelerated bone loss. In order for bones to maintain their structural integrity, large numbers of new cells must be continuously available. Cells responsible for bone formation are called osteoblasts and those responsible for bone resorption are called osteoclasts. The regulation and/or proliferation of these cell types comes under local and systemic factors in the body. Some of those factors include calcium levels, phosphates, alkaline phosphatase, and collagen matrixes.

Osteoblasts are responsible for bone mineralization and synthesize the bone matrix with the enzymatic help of alkaline phosphatase. Bones become mineralized and strong as calcium is incorporated into the matrix with growth. Osteoblasts become osteocytes as they are surrounded by bone matrix and the number of osteocytes is relatively constant for any given bone during bone forming growth cycles. Approximately 5% to 10% of existing bone is replaced every year (Tam, 1989), differing from bone to bone.

Osteoclasts resorb bone through an attachment zone called a clear zone or a sealing zone. Bone mineral is resorbed in this resorption zone area through acidification processes (Tam, 1989). Therefore, the total of mineralized, fully developed bone is kept relatively constant through the actions of bone-forming osteoblasts and bone resorbing osteoclasts, so that bones do not become over-mineralized or under-mineralized over an individual's lifetime. However, metabolic bone conditions or diseases can disrupt these normal balances.

## PAGET'S DISEASE OF BONE

Paget's disease is a skeletal disorder in which there is a marked focal over-growth (proliferation) of the normal cellular components of bone. The bones involved vary from patient to patient but bones that are often affected include the bones of the jaws and skull, tibia, and fibula.

The cause of Paget's disease remains undetermined, although virus particles of the paramyxoviridae family have been found in many patients. No other etiologic agents have been described to date.

The incidence of Paget's disease is difficult to determine with certainty as many patients are diagnosed when seeking treatments for other conditions. The incidence in the adult population over 40 years of age, from autopsy data, may be 3% to 4% of individuals in countries with the highest incidence, namely England, Australia, New Zealand, and the United States.

## Pathophysiology

Paget's disease develops due to increased osteoclastic activity resulting in patchy, lytic areas in the affected bones, which initially may be bones of the skull. The osteolytic processes may involve the lower-extremity long bones, with appearance of osteosclerotic lesions noted on x-ray. The osteosclerotic phase may be the response of osteoblasts to the increased resorption of bones from the actions of the osteoclasts.

The disease causes few symptoms early in the condition. The most common complaints in symptomatic patients include pain in bone(s) and deformity of involved bones. The pain may range from mild to severe, from intermittent to persistent. Persistent pain may be associated with nerve impingement and/or degenerative arthritis. Bone deformities range from enlargement, most noticeable in the skull, facial bones, clavicles, and extremities, to bowing of the tibia and fibula. A common symptom is an increase in skin temperature over the affected bone.

Diagnosis of Paget's disease is often made from the roentgenographic evidence, with the osteolytic and/or osteosclerotic lesions noted. Diagnosis may also be made related to the marked enlargement of the skull and facial bones.

Treatments include administration of calcitonin over several months to decrease the action of osteoclasts.

At times patients with Paget's disease develop pathological fractures related to the osteolytic bones, and the appearance of malignant osteogenic sarcoma, which occurs in about 1% of persons with Paget's disease. Degenerative arthritis is the most common complication of this disease.

The nursing care of persons with Paget's disease is given with osteomalacia, p. 235.

## OSTEOMALACIA

Osteomalacia is a disease of adults in which bones lose their mineralization after growth has been completed. Osteomalacia is the adult form of rickets. It is caused by deficiencies of calcium, phosphorus, or both, or inadequate vitamin D intake. These inadequacies result in loss of mineralization of bones when replacement is required because of normal catabolic functions. The balance of bone growth and resorption is disrupted.

Symptoms of osteomalacia include softening and deformation of skeletal bones due to the failure of mineralization and the bones' lack of rigidity. Pathological fractures are common. Marked deformities of bones of the lower extremities affect their ability to bear normal weights, and deformities progress. If deficiencies in needed minerals and vitamin D become severe, the spinal column develops curvatures and the pelvic bones flatten, causing severe, incapacitating pain.

Diagnosis of osteomalacia is made from the patient's history, physical examination, x-rays, and serological studies.

Treatments involve administration of calcium, phosphorus, and vitamin D. Monitoring utilization of replacements is also done. Exposure to sunlight is necessary for the metabolism of vitamin D in the body. Over time, with proper intake and utilization of the minerals and vitamin D, osteomalacia should become reversed.

The nursing care process for osteomalacia is given on p. 235.

## OSTEOPOROSIS

Osteoporosis is a systemic reduction in the density and mass of bones which occurs when the balance of bone formation and resorption is disturbed. It is mistakenly called the "thin bone disease," but patients with osteoporosis do not have thinner bones; their bones are just smaller than they should be. As a result, the bones are unable to bear normal body weights, become deformed, and can fracture more easily.

### Pathophysiology

Bone resorption is under the control of osteoclasts, parathyroid hormone, and steroid hormones, such as estrogens and androgens. Hormones also affect the action of osteoblasts to slow bone formation. As people age, less estrogens and androgens are produced, leading to increased bone resorption and less bone mass (see Table 9.1). The bone mass that remains is fully mineralized; there is just less of total bone mass. Less total bone mass (less bone density) increases the risk of bone fractures.

Women over age 50 (at menopausal age) develop osteoporosis twice as rapidly as males, who develop it at much later ages and in much smaller numbers—only about 2% of males over 50 have measurable osteoporosis, whereas 30% of women over 50 do. Postmenopausal acceleration of loss in women produces a reduction in total skeletal mass amounting to 20% to 30% over a 20-year period (Avioli, 1987).

**Table 9.1** Substances That Regulate Bone Formation and Resorption

### Regulators of Bone Formation

| | | |
|---|---|---|
| A. | Hormones | |
| | Parathyroid hormone (PTH) | |
| | Calcitonin | Steroids |
| | Prostaglandins | Thyroid |
| | Glucagon | Estrogens |
| | Epinephrine | Androgens |
| | Norepinephrine | 1, 25–Dehydroxy–vitamin D |
| | Insulin | Somatostatin |
| | Calcium, phosphate, and fluoride ions | |
| B. | Bone Growth Factors | |
| | Epidermal growth factor (EGF) | |
| | Fibroblast growth factor (FGF) | |
| | Platelet derived growth factor (PDGF) | |
| | Transforming growth factor (TGF) | |
| | Insulin-like growth factor (IGF) | |
| | Exercise | |

### Regulators of Bone Resorption

| | |
|---|---|
| A. | Prostaglandin $E_2$ |
| | Vitamin A |
| | Vitamin D metabolites |
| | Lymphokines |
| | Interleukin I |
| B. | Bone Resorbing Factors |
| | Osteoclast activating factors |
| | Colony-stimulating factors |
| | Tumor necrosis factor |
| | Osteocalcin |
| | Osteonectin |
| | Bone morphogenetic protein |

Osteoporosis related to disuse and immobility, may also develop in younger persons especially in paraplegics or quadriplegics whose demineralization is related to lack of muscle activity and calcium loss from bones.

Fractures of the distal radius, hip (femoral neck), vertebral body (crush or compression fracture) become increased risks with increasing age. Minor trauma such as a twist or unexpected turn can result in a fracture in older women. Arthritis, Parkinson's disease, fainting, or transient ischemic attacks can also lead to falls and fractures.

Symptoms of osteoporosis may be subtle and varied until the condition becomes pronounced. One of the most noticeable symptoms is acute back pain related to vertebral compression or wedging with resultant nerve compression. Physical symptoms also include increased kyphosis and mild respiratory compromise. A fracture in the distal radius or proximal femur may also be a signal of osteoporosis, as may be loss of height associated with kyphosis.

Diagnosis is made from the patient's health history and menstrual status, if a woman, physical examination with noticeable kyphosis, serologic studies showing elevated calcium levels, and low levels of alkaline phosphatase. Radiologic studies including single- or dual-photon absorptiometry and quantitative computed tomography also show relative amounts of bone mass and can show some compression fractures of vertebrae.

Treatments include diets high in protein and calories to aid bone formation and boost daily dietary intake of vitamin D and calcium to maintain normal blood levels of calcium. Intake of a combined estrogen-progestin tablet (estrogen, 0.625 mg/day for 25 days, with medroxyprogesterone, 10 mg for last 10 days of cycle). Because of the increased risk of endometrial and breast cancer and cardiovascular complications, some patients opt not to take the hormonal replacements. Some patients are now being treated with etidronate (Didronel), which has been shown to strengthen bones and help prevent fractures.

Moderate exercise programs such as walking, swimming, and bicycle riding have been stressed to increase retention of calcium in bones.

## NURSING PROCESS

## NURSING DIAGNOSIS

### *IMPAIRED PHYSICAL MOBILITY RELATED TO WEAKENED BONES FROM PAGET'S DISEASE, OSTEOMALACIA, OR OSTEOPOROSIS*

Assessment

1. Assess gait, mobility, posture, and strength.
2. Assess for kyphosis, deformed bones, misshapen or excess bone structures (Paget's disease).
3. Assess for presence, degree, and amount of pain when ambulating, standing, or sitting.

## Expected Outcomes

The patient will:

- have increased or adequate physical mobility.
- have increased bone strength and mass following treatments.
- have fewer pain episodes following treatments.
- have reduced risk of bone fractures.

## Nursing Interventions

1. Assist patient to change positions as needed.
2. As needed or ordered, teach patient use of a cane or crutches to increase stability when ambulating.
3. Assist patient with ROM exercises to maintain muscle strength.
4. Monitor physical therapy program and benefits as needed.

## Evaluation

The patient had:

- satisfactory mobility over time and with treatments.
- increased bone strength and mass following treatments (medications) and diet.
- had less pain following medications and diet replacements.
- had lessened risk of bone fractures after treatments.

## NURSING DIAGNOSIS

*POTENTIAL FOR INJURY (RISK OF FRACTURE) RELATED TO WEAKENED BONES, LESS BONE MASS, AND DEFORMED MASS*

## Assessment

1. Assess shape of bones throughout body.
2. Assess posture and position of feet, legs, and arms when ambulating.
3. Assess patient's concerns or fears about possible fractures.

## Expected Outcomes

The patient will:

- have reduced risk of fractures following treatments.
- have more normally-shaped bones and improved posture following treatments.

## Nursing Interventions

1. Instruct patient to maintain a safe home environment, e.g., no long, uncovered, or loose cords or small, loose rugs; instruct patient how to rise and sit.
2. Administer ordered diet; instruct patient on high-calcium foods (see Table 9.2) and increased intake of vitamin D and their effects in the body.
3. Administer ordered medications promptly; discuss expected and side effects of medications.
4. Discuss physical therapy program or exercises to increase calcium retention.
5. Discuss purposes of estrogen-progestin regimen and expected or side effects and risks associated with this regimen (see p. 235).
6. For Paget's disease, administer calcitonin as ordered; discuss expected and side effects.
7. Discuss symptoms, such as increased pain and inability to bear weight, if present, to report to physician.

## Evaluation

The patient had:

- less risk of fracture following exercises and treatments.
- more normally-shaped bones and straighter posture following treatments.

**Table 9.2** Calcium Content of Selected Foods

| Food | Serving Size | Calcium (mg) |
| --- | --- | --- |
| Milk, 2% | 1 cup | 297 |
| Milk, skim | 1 cup | 296 |
| Milk, nonfat, dry | 1 tbsp | 52 |
| Yogurt, low fat, plain | 1 cup | 400 |
| Cheese, cottage | 1/2 cup | 90 |
| Cheese, cheddar | 1 oz | 213 |
| Cheese, Swiss | 1 oz | 262 |
| Ice cream | 1/2 cup | 97 |

(continued)

**Table 9.2** (Continued)

| Food | Serving Size | Calcium (mg) |
|------|------------|-------------|
| Ice milk | 1/2 cup | 102 |
| Broccoli | 1 stalk | 158 |
| Salmon, canned with bones | 3 oz | 167 |
| Spinach, cooked | 1 cup | 167 |
| Tofu, bean curd | 3 1/2 oz | 128 |
| Beans, red kidney | 1 cup | 74 |
| Beans, navy, cooked | 1 cup | 95 |
| Muffin, bran | 1 muffin | 57 |
| Shrimp, canned | 3 oz | 100 |
| Molasses, blackstrap | 1 tbsp | 135 |
| Milk chocolate bar | 1 oz | 65 |
| Collard greens, cooked | 1 cup | 289 |
| Farina, cooked | 1 cup | 147 |

## NURSING DIAGNOSIS

### PAIN RELATED TO ABNORMAL BONE GROWTH AND SHAPE, NERVE IMPINGEMENT, OR DEGENERATIVE ARTHRITIS

#### Assessment

1. Assess site(s) of pain.
2. Assess characteristics, duration, and severity of pain.
3. Assess associated symptoms such as numbness and inability to bear weight.

#### Expected Outcomes

The patient will:

* experience relief of pain with medications.
* have no progression of bone abnormalities.

#### Nursing Interventions

1. Assist patient to position of comfort; encourage patient to change position q 2–3 hours.
2. Administer analgesics as ordered; monitor results of medications.

3. Apply back support if ordered; teach patient how to apply back support.
4. Massage neck and back to relax sore or aching muscles.
5. Monitor effects of use of ambulatory aid (cane or crutches).
6. Monitor effects of physical therapy.

## Evaluation

The patient had:
* satisfactory pain relief with analgesic administrations.
* no increases in bone abnormalities following treatments.

## GOUT

Gout is a hereditary disease in which overproduction or decreased excretion of uric acid and urate salts leads to high levels of uric acid in the blood. Gout is caused by a lack of the enzyme needed to completely metabolize purines for renal excretion. It is the incomplete metabolism that causes the uric acid buildup. Uric acid is a breakdown product of purines.

## Pathophysiology

Urate salts that are not excreted by the kidneys build up in body tissues because of high blood levels. Tissues of the ears, kidneys, and joints are most commonly affected by these deposits. Such deposits are called tophi. Urate crystals are very sharp, pointed substances which cause irritation and inflammation in the joints where they are deposited. One joint that is frequently affected is the first metatarsal joint of the great toe, where the urate crystals can cause severe, excruciating pain. Other commonly affected joints are the wrists and the metacarpal joints. Affected joints become inflamed, hot, deformed, edematous, and very painful.

Men are more afflicted with gout than women, and children are rarely affected. Secondary gout can develop from increased cell destruction or breakdown from drug therapies for malignant diseases such as leukemia.

Symptoms of gout include sudden, excruciating pain episodes, deformed, inflamed joints, and deposits of tophi in various tissues. Only during acute attacks is the body temperature elevated, and blood pressure can become elevated during an acute episode.

Diagnosis is made from the patient's history, presence of visible tophi, and hot, inflamed, deformed joints. Serum uric acid levels are elevated above normal (normal: men, 3.9–7.8 mg/dl; women, 2.5–6.8 mg/dl). Radiologic studies show cystlike, punched-out areas under cartilage layers. Aspiration of joint fluid reveals the characteristic urate crystals.

Treatments for acute attacks include the administration of colchicine (colsalide), 1 mg po followed by 0.5 mg tablet every hour until diarrhea occurs or the pain is relieved (dosage is limited to 8 mg during an acute attack). Acute attacks can be prevented by administration of probenecid (Benemid) or allopurinol (Zyloprim) given daily in individualized doses, and intake of a low-purine diet (see Table 9.3). Joint pain can be relieved by mild analgesics such as aspirin every 4 hours except during acute attacks. Ice bag application over an inflamed joint may help ease inflammation during an acute attack, as does bed rest or nonweight bearing on affected joints.

**Table 9.3** Purine Content of Foods

| High (150–1,000 mg/100 g) | Moderate (50–150 mg/100 g) | Negligible |
|---|---|---|
| Herring | Chicken | Vegetable soups |
| Sardines | Crab | Butter |
| Mussels | Salmon | Refined cereals |
| Liver | Veal | Eggs |
| Sweetbreads | Mutton | Fruits |
| Kidney | Bacon | Vegetables |
| Venison | Pork | Cheese |
| Goose | Beef | Milk |
| Meat soups | Ham | Sugar |
| Anchovies | Lentils | |
| Brains | Whole-grain cereals | |
| Heart | Beans | |
| | Spinach | |
| | Asparagus | |
| | Cauliflower | |

## NURSING PROCESS

## NURSING DIAGNOSIS

### PAIN (ACUTE, SEVERE) RELATED TO JOINT INFLAMMATION AND URATE DEPOSITS

#### Assessment

1. Assess joint(s) for signs of inflammation: reddened, hot, edematous, painful, deformed joint(s) with evidence of tophi.
2. Assess ear cartilage for presence of tophi.
3. Assess for history of gout in other family members.
4. Assess for systemic symptoms such as nausea, headache, and fever.

## Expected Outcomes

The patient will:

- have relief of pain with medications and treatments.
- have relief of joint inflammation.
- have few acute episodes of pain with daily medications.
- regain physical mobility once pain is relieved.

## Nursing Interventions

1. Assess characteristics of patient's pain, its duration, and sites and systemic symptoms.
2. Position patient as comfortably as possible with affected joint(s) elevated on pillow.
3. Apply ice bag to site(s) to lessen inflammation.
4. Administer ordered medication; usually colchicine 0.5 to 1 mg/hr until patient has relief of pain or diarrhea—may give up to 8 mg total dose. This drug helps excretion of urates.
5. Administer nonnarcotic analgesic such as aspirin for headache and joint pain.
6. Prepare patient for long-term medication with antigout medication when ordered.
7. Assist to use ambulatory aid such as cane or crutch during acute attack of pain if weight bearing is permitted.

## Evaluation

The patient:

- experienced relief of acute pain with medication.
- had lessened joint inflammation over time and with long-term medications.
- had fewer acute episodes with long-term medications.
- regained physical mobility when pain relieved.

## NURSING DIAGNOSIS

### ALTERED NUTRITION RELATED TO INCOMPLETE PURINE METABOLISM

## Assessment

1. Assess for intake of high-purine foods as listed in Table 9.3.
2. Assess for food likes and dislikes.

## Expected Outcomes

The patient will:

- reduce or eliminate intake of high-purine foods.
- have dietary intake of nutritional foods.

## Nursing Interventions

1. Assess intake of foods with or without purines and for food likes and dislikes.
2. Seek consultation with the dietitian for foods low in purine.
3. Teach patient about purine restrictions and proper nutritional guidelines.
4. Monitor patient's selection from menus.

## Evaluation

The patient:

- chose low-purine foods from menus.
- chose nutritional foods according to suggested guidelines.

## BIBLIOGRAPHY

Avioli, L.V. (Ed.) (1987). *The osteoporotic syndrome.* Orlando, FL: Grune & Stratton.

Beltran, J. (1990). *MRI musculoskeletal system.* Philadelphia: Lippincott.

Berg, E., & Moyle, D.D. (1988). Osteoporosis: An overview of causes, prevention, and therapy. *Journal of Musculoskeletal Medicine, 5*(1), 64–81.

Betts, K. (1988). Women should know risks of taking estrogen for osteoporosis. *Oncology Times, 10*(9), 7,27.

Gulanick, M., Klopp, A, & Galanes, S. (Eds.) (1986). *Nursing care plans, nursing diagnosis, and intervention.* St. Louis: Mosby-Yearbook.

Lane, J.M. Healey, J., Bansal, M., & Levine, B. (1988). Overview of geriatric osteopenic syndromes. II. Clinical presentation, diagnosis, and treatment. *Orthopaedic Review, 17*(2), 1231–1236.

Licata, A.O. (1988). Some thoughts on osteoporosis in women. *Cleveland Clinic Journal of Medicine, 55*(3), 233–238.

McCance, K.L., & Huether, S.E. (1990). *Pathophysiology.* St. Louis: Mosby-Yearbook.

Niewoehner, C.B. (1989). Prevention of osteoporosis. *Journal of Musculoskeletal Medicine, 6*(5), 57–66.

Simmons, J.V., & Norwood, S.M. (1987). Calcitonin and osteoporosis: New mechanisms of pathophysiology. *Orthopaedic Review, 16*(10), 26–32.

Stewart, E.L. (1988). Calcium intake and osteoporosis. *Your Patient and Fitness, 1*(2), 12–14.

Stulberg, B.N., & Watson, J.T. Management of orthopedic complications of metabolic bone disease. *Cleveland Clinic Journal of Medicine, 56*(7), 696–703.

Tam, C.S., Heersche, J.N.M., & Murray, T.M. (1989). *Metabolic bone disease: Cellular and tissue mechanisms.* Boca Raton, FL: CRC Press.

Woolf, A.D., & Dixon, A.S.J. (1988). *Osteoporosis: A clinical guide.* Philadelphia: Lippincott.

# 10

# NURSING CARE OF PERSONS IN CASTS

The focus of this chapter is on the factor of *immobility* as one requirement to permit the bridging, consolidation, and mineralization at the fracture site to become sufficiently strong for gradual resumption of use. The use of casts to maintain relative immobility of the fractured fragments is the topic of this chapter.

A cast is one of the major methods of providing the necessary immobility for the time needed for bone union. Other methods are one or another type of traction, external fixation, or surgical intervention and internal fixation. The cast has many advantages over the other methods: it is relatively easy to apply, requires minimal care, encases the tissues after it dries, doesn't require hospitalization, and the patient can be active, mobile, and engaged in many of life's usual activities while the fractured bones are immobilized. In addition, a cast is less expensive than the other methods of immobilization.

Decisions about the use of a cast for the treatment of a particular fracture involve both the physician and patient. Discussions of the injury, preparation for casting, and postcast care permit the patient to participate as actively as desired in goal-setting. Cost factors may or may not be included in the discussion with the patient and family members before application. Nursing personnel can be included in these discussions as active participants in preparing the patient, and then can follow through in assisting during the application of the cast and in carrying out the postcast care.

A cast is an externally applied structure made of gypsum (plaster of paris), fiberglass, plastic, or varieties of cast tapes. A cast may be applied to aid healing of an injury or fractured bone while holding the tissues in specific anatomical positions, or to assist with realigning malpositioned structures and tissues, such as club foot, congenital hip dislocation, or dysplasia. The firmness of the cast helps overcome rotational forces, muscle tension, or muscle tone for the time required by the particular condition to regain alignment, bony union, or joint stability. Once it dries, the cast will hold the tissues as they are placed inside the cast; therefore, it must be applied carefully and properly.

A cast can be applied to a leg or forearm, referred to as a *short leg* or *short arm* cast; to the entire lower or upper extremity, referred to as *long leg* or *hanging cast,* respectively; to the body, encircling the thorax and pelvis, referred to as a *body cast;* to the chest, neck, and head with openings for the arms, ears, and face, referred to as a *minerva jacket;* and to the pelvis and one or both legs, referred to as a *hip spica* or *spica* cast.

## Procedures

### APPLICATION OF A CAST

#### Materials Needed

Materials are usually arranged on shelves or portable carts for easy accessibility (Figs. 10.1, 10.2, 10.3, and 10.4), and include:

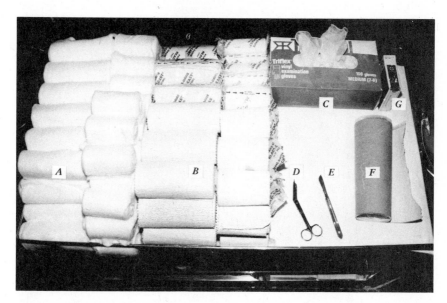

**Figure 10.1** Cart containing supplies for application of a plaster cast: (a) sheet wadding in two sizes; (b) plaster rolls in three sizes; (c) gloves; (d) scissors to cut sheet wadding and plaster; (e) scalpel to trim plaster; (f) felt for padding; (g) pail, only partially visible, for water to wet plaster rolls.

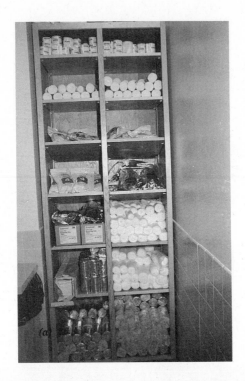

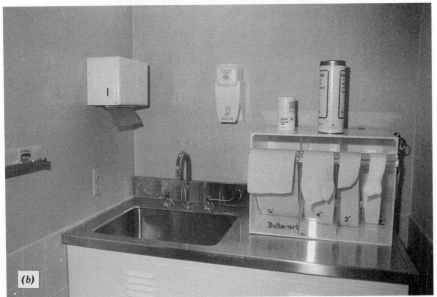

**Figure 10.2** (a) Shelves and (b) accessory supplies and sink used for cast materials and cast applications.

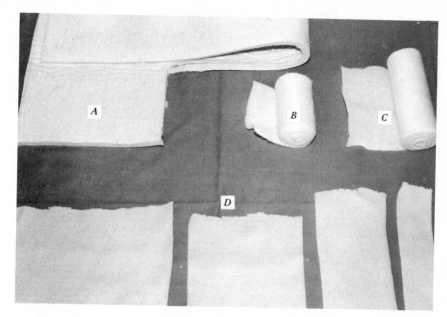

**Figure 10.3** Types of padding under plaster of casts: (a) felt that can be cut to size; (b, c) sheet wadding; (d) various sizes of stockinette.

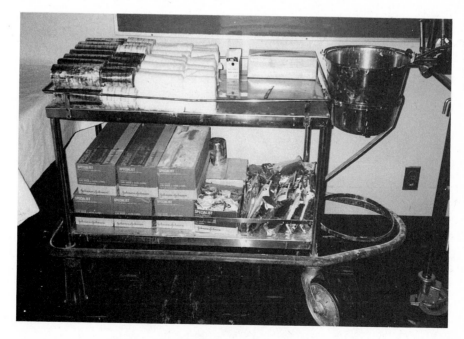

**Figure 10.4** Portable cart for cast application.

- Plaster rolls—rolls of 2, 3, 4, and 6 inches, or
- Fiberglass rolls of 3, 4, or 6 inches
- Padding—felt in several widths and thicknesses, stockinette, sheet wadding, webril, or spandex rolls
- Plastic-lined pail
- Gloves and apron
- Scissors
- Floor covering, such as paper or plastic
- Cast cutter (if old cast is to be removed)
- Water (warm to hot) to aid setting of plaster or fiberglass
- Fracture table, cart, or comfortable chair for patient

## Responsibilities of the Physician Before Application of a Cast

- Examines the patient and orders radiologic and other studies.
- Discusses purposes and advantages of treating the patient's injury with a cast.
- Explains the type and size of cast to be applied.
- Explains how cast will be applied.
- Orders medications required, such as muscle relaxants and analgesics.
- Secures the signed informed consent

## Responsibilities of Nursing Personnel Before Application of a Cast

- Clarifies procedure to decrease patient's anxiety. If the patient is a child, uses language, toys, or games appropriate to the age of the child. The nurse also may incorporate or use suggestions from the parents to calm the child.
- Checks the skin for open areas, lesions, rash, edema, and deformity. Skin cleansing must be done gently and carefully to prevent additional trauma. Surgical wounds should be closed and covered with sterile dressings to prevent infection.
- Assesses patient's vital signs.
- Administers muscle relaxant or analgesic medications as ordered.
- Gathers materials for the cast application.
- Positions the patient comfortably and properly for the cast application.

## Responsibilities of the Physician During Application of a Cast

- Performs a reduction of the fracture site.
- Covers the skin surfaces with pieces of felt, stockinette, sheet wadding or other covering to protect the skin.

- Puts on gloves to protect hands from plaster or fiberglass. Fiberglass "slivers" can irritate the skin.

- Applies the dampened plaster or fiberglass rolls smoothly and evenly to the desired areas. The material is smoothed to fit the contour of the skin surfaces. Tucks may be taken in the rolls to make a smooth cast surface, and each turn of the roll overlaps the preceding one by approximately one-half its width so that no two turns directly overlap, which could cause undue pressure in that area. Joint areas are covered while in moderate or full flexion by using partially overlapping figure-of-eight turns. If additional strength is needed for support around joints, longitudinal strips of wet plaster or fiberglass are incorporated into the cast in those areas.

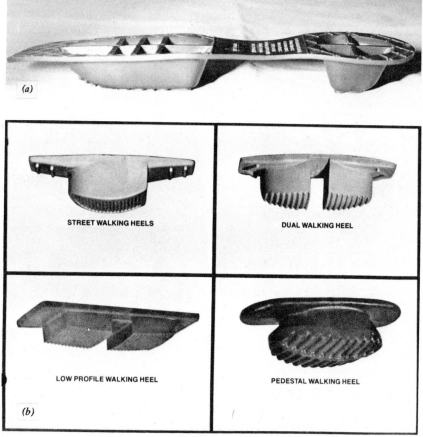

*(a)*

STREET WALKING HEELS

DUAL WALKING HEEL

LOW PROFILE WALKING HEEL

PEDESTAL WALKING HEEL

*(b)*

**Figure 10.5** Types of walking heels for casts.

- Completes the cast by placing a walking heel in the sole area of a leg cast if weight bearing will be permitted (see Fig. 10.5); "finishes" the cast by turning down the ends of the lining material over the plaster or fiberglass, then covering the turned-down edges with another turn of the cast material to create a smooth edge against the skin and secures the end of the lining material (see Figs. 10.6, 10.7, and 10.8).

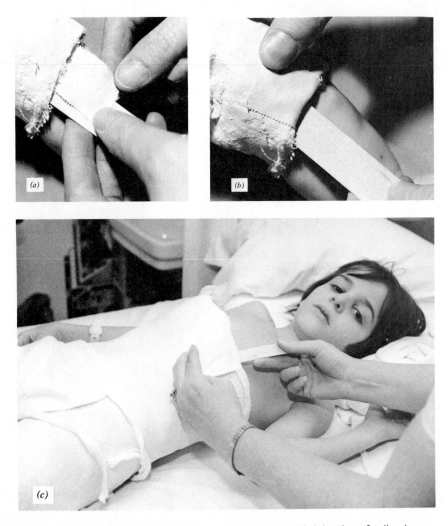

**Figure 10.6** Petaling a cast after it is dry and trimmed: (a) strips of adhesive are placed under the edge of the cast and (b, c) are held in place with a tongue blade while the upper edge is folded over the edge of the cast. After the edges are covered, the outer edges of the adhesive are covered with an encircling strip of adhesive to keep the adhesive strips in place.

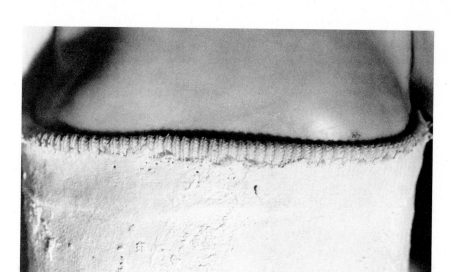

**Figure 10.7** Petaling done at time of application of plaster. The stockinette is folded back over the edges of plaster, and the edge is covered with plaster. This type of petaling can be done if the cast needs no trimming.

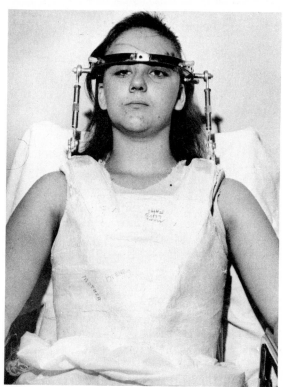

**Figure 10.8** Halo traction with vertical braces stabilized in the plaster cast. The traction and cast hold the cervical vertebrae immobile following a fracture.

- A special cream may be used to smooth and fill the rough edges of the fiberglass. The cast is full strength in 3–5 minutes.
- If the cast is applied with cast tape, it is applied similarly to plaster. The cast tape adheres to the previous turn and is stable in approximately 15 minutes.
- If the physician applies a cast with fiberglass materials, he or she will wear gloves and a gown for protection; the fiberglass is irritating to the skin and hard on clothing.
- The fiberglass material is dampened or warmed according to the manufacturer's directions, applied to the areas desired, and then covered with dampened elastic bandages to help mold the fiberglass over the skin surfaces, or a special cream may be used to smooth and fill the rough edges of the fiberglass. The fiberglass cast is set or cured in 3–5 minutes and, if used, the elastic bandages are then removed.

## Responsibilities of Nursing Personnel During Application of a Cast

- Holds the affected tissues in the desired position.
- Offers support and comfort to the patient as needed.
- Wets the plaster rolls and removes excess water from the roll by squeezing gently.
- Supplies the dampened rolls to the physician continuously to facilitate the application of the cast.
- Assists the physician with the cast finishing or trimming as needed.
- Stays with the patient during the time for initial plaster, cast tape, or fiberglass curing.
- Assists with moving the patient to the hospital room or prepares the patient for discharge.

## Nursing Responsibilities in the Immediate Postcast Period

- Applies ice bags to lessen bleeding into the injured tissues in the cast.
- Positions the patient and the damp cast on a firm, smooth surface. Places pillows without plastic covers under joints to maintain the proper degree of flexion without strain, being sure to handle the cast with the palms of the hands to prevent pressure areas in the cast from fingertips and lifting the cast at two joints to prevent undue stress at the injury site.
- Explains the warmth felt by the patient as the plaster sets and dries. The warmth is due to the chemical reaction of the calcium sulfate (gypsum) and the water of hydration which causes the cast to feel hot, even though damp. A plaster cast is considered "unset" for at least an hour, during which it should be carefully handled to avoid breaking or bending.
- Explains the need to keep the casted areas uncovered to facilitate drying of the plaster. Care should be taken to maintain the patient's modesty and privacy with appropriate drapes and covering.

- Explains that the drying period of large plaster casts may be 48–72 hours or longer, depending on the humidity and temperatures. Drying may be aided by the use of fans (if there is no break in the skin), exposure to sunlight, or low-wattage light bulbs.
- Provides home care instructions to the patient and family if the patient is to be discharged (see p. 276 for home instructions).

## NURSING DIAGNOSIS

### POTENTIAL FOR INJURY RELATED TO THE PRESENCE OF A DAMP CAST

#### Assessment

1. Observe the shape and size of the cast in order to note if cast should become deformed or break before dry (see Fig. 10.9).
2. Assess tissues above and below the cast for edema, temperature, pressure into skin, or rough edges of the cast (see Fig. 10.10).
3. Assess color of tissues above and below cast.
4. Assess person's reaction to the presence of the cast, complaints of pain or discomfort or concerns for self-care.

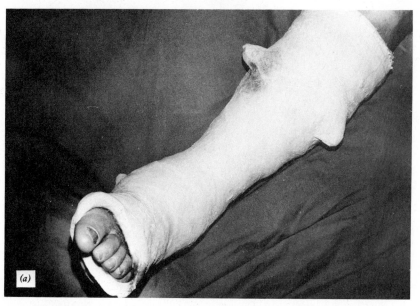

(a)

**Figure 10.9** (a) Short-leg cast incorporating Steinmann pins through the upper tibia and fibula and the calcaneus bone of the heel to immobilize midshaft fractures of the tibia and fibula:

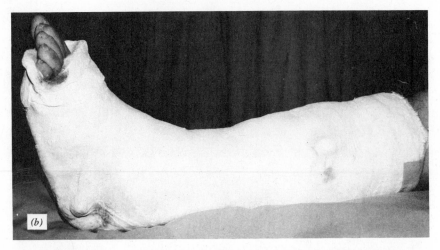

**Figure 10.9** (b) Lateral view of same patient's leg showing drainage.

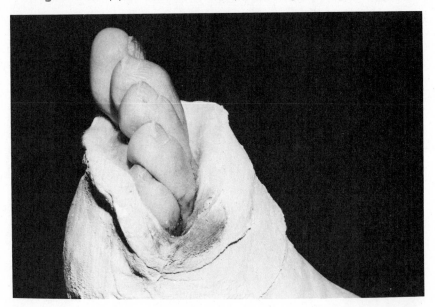

**Figure 10.10** Close-up view of the toe area of the short-leg cast. Note that all toes are visible and can easily be counted. The toes are free of pressure from the cast.

## Expected Outcomes

The patient will:

- maintain proper position while the cast is damp or uncured.
- assist with turning.
- move the fingers or toes of the affected extremity.

- have only minimal to moderate edema.
- have pain relief from medication and repositioning.
- participate in self-care as able.

## Nursing Interventions

1. Explain the positions and turning required or necessary because the cast is damp or uncured.

2. Keep the casted extremity elevated on a pillow or in a sling to aid venous return and to lessen pressure on joints.

3. Support the cast under two joints when turning or repositioning the patient and cast to prevent unsafe pressure on a wet cast or "levering" action of joints on soft tissues around the injury area.

4. Use the palms of the hands, not the fingertips, under the cast when lifting the cast to avoid creating pressure points inside the cast with the fingertips.

5. Keep encased areas uncovered for 24–72 hours, depending on the humidity and thickness of the plaster.

6. Keep fans (if used) from falling or vibrating off stands or tables by using a firmly based fan. A fan should not be used if there is an incision or open wound (even though covered by a dressing), because the fan could cause organisms to be blown under the cast, where they could lead to an infection. Also, use of a hair dryer on low temperature is controversial for the same reason. The temperature of the hair dryer may also cause bleeding and could possibly cause a burn.

7. Keep the room temperature warm enough to aid drying, but not so high that the patient perspires under the cast. Room temperatures of 72–76°F are usually satisfactory.

8. Turn the patient every 3–4 hours to promote even drying of all parts of the cast.

9. Perform neurovascular checks usually ordered for every hour to ascertain local effects of cast on tissues. Neurovascular checks include the following eight checks:

   a. Observe capillary refill by compressing the nail of a finger or toe, release, and count the seconds until the nail turns pink. Normal refill is 2–4 seconds. Report if refill is 6 seconds or longer, as the arterial or capillary circulation is too sluggish.

   b. Observe the color of the encased tissues and compare with like tissues on the opposite side of the body. The encased tissues will appear slightly paler than tissues on the other side.

   c. Feel the temperature of both extremities or like tissues on both sides of the body. The encased tissues will be slightly cooler.

d. Observe for the presence of and amount of edema (see Fig. 10.11). The affected tissues may be slightly to moderately edematous, but the skin should not be tight. If the tissues are severely edematous, venous stasis may be present, or there may be excessive tissue trauma preventing satisfactory venous return. Measure the circumference of the edema-

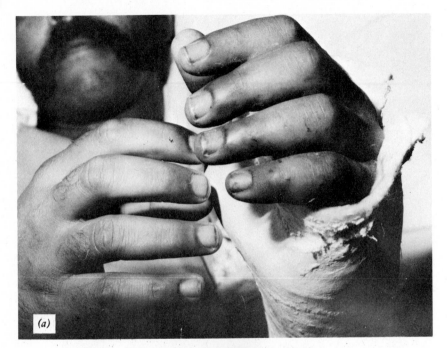

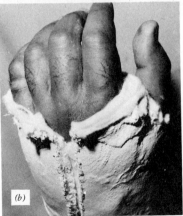

**Figure 10.11** (a) Comparison of "like" tissues during neuro-vascular checks. (b) Cast is being cut because of severe edema of fingers and the patient's complaints of numbness and tingling.

tous area (if the cast is not in the way) and compare with opposite-side tissues for assessment of amount of edema.

e. Ask the patient to describe feelings of the tissues in the cast. Ask if fingers or toes feel numb, tingle, feel like "pins and needles," or feel as if they are asleep. Decreased or altered sensations are indications of nerve pressure and should be reported.

f. Ask the patient to move the fingers or toes (or other tissues) contiguous to the encased tissues. The patient should be able to actively move the parts but may have some soreness or pain with active movement, unless there has been nerve damage.

g. Ask the patient about the amount of pain and changes in function experienced. Pain may be reported as being dull or aching, but the patient should not complain of a sudden increase in the amount or degree of pain, which could signify loss of reduction or hemorrhage into the area. The patient also should not be able to use the part(s) as freely as before the cast and should not be able to bear weight without the support of the cast, and walking aid, if allowed weight bearing.

h. Compare the encased side or tissues with like tissues on the opposite side to note any differences as signs to record and report (see Neurovascular Checks Flow Sheet, Fig. 11.18, p. 301).

10. Keep the lower extremity elevated to heart level. Elevation should not exceed the patient's central venous pressure (see p. 111 for rationale) (see Fig. 10.12).

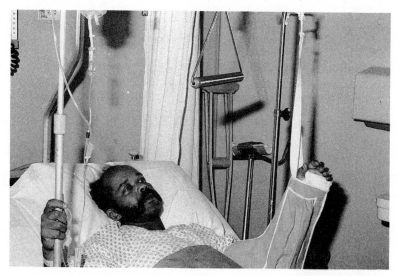

**Figure 10.12** Elevation of the patient's forearm cast by placing the extremity in a sling and elevating by attaching the sling to an intravenous pole. The patient's elbow should be supported with pillows to lessen muscle strain.

11. Apply ice bags to the damp cast to lessen bleeding and edema formation.

12. Record the patient's reactions, comments, and complaints, as well as all results of the neurovascular checks on the patient's chart.

## Evaluation

The patient:

- participated in turning and repositioning during the drying period.
- experienced pain relief over time with medications.
- moved digits actively and had normal neurovascular checks.
- participated in self-care as able.

## NURSING DIAGNOSIS

*IMPAIRED PHYSICAL MOBILITY RELATED TO INJURY AND PRESENCE OF A CAST*

### Assessment

1. Assess the amount of movement or limitations imposed by the injury, size of the cast, or muscles/joints in the cast.

2. Assess the ROM exercises to unaffected muscles.

3. Assess the patient's ambulation, use of an ambulatory aid with weight-bearing restrictions, as ordered.

### Expected Outcomes

The patient will be

- able to perform ROM exercises and muscle-setting exercises actively every 2–3 hours.
- ambulatory with an ambulatory aid as required for weight-bearing restrictions.

### Nursing Interventions

1. Explain the purposes and techniques for ROM exercises and muscle-setting exercises.

2. Assist the patient to turn every 3–4 hours to relieve pressure on tissues and to increase perfusion.

3. Assist the patient with range of motion (ROM) exercises to unaffected tissues.

4. Keep the side rails up when the patient is unattended to avoid accidental loss of balance or falls from the bed due to a large or cumbersome cast.

5. If only an extremity is in the cast and the patient is to be up, assist the patient up in a chair or to ambulate with use of a walker, cane, or crutches if the patient is to limit weight bearing. Apply a sling for an upper extremity with a cast to provide support and comfort.

6. Encourage the patient to perform active quadriceps, triceps, biceps, and gluteus setting exercises to maintain muscle strength and joint function.

## Evaluation

The patient:

- maintained muscle/joint ROM and strength through the planned exercise program.
- ambulated up and down stairs safely with crutches.
- could apply a sling for an upper extremity in a cast.

## NURSING DIAGNOSIS

### POTENTIAL FOR IMPAIRED GAS EXCHANGE RELATED TO A BODY OR SPICA CAST

## Assessment

1. Assess respiratory functions, breathing or chest excursions, rates and depth of respirations, and breath sounds.
2. Assess for presence of cough, production of sputum, and elevated temperature.
3. Assess use of respiratory aid.

## Expected Outcomes

The patient will:

- perform deep breathing and coughing exercises every 2–3 hours.
- use the respiratory aid every 2–3 hours.
- have normal breath sounds in all lobes.
- have normal peripheral perfusion and oxygenation.

## Nursing Interventions

1. Explain the purposes and techniques for doing deep breathing and coughing exercises and using a respiratory aid or incentive spirometer to increase compliance and understanding.

2. Assist the patient to do deep breathing and coughing activities every 1–2 hours to aid in pulmonary ventilation, perfusion, and clearing of respiratory passages.

3. Assist the patient to use a respiratory aid such as the Respirex or Triflow as incentive spirometer if ordered to maintain or increase respiratory depth.

4 Auscultate breath sounds every 4 hours to determine respiratory depth and adequacy.

5. Observe respiratory rates, rhythms, and depth for evidence of adequacy or beginning difficulty with air exchange.

6 Observe overall body color for adequacy of oxygenation. Color should be pink.

7. Assist the patient to change positions to increase perfusion.

## Evaluation

The patient:

- performed pulmonary exercises, coughing, and use of a respiratory aid every 2–3 hours with occasional reminding.

- maintained adequate pulmonary perfusion and oxygenation.

- had normal breath sounds in all lobes.

- had normal peripheral perfusion.

## NURSING DIAGNOSIS

### DEFICIT IN SELF-CARE, HYGIENE, TOILETING, OR GROOMING RELATED TO A LARGE CAST

## Assessment

1. Assess the patient's understanding of self-care needs.
2. Assess ability to do self-care.

## Expected Outcomes

The patient will:

- use assistance with and participate in self-care as permitted by the cast and injury.
- regain independence in hygiene, toileting, and grooming as permitted by the cast and injury.

## Nursing Interventions

1. Explain the modifications or limitations imposed on hygiene, toileting, and grooming to maintain the integrity of the patient's tissues, as well as the integrity of the cast, as, for example, the need to cleanse the tissues outside the cast gently and thoroughly, keep the cast dry and water-free (if plaster), and keep powders or lotions from under the cast if using these aids to maintain skin tissues.
2. Teach use of bedpan and urinal if needed.
3. Assist the patient with the bath or shower and oral hygiene as needed.
4. Assist the patient to maintain personal hygiene by assisting with shaving, nail care, application of makeup, and use of other personal hygiene materials.
5. Assist with hair care and shampooing hair if assistance is needed. Assist to dry the hair to prevent exposure to dampness and cooling.
6. Encourage the patient to use own gown, shirts, or their personal clothing as permitted by the cast and injury.

## Evaluation

The patient:

- bathed and groomed self with minimal assistance.
- kept the cast dry and clean.
- performed toileting activities with assistance.

## NURSING DIAGNOSIS

### ALTERATION IN COMFORT RELATED TO ACUTE PAIN

## Assessment

1. Assess for presence and extent of pain, location and type of pain (burning, stabbing, aching, throbbing, or other [see p. 262 for assessment parameters]).

2.  Assess intensity of the pain—its duration, pattern, and effective relief measures.

3.  Assess patient's understanding of the meaning of pain.

## Expected Outcomes

The patient will:

-   understand the causes for acute pain.

-   have the pain relieved by medication, massage, and positioning.

-   have physical and emotional rest.

## Nursing Interventions

1.  Explain pain mechanisms and the causes and purposes of acute pain to increase the patient's understanding.

2.  Ask the patient to describe the type, location, intensity or severity, and duration of the pain to assure the patient of your concern and interest in the pain experiences.

3.  Ask the patient to explain pain relief measures used, what makes the pain worse, what he/she wants done now to ease the pain.

4.  Offer and administer ordered narcotics/analgesics every 3–4 hours around the clock as needed to conserve energy needed for recovery. Patients in pain dissipate valuable energy trying to find comfortable positions and worrying about achieving pain relief.

5.  Ask the patient if the medication has relieved or controlled the pain. Asking such questions assures the patient that comfort is a mutual patient-nurse goal.

6.  Reposition the patient to rest muscles or relieve pressure and increase tissue oxygenation to ease some pain.

7.  Massage sore or tired muscles to increase circulation and aid removal of wastes and irritants from muscles. Secure an order for a nonnarcotic analgesic or muscle relaxant medication if needed as pain decreases or abates. Pain is lessened when muscles relax and the patient is less tense.

8.  Offer and administer sedatives at bedtime with the narcotic or analgesic to help assure long, restful sleep from the synergistic action of the medications.

9.  Explore the patient's understanding of the meaning of pain to him or her.

## Evaluation

The patient:

- indicates that the pain is tolerable, decreased, or relieved.
- shows evidence of pain relief by assisting with repositioning, resting, and sleeping at night and no moaning, guarding, wincing, or reluctance to move.
- verbalizes understanding of causes of acute pain.

## NURSING DIAGNOSIS

### POTENTIAL FOR ALTERATION IN SKIN INTEGRITY RELATED TO CAST AND DECREASED MOBILITY

## Assessment

1. Assess all skin surfaces outside the cast for evidence of integrity or pressure areas.
2. Assess the cast edges for roughness or tightness.
3. Assess for odors or drainage from inside the cast.

## Expected Outcomes

The patient will:

- retain intact skin surfaces with pink color and no edema, pressure areas, or decubiti.
- have no odors or drainage from skin surfaces.

## Nursing interventions

1. Explain the need for and purposes of making frequent observations of the skin surfaces.
2. Observe the skin surfaces outside the cast for signs of circulatory compromise, such as whiteness, bluish discoloration, or excessive redness. A white color is indicative of decreased arterial perfusion; a bluish color indicates venous stasis; and redness indicates increased arterial perfusion or first signs of inflammation.
3. Gently massage around bony prominences every 4 hours to maintain proper circulation.
4. Reposition the patient every 3–4 hours as needed to relieve tired tissues and increase perfusion in dependent tissues (see Fig. 10.13 and 10.14).

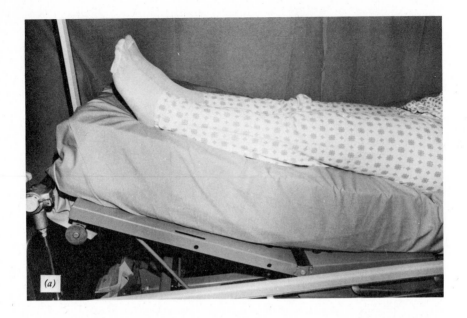

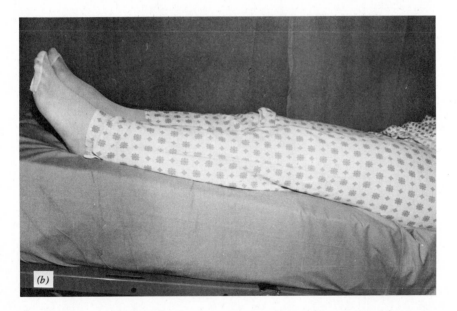

**Figure 10.13** (a) Improper elevation of the foot of the bed. Sagging of the mattress in the knee gatch area can cause hyperextension of the knee. (b) Proper elevation of the foot of the bed and knee gatch. The knee gatch should only be elevated to straighten the mattress.

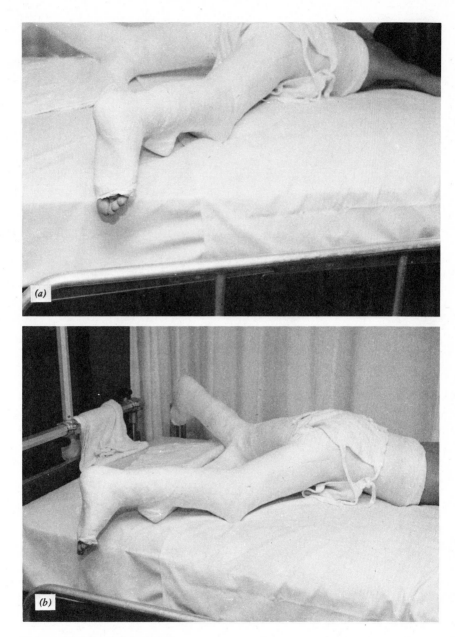

**Figure 10.14** (a) A patient in spica cast turned to the abdomen. Note that toes are off the bed to prevent pressure. (b) Same patient on abdomen. Small pillows should be placed under the pelvis and groin area to lessen pressure, and a small pillow should be placed under the leg to support the leg and foot on both sides of the cast.

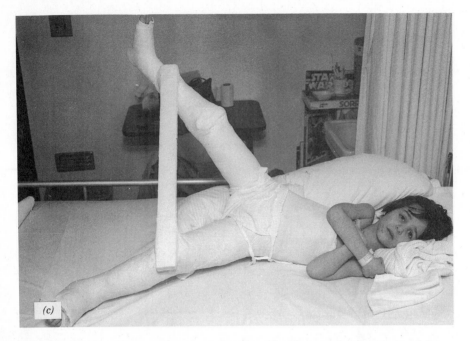

**Figure 10.14** (c) *Same patient turned to the side. The crossbar is only to add stability to the cast. It should not be used for lifting, because it could loosen and potentially cause an injury if the patient were dropped.*

5. Keep the bed linens clean, dry, and wrinkle-free to prevent abrasions or maceration of skin surfaces.

6. Apply cornstarch or talc to skin surfaces for comfort and to facilitate moving. Powders decrease friction, making moving easier.

7. Check the edges of the cast for roughness or unfinished edges. Petal the edges with adhesive strips to decrease the possibility of rough edges causing a skin abrasion (see Fig. 10.6 for petaling).

8. Sniff the cast ends to detect any odors and check around the cast for any drainage, which could signify a developing pressure area or infection. The cast may need to be "windowed" to determine the source of the odor or drainage.

## Evaluation

The patient had:

- intact skin surfaces outside and inside the cast, therefore no decubiti.
- no drainage or infection under the cast.
- adequately perfused, pink tissues with capillary refill in 2–4 seconds.

# NURSING DIAGNOSIS

## *POTENTIAL FOR ALTERATION IN NUTRITIONAL INTAKE OR UTILIZATION OF FOODSTUFFS*

### Assessment

1. Assess appetite, nausea, vomiting, and amount of food eaten.
2. Assess quality of foods eaten for simple or complex carbohydrates, proteins, fats, vitamins, and minerals.
3. Assess ability or problems caused by cast in patient's feeding self, or if assistance is needed.

### Expected Outcomes

The patient will

- have daily intake of high biologic value proteins, 50–55% carbohydrates of total caloric intake, and 20–30% fat intake of daily diet.
- have daily intake of essential vitamins and minerals.
- have 3000 cc of fluid intake daily.

### Nursing Interventions

1. Explain the dietary needs and food groups to aid the patient's understanding, cooperation, or participation.
2. Assist the patient to select foods high in protein, vitamins, minerals, and, if necessary, calories to provide foodstuffs necessary for cellular healing and to maintain nutritional balances. Proteins should be of high biologic value (complete proteins), and carbohydrates should make up 45–55% of the daily caloric intake to provide the fuel for energy needs. Fiber should also be increased for bulk, and the fluid intake should be increased to aid in preventing constipation and to maintain urinary output. Fluid intake should be a minimum of 2,500–3,000 ml and should include milk to provide calcium intake needed for solid bone healing.
3. Assist patient to a comfortable position for eating; cut foods if needed, and open cartons; feed patients unable to feed themselves.

### Evaluation

The patient had:

- intake of sufficient carbohydrate, protein, fat, vitamins, and minerals to maintain weight and health.

- no nausea or vomiting.
- 3,000 ml fluid intake daily.

## NURSING DIAGNOSIS

*POTENTIAL ALTERATION IN BOWEL OR BLADDER ELIMI-NATION RELATED TO THE PRESENCE OF THE CAST OR BACK-LYING POSITION*

### Assessment

1. Assess the patient for usual bowel and bladder habits.
2. Assess urinary output for color, burning, urgency, frequency, or other complaint.
3. Assess for amount, color, and character of the stool.
4. Assess likes and dislikes for fluid intake.

### Expected Outcomes

The patient will have:

- urinary output consistent with daily intake.
- clear, painless urination.
- a soft, brown, formed stool at least every other day.
- a daily fluid intake of 3,000 ml.

### Nursing Interventions

1. Provide privacy for toileting efforts and provide the urinal or bedpan if patient is on bed rest. Allow sufficient time for elimination efforts to help the patient maintain usual patterns of elimination.
2. If allowed up, assist the patient to the bathroom or bedside commode to facilitate elimination. Provide for privacy with curtains or screens.
3. Ask the patient about any straining, soreness, or other concerns when having a bowel movement to determine if other interventions are needed.
4. Ask the patient about any voiding difficulties, such as burning, frequency, urgency, or hesitancy, or other complaints to determine if a urinary infection is present.
5. Examine the color, consistency, and amount of stool; examine the color, clarity, and amount of urine.

6. Assist the patient to achieve a fluid intake of 2,500–3,000 ml to aid bowel and urinary elimination by providing fluids of the patient's choice or likes.

7. Provide fluids with acid ash (cranberry and prune juices) to lessen possibility of development of renal calculi.

8. If constipation becomes a problem and is unrelieved by dietary changes or increased fluid intake, request an order for a stool softener, laxative, or suppository from the physician. Constipation is a common concern of persons with limited mobility.

9. Assess the patient's complaint of costovertebral angle (CVA) pain as a possible sign of renal or urinary infection. Check the patient's temperature, secure a urine specimen, and notify the physician.

## Evaluation

The patient:

- voided clear, yellow urine without complaints.
- had output consistent with intake.
- had bowel output of soft, formed, brown stool without straining or tenseness.
- had daily fluid intake of 3,000 ml.

## NURSING DIAGNOSIS

### POTENTIAL DEFICIT IN DIVERSIONAL ACTIVITIES RELATED TO CAST LIMITATIONS OR PARTICIPATION IN USUAL SOCIAL ACTIVITIES

## Assessment

1. Assess activity likes and dislikes and usual social activities.
2. Assess muscle strengths and weaknesses for particular games or activities, such as puzzle construction, card holding, or throwing dice.

## Expected Outcomes

The patient will:

- participate in social activities using muscles and joints as able.
- have social activities that are active, rather than passive, to maintain muscle functions.
- engage in meaningful social activities to regain usual roles in the family and community.

## Nursing Interventions

1. Assist the patient to engage in active diversional activities that use muscles and joints not in the cast. Avoid passive activities that lessen muscle use and lessen muscle strength.

2. Seek consultation with physical and occupational therapists to have the patient do exercises and activities to increase or maintain muscle strength and use.

3. Encourage the patient to interact, play games, work puzzles, and do other active exercises to maintain muscle use.

4. Encourage the patient to return to usual meaningful activities as able with the cast.

## Evaluation

The patient:

- used physical and occupational therapies to increase or retain muscle/ joint strength.

- engaged in social activities actively to regain or maintain muscle/joint strength.

- used meaningful social activities to return to usual roles in the family and community.

## CAST SYNDROME

Cast syndrome is a serious complication that most often occurs in patients in body casts or hip spica casts, although it can also occur to any patient who has an arm or leg cast. Cast syndrome is a series of events that lead to severe small intestinal ileus as a consequence or cause of loss of blood flow through the superior mesenteric artery. From abnormal bending or kinking of the mesenteric artery caused by the patient's position of hyperextension in the cast, the blood supply is decreased leading to stasis, increased putrefaction, and ileus. Ileus can also be caused by excessive aerophagia or air swallowing by an anxious or nervous patient, and the development of gastric and intestinal ileus produces cast syndrome; the patient does not need to be in a body or spica cast to produce the symptoms.

Symptoms of cast syndrome include the patient's complaints of feeling bloated, full of air and gas, feeling as if the cast is so tight they cannot take a deep breath, and feeling nauseated. If the ileus progresses, the patient becomes more frightened or anxious and dyspneic. The vital signs show elevations in blood pressure, pulse, and respiration, accompanied by normal temperatures or low-grade fever. Anxiety increases unless the condition is relieved, and the cast may need to be bivalved. Other treatments include relieving the ileus by giving nothing by mouth, repositioning or turning the patient, inserting a nasogastric tube to relieve the ileus, administration of a sedative (often diazepam [Valium]), administration of intravenous fluids, and bivalving the cast (even if not a spica or body cast). The bivalved cast is taped together firmly but more loosely until the ileus is relieved, when the cast is repaired with new applications of cast material. If the ileus becomes severe, surgery may be necessary to repair intestinal obstruction and intestinal necrosis resulting from the interrupted blood supply. Fluids are administered intravenously to maintain blood volume during the period of acute ileus.

Bivalving casts may be done for reasons other than ileus and cast syndrome. They may be bivalved to check dressings and incisions, to relieve marked edema or severe pain, and to permit use of either the anterior or posterior shell to help maintain the required position or degree of immobility desired. The bivalved cast is then either used as one shell or the two pieces may be taped or replastered together to provide more stability for the patient.

## PATIENT TEACHING AND DISCHARGE PLANNING FOR HOME CARE IN A CAST

## NURSING DIAGNOSIS

### KNOWLEDGE DEFICIT RELATED TO DISCHARGE AND HOME CARE NEEDS

#### Assessment

1. Assess patient's and home caretakers' knowledge of discharge plans and home care preparations (see figs. 10.15 and 10.16).
2. Assess family's understanding and readiness to assist the patient with home care as needed.
3. Assess need for supplies and equipment for home care.

#### Expected Outcomes

The patient will:

- learn self-care, if able, for home care.
- have supplies and equipment provided for home care.
- utilize family members for assistance with self-care.
- verbalize signs and symptoms of complications to report to the physician.

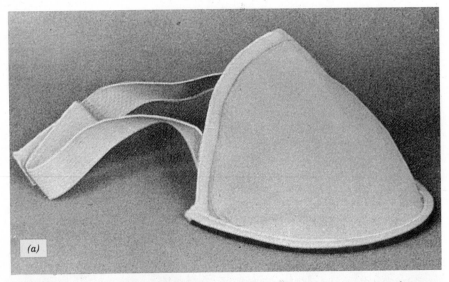

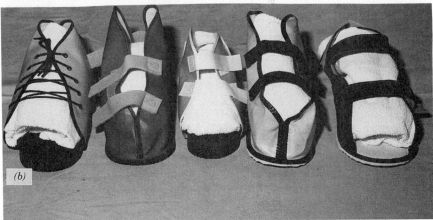

**Figure 10.15** (a) Toe covering for warmth. (b) Shoes for warmth and protection while in a cast.

## Nursing Interventions

1. Instruct the patient and family members in home care, as required. Provide instructions verbally and in written form for perusal and clarification.

2. Instruct the patient about steps (all previously mentioned in this chapter) to maintain an intact cast, ROM and muscle-setting exercises, activities to maintain skin integrity, proper nutrition, bowel and bladder elimination, pain relief, nighttime sedation, and pulmonary exercises.

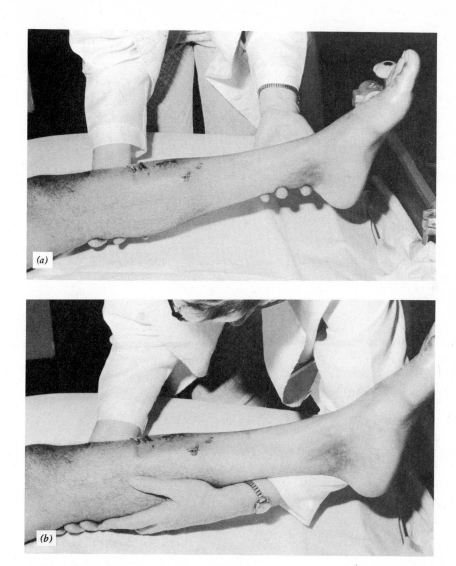

**Figure 10.16** (a) Lifting the leg by supporting a joint in each hand. (b) Supporting entire leg and joints with one hand and arm. Note that the proximal and distal joints are both supported to prevent hyperextension of either joint.

3. Discuss sexual activities and positions if needed because of a cumbersome spica cast to decrease concern or fear related to sexual intercourse.

4. Observe the patient's ambulation, ascending or descending stairs, and sitting or rising from a chair to ascertain the patient's ability and safety.

5. Instruct the patient and family members in proper application and elevation of an extremity in a sling (see fig 10.17).

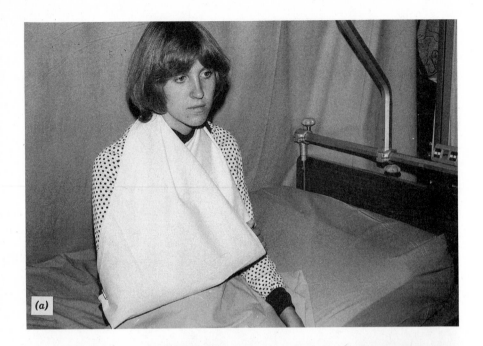

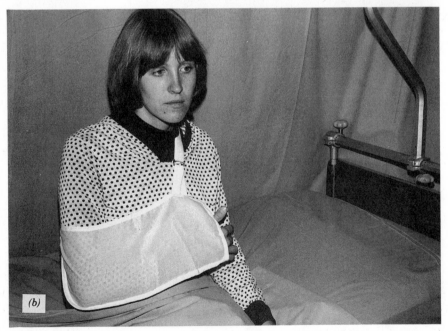

**Figure 10.17** (a) Cloth sling to support arm and forearm.; (b) Commercially available sling.

6. Instruct the patient and family members about signs or symptoms to report to the physician including such things as increasing amounts of soreness or pain, increased swelling, numbness, tingling or burning, inability to move tissues around cast, change in color, white or red or discolored areas, change in temperature, coolness of digits or warm or hot areas, foul odor or drainage, and cracks or breaks in the cast.

## Evaluation

The patient

- verbalized self-care steps and manipulated supplies or equipment correctly.
- verbalized methods to maintain the integrity of the cast.
- used ambulatory aids correctly and safely in walking and stair climbing.
- verbalized signs and symptoms to report to the physician.

## Procedures

### CUTTING AND REMOVING A CAST*

#### Materials Needed

- cast cutter
- scissors with blunt ends

#### Techniques

- Explain that the cast cutter is noisy while cutting through the cast material.
- Explain that the blade of the cutter will not cut the patient's skin because of the protective lining (stockinette, felt, or sheet wadding) and that the blade is withdrawn when through the plaster or other cast material.
- Depress the cutter blade into the cast along a lateral or anterior surface of the cast until the blade cuts through the cast in that area.
- Continue to cut the cast from end to end lengthwise.
- Gently wedge the scissors into the cut areas and spread the blades to widen the cut along the length of the cast.

..................................

*Only physicians, specially trained nurses, or orthopaedic technicians should cut casts, either in an emergency or routinely.

- Cut (bivalve) both sides of a large cast, such as a body or spica cast.
- Cut the underlying skin coverings through the length of the cast.
- Slide the cast and the skin coverings off the skin areas.

## Post-cast-removal Care

- Explain to the patient that the muscles and joints that were in the cast will be weak and sore, and that use and movement should be begun moderately with rest periods taken.
- Explain that there may be mild to moderate soreness or pain with reuse and that use of a nonnarcotic analgesic every 4 hours for 24–48 hours should relieve the pain. Generally, it takes twice as long to regain full functions as the part was in a cast; thus a recovery time of 2–3 months is normal for tissues in a cast for 6 weeks.
- Explain skin care following removal of the cast:
  - Have the patient liberally apply full-strength solution of cold-water wash with enzymes, such as Woolite® or Delicare®, to the skin areas that were in the cast and to let it remain on the skin for at least 20 minutes. The enzymes loosen dead cells and fatty or crusty lesions without injuring the underlying cells.
  - Following the loosening period, have the patient immerse the area in warm water or in a bathtub, and gently rinse off the loosened cells and debris, being careful not to scrub or use fingernails, which could abrade the skin surfaces.
  - Rinse the area with clear water.
  - Pat the skin areas dry with a towel, again taking care to dry the skin gently, because it is quite tender.
  - Have the patient apply a moisturizing skin lotion to the area to maintain the cells' integrity.
  - Instruct the patient to repeat the above steps in 24 hours, after which only the usual skin cleansing is needed.
- Explain that the tissues may develop some edema which at times may become marked.
  - Instruct the patient to elevate the affected tissues as often as possible for the next 24–48 hours.
  - If the edema becomes marked, instruct the patient to use ice to lessen the edema or to have the tissues wrapped with elastic bandages. Usually the edema abates with moderate use and elevation.

## BIBLIOGRAPHY

Benz, J. (1986). The adolescent in a spica cast. *Orthopaedic Nursing, 5*(3), 22–23.

Farrell, N.A. (1985). Cast syndrome. *Orthopaedic Nursing, 4*(4), 61–64.

Gulanick, M., Klopp, A., & Galanes, S. (Eds.). (1986). *Nursing care plans, nursing diagnosis, and interventions.* St. Louis: Mosby-Yearbook.

Kim, M.J. McFarland, G.K. & McLane, A.M. (1991). *Pocket guide to nursing diagnoses* (3rd ed.). St. Louis: Mosby-Yearbook.

Mourad, L. (1991). *Orthopedic disorders.* St. Louis: Mosby-Yearbook.

Renshaw, T.S. (1986). *Pediatric orthopedics.* Philadelphia: Saunders.

# 11

# USE OF TRACTION FOR TREATMENT OF ORTHOPAEDIC CONDITIONS

Traction is the use of pull to exert force indirectly or directly to bones to overcome deformity or to help restore alignment following trauma. Sufficient weight (pull) must be used to overcome muscle spasms, shortening, overriding and/or angulation of bones to bring them back into their desirable anatomic positions.

There are two forms of traction—*skin* or *skeletal* traction. Skin traction is applied to the skin surfaces and indirectly to the bones, whereas skeletal traction is applied directly to the bones via a nail or pin(s) drilled through the skin and bones.

## PRINCIPLES OF SKIN TRACTION

Many strategies are used in the various skin tractions to maintain the integrity of the skin and underlying tissues. These are based on the following principles:

- Skin traction is maintained for relatively short periods (as compared to skeletal traction), in order to prevent loss of skin attachments (epidermis is "loosely" attached to subcutaneous tissues).
- Skin traction uses 2–4 kg (5–10 lb) of weight as the maximum weight. Less weight is used for very young or elderly persons.
- Skin traction might be intermittent to allow tissue inspection or rest to the parts. It is applied over large areas of skin to distribute the load more efficiently.
- Skin traction is an effective means to treat muscle spasm or overriding or shortening of fractured bones, to relieve pain in inflammatory conditions, and to help lessen flexion contractures.

- Skin surfaces should be intact, carefully washed and dried, and, unless excessively hairy, should not be shaved before traction is applied. Nicks or cuts may result from shaving and become inflamed under the traction.
- Pressure on skin/soft tissues over bony prominences must be avoided by covering them with padding before the traction is applied.
- Muscles and joints should not remain in full extension for extended periods. Full extension weakens muscles, ligaments, and tendons and may cause posttreatment arthritis.
- The amount of weight used for skin traction should be sufficient only to overcome the muscle spasm yet leave enough tone in the muscles to help hold the bone ends for healing if traction is being used for fracture treatment. Too much weight may cause distraction (pulling apart of bone ends), which could delay healing or result in nonhealing (nonunion). Persons with large muscle masses require more weight to overcome muscle spasm. Injuries to stronger (femoral) muscles require more weight to overcome the muscle spasm.
- Skin traction can be applied intermittently to treat nonfracture inflammatory conditions. The amount of weight for skin tolerance is frequently sufficient to ease inflammatory conditions in underlying soft tissues (muscle spasm, nerve pressure, arthritic pain, and others).
- Skin traction might not allow for enough weight to exert sufficient pull on fractured bones that are severely overriding, angulated, or have soft tissues between the fractured ends. Treatment with skeletal traction or surgery may be needed for those conditions.
- Dark-complexioned persons (brown or black hair, brown eyes, olive skin) have greater "tissue integrity" than light-skinned, freckled, or blue-eyed persons; therefore, they have greater tolerance to skin traction (thought to be due to melanocyte activity). There are also variations in skin tolerances in the very young, elderly, diabetic, or persons with connective tissue diseases involving the skin or underlying tissues.

## TYPES OF SKIN TRACTION

The commonly used forms of skin traction are Buck's extension, Bryant's (called Gallows in England), Russell's, modified Russell's, pelvic belt (pelvic girdle), head halter, pelvic sling, Cotrel's, and Dunlop's. All but Bryant's are used for adults. Bryant's traction is used for children under 18 kg (40 lb) to treat fractures of the femur, and the techniques are described in pediatric orthopaedic nursing texts.

The specific type of skin traction used depends on the type of injury; the area, bones, and tissues injured; the effects of gravity and muscle action; and the purpose for the use of the particular type of skin traction.

Briefly, the descriptions below explain the various types of skin tractions used for adults.

## Buck's Extension

Buck's extension involves application of a foam rubber boot or adhesive strips on the lateral surfaces of one or more extremities, with the strips held in place by elastic bandages. Weights are attached to a spreader connecting the distal ends of the adhesive strips or the boot. This traction is used for arthritic conditions of the extremities and, prior to surgery, for hip fractures to help maintain immobility and decrease trauma (Fig. 11.1).

## Russell's Traction

Russell's traction is a modification of Buck's extension with the addition of a sling under the affected knee; the sling is attached to a rope and pulley with the rope running to an arrangement of three pulleys attached to the bed frame and the adhesive strips as shown in Fig. 11.2a. The arrangement of the ropes, pulleys, and knee sling distributes the pull more effectively throughout the entire limb. It also uses Newton's third law of thermodynamics, which states that for every force in one direction, there is an equal force in the opposite direction; thus, the pull is doubled to the limb without adding additional weight to the weight holder (Fig. 11.2b). Because of the distribution throughout greater skin areas, the increased pull is more efficient and less injurious to the skin tissues. With 5 lb of weight, 10 lb of pull is accomplished with Russell's traction. Russell's traction is used for the same purposes as Buck's extension, as well as for acetabular conditions. Split Russell's traction is a variation of "classic" Russell's (see Fig. 11.3).

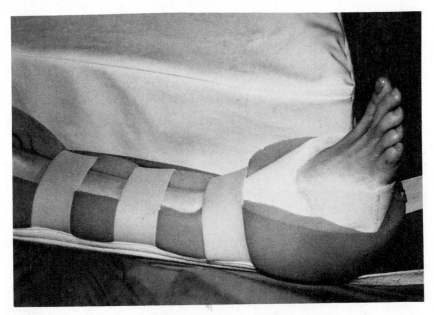

**Figure 11.1** Buck's extension with a traction boot. The patient has a heel protector in place.

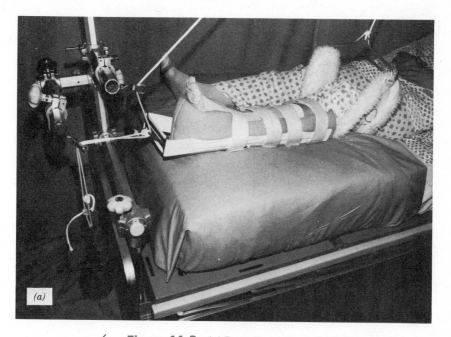

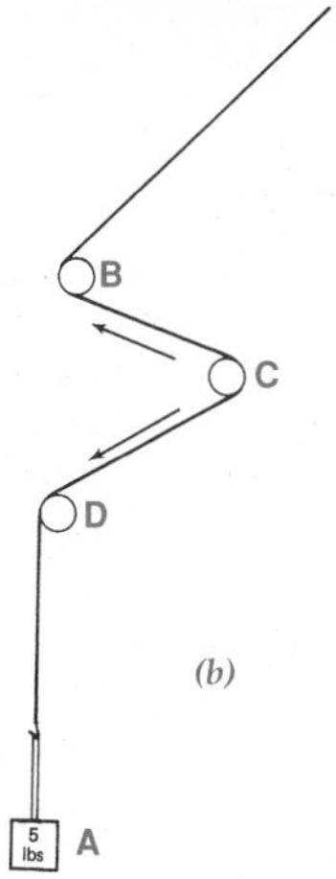

**Figure 11.2** (a) Russell's traction. (b) Pulley arrangement that doubles the amount of pull in Russell's traction. Arrows indicate pull in opposite direction.

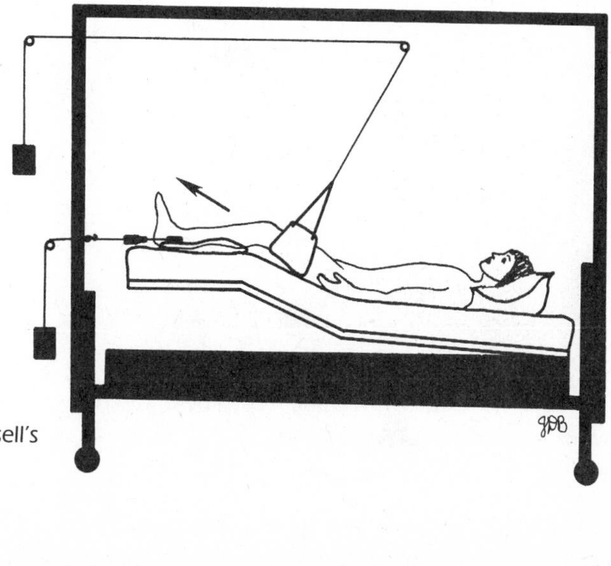

**Figure 11.3** "Split" Russell's traction.

## Pelvic Belt (Girdle)

A belt or "girdle" is placed around the pelvic area; a long strap on each side of the belt is attached to a large spreader bar at the patient's feet, with weights connected to the spreader bar. The amount of weight usually varies from 20–30 lb. This traction is used to overcome the muscle spasms that may accompany low back pain, herniated nucleus pulposus (ruptured disc), or other lumbar back conditions (Fig. 11.4).

## Head Halter

A soft halter is fitted over the head and chin. Side straps are attached to a spreader bar with ropes and weights attached to the spreader (see Figs. 11.5a–c). This traction is used to treat arthritic conditions of the cervical vertebrae and muscles. It should not be used for fractures of the cervical vertebrae, except to maintain immobility prior to insertion of skeletal tongs.

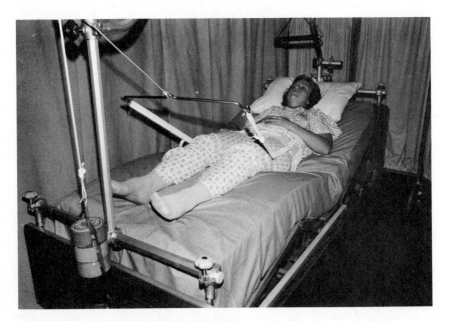

**Figure 11.4** Pelvic belt traction with straps to one spreader bar. Note the pressure over the trochanteric region by this narrow spreader bar. Each rope may be attached to a separate pulley on each side of the bed frame bar to lessen pressure on the sciatic nerve.

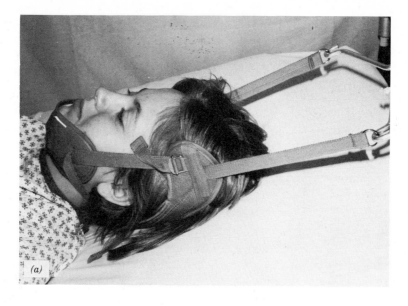

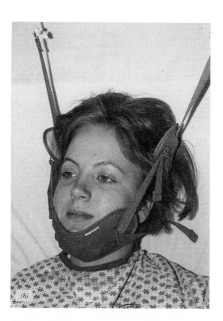

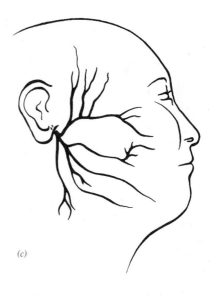

**Figure 11.5** Cervical head halter traction with one spreader bar. Note that ears are clear of the halter. Pull comes from the occipital area of the halter. The head of the bed may be elevated (per doctor's preference) for countertraction. (b) Straps of the head halter are attached to separate pulleys to lessen pressure on the facial nerve. (c) Distribution of the facial nerve.

### Pelvic Sling

This treatment is really a suspension rather than a traction, but it is generally included as a form of skin traction. A sling or hammock is placed under the lower back and buttocks, with metallic bars threaded through sewn areas at the ends of the sling. These metallic bars are fitted into a heavy spreader bar, which is attached to rope and pulleys to suspend the buttocks slightly off the bed. A pelvic sling may be used for treating fractures of one or more pelvic bones—so called "open book" fractures of  . the symphysis pubis—although recently it has been replaced by use of external fixators (see Figs. 11.6a-b).

### Cotrel's Traction

Cotrel's traction is a combination of head halter used simultaneously with pelvic belt traction to the pelvis. It is used to help overcome muscle actions to assist in overcoming scoliosis curvature before surgical correction (see Fig. 11.7).

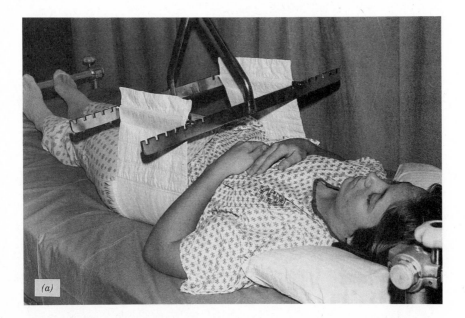

**Figure 11.6** (a) Weil pelvic sling suspension. Sling is padded to lessen pressure. Approximately 14–17 kg (30–35 lbs) weight is needed to lift the buttocks slightly off the bed.

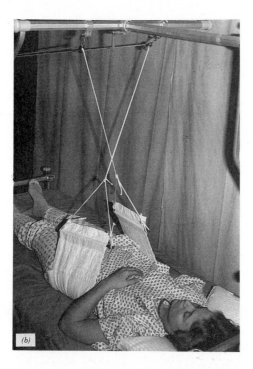

(b)

**Figure 11.6** (b) Alternate form of pelvic sling application that provides greater compression for bilateral fractures of the pelvis.

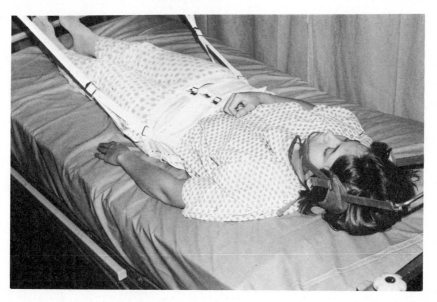

**Figure 11.7** Cotrel's traction, which combines pelvic belt and cervical head halter traction for treatment of scoliosis or other conditions of the vertebral column.

## Dunlop's Traction

Dunlop's traction is basically Buck's extension applied horizontally and vertically to the humerus and forearm, respectively. It is used to treat fractures of the humerus with the vertical forearm portion merely being a means to help hold the forearm upward to maintain proper direction for the humeral traction (see Fig. 11.8).

Generally, each type of skin traction mentioned above has its "classic" position used in the majority of persons. Variations may be required for a particular condition or individual injury.

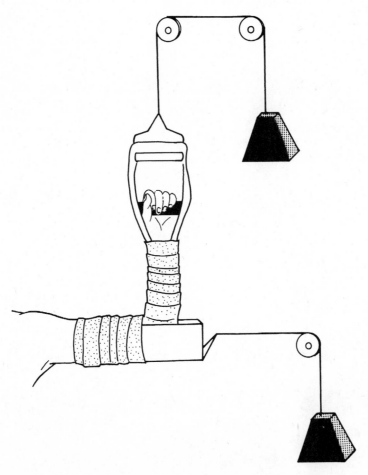

**Figure 11.8** Dunlop's side arm traction, used for treatment of supracondylar fractures of the humerus.

The amount of weight used for each type of skin traction varies with the type and the specific tissues involved. In addition, the amount of skin surface area involved with the traction influences the amount of weight used. If the weight is distributed over larger areas, more weight is usually used; for example, with pelvic belt traction, 25–35 lb of weight may be used; conversely, 5–7 lb of weight is all that the skin of an arm or leg can tolerate without excess pull on the epidermal tissues, which could lead to irritation or open lesions. Epidermal layers can also lose their underlying skin attachments because of their "loose" attachments. Loss of these underlying attachments can lead to disruption of perfusion caused by circulatory disruption. Therefore, the type of skin traction to be applied and the tissues and the area to be in traction are vital considerations in patient care. Also the age and overall health of the person must be considered for each type of traction, as concomitant health alterations might contraindicate the use of a specific type of skin traction. Diabetes or severe peripheral vascular disease would cause concern when Buck's extension or Russell's traction is being considered.

## Procedures

### APPLICATION OF SPECIFIC TYPES OF SKIN TRACTION

Nurses may initiate each of the specific types of skin traction or may assist the physician or a technician with the application. Nurses remove patients from traction and reapply the traction according to physician's orders, the patient's responses, and institutional policies.

#### Materials Needed for All Types of Skin Traction

- weights (have 1, 2, and 5 lb weights available)
- rope—nylon on rolls
- weight holder(s)
- spreader bars or spreader "shoe"
- pulleys
- bed frame with additional bars

#### Additional Materials Needed for Buck's Extension or Russell's Traction

- Skin-Trac boot or Buck's boot
- adhesive strips, foam rubber, or elastic adhesive strips
- elastic bandages or similar elastic wraps
- thromboembolic hose, if requested by physician

- knee sling for Russell's traction
- heel protectors (optional)

To establish Buck's extension traction:

- Check skin areas to be placed in traction for cleanliness, presence of open lesions or raised areas such as moles or blisters. Traction should not be applied over open, blistered, or irritated skin.

- Apply thromboembolic hose to one or both legs, if ordered.

- Place the Buck's boot under the affected leg; check for appropriateness of size.

- Close the pressure-occlusive straps, beginning with the distal strap, and proceed up the leg, using care to avoid closing the straps too tightly.

- Tie the rope to the attachment on the end of the Buck's boot and attach the weight holder to the other end of the rope.

- Slowly add the ordered amount of weight to the weight holder.

- Lower the weight holder and weights till the rope is taut over the pulley.

- Adjust the patient's position in bed so the pull is direct and straight. The leg in traction should be on the mattress *without a pillow* under the leg, because the pillow would cause friction, thereby decreasing the effectiveness of the traction. The knee gatch may be slightly elevated for comfort and countertraction (Figs. 11.9 and 11.10).

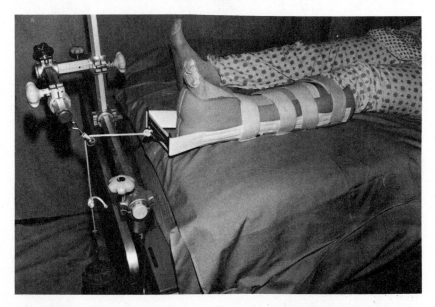

**Figure 11.9** Buck's extension with the knee gatch slightly elevated for countertraction and comfort. Note that the rope is riding freely in the pulley.

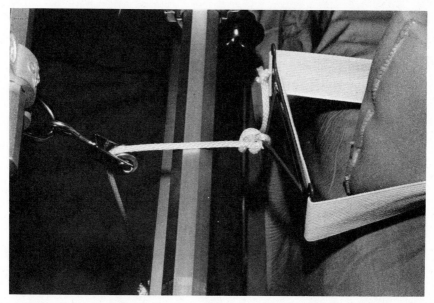

**Figure 11.10** Improper Buck's extension. The patient's heel is off the edge of the mattress, which will cause pressure on the calf. The rope is resting on the crossbar, causing friction, which lessens the effectiveness of the traction.

If a Buck's boot is not used, the techniques are to:
* Apply the adhesive strips to the lateral surfaces of the affected leg.
* Cover the strips and the leg with elastic bandages beginning at the foot and wrapping up the leg to just below the knee. Use even pressure, and avoid exerting pull to the bandage, which could make it become too tight.
* Attach the shoe to the distal ends of the adhesive strips.
* Lower the weight slowly until the rope is taut over the pulley.
* Adjust the patient's position (as above).

To apply Russell's traction:
* Check and prepare the skin as described on p. 279.
* Apply the Buck's boot or adhesive strips and bandage as for Buck's extension.
* Place knee sling under affected knee and hook sling to spreader bar.
* Attach a rope to the spreader bar; thread it over an overhead pulley on the bed frame, then to the upper pulley on the frame at the end of the

bed; and continue to thread the rope through the shoe of the adhesive strips or in the appropriate area in the Skin-Trac boot, then over the lower pulley (see Fig 11.2).

- Tie the rope to the weight holder.
- Apply the ordered amount of weight on the holder.
- Slowly lower the weighted weight holder until the rope is taut over all pulleys.
- Check the patient's position, the knee sling, all the pulleys, and the rope. The rope should move freely over the pulleys.

## Additional Materials for Pelvic Belt Application

- Pelvic belts or "girdles" of several sizes
- Large-size spreader bar

To apply pelvic belt traction:

- Place the belt under the patient's buttocks.
- Adjust the belt so the top is above the iliac crests in front and the posterior iliac spines in the back.
- Close the belt, beginning with the lower straps.
- Attach a rope to each of the lateral straps of the belt.
- Attach the rope to large spreader bar at the foot of the bed, or tie each strap to a rope over separate pulleys, then attach to a weight holder on each side of the foot of the bed. (Separate attachments are used for obese patients to prevent pressure over the sciatic nerve.) (See Figs. 11.4 and 11.11.)
- Attach a weight holder to the spreader bar(s).
- Apply ordered amounts of weights—possibly 25–30 or more pounds.
- Adjust the patient's position in bed to the Williams position, if ordered. This position involves elevating the head of the bed 45° and the knee gatch 45°. This position aids in relaxation of lumbosacral muscles (see Fig. 11.12).

## Additional Materials Needed for Pelvic Sling Application

- pelvic sling with lamb's wool lining
- spreader bar specifically made for this traction
- metallic crosspieces

To apply a pelvic sling:

- Place the sling under the patient's buttocks. Patient may be turned to the side to aid in placing the sling in the proper position.

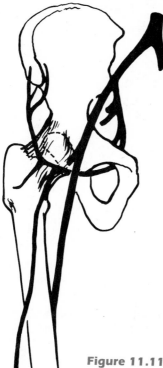

**Figure 11.11** Course of the sciatic nerve from the lumbosacral/ vertebral area down the posterior buttock and thigh.

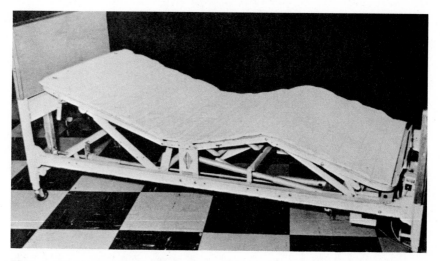

**Figure 11.12** Bed in Williams position for pelvic belt traction. This position flexes the knees and hips to relax the gluteal and lumbosacral muscles.

- Insert the metallic crosspieces in the slots in the sling, being careful to have the crosspieces in the slot on either side that is equidistant from the center (Fig. 11.6a).

- Attach the spreader specifically designed for the sling to a rope and pulleys on the bed frame.

- Attach the weight holder and weights to the rope (the spring mechanism on the spreader will automatically cause the spreader to be pulled up to the pulley and the weights attached to the rope).

- Secure assistance of another nursing person (needed to secure the sling to the spreader). Position the second person on the opposite side of the bed.

- Lower the spreader to just above the sling, and hold with one hand or spring mechanism will pull it back up.

- Place metallic pins holding sling in slots of spreader, taking care to have both sides of the sling in slots equidistant from end of spreader (Fig. 11.6a). Both personnel should insert the sling at the same time to avoid shifting the patient "off center."

- Allow the spreader bar to rise slowly by its spring mechanism until sling is taut. The patient's buttocks should be just off the bed if sufficient weight has been applied; if the buttocks are still on the bed, more weight should be added to raise the sling.

To remove the sling, *without releasing weights\**:

- Grasp the top of the spreader bar and pull the spreader bar down slowly toward the patient's abdomen until the sling is loosely remaining in the spreader.

- While holding the spreader bar in the descended position, unhook the sling from one side of the spreader, being careful to lay the sling with its metal crosspiece on the bed to prevent injury to the patient (see Fig. 11.13).

- Unhook the crosspiece on the opposite side of the spreader bar and lay it on the bed.

- Slowly let the spreader bar rise until the spring mechanism reaches the pulley to hold the spreader bar securely.

- Remove the two crosspieces from the sling and turn the patient to the side to remove the sling from the bed if desired.

......................................

*If the weights are inadvertently lifted while the spreader bar and sling are in place, the spreader bar will descend toward the patient's abdomen and can cause injury. Thus, the sling is removed with the weights holding the spreader bar in place.

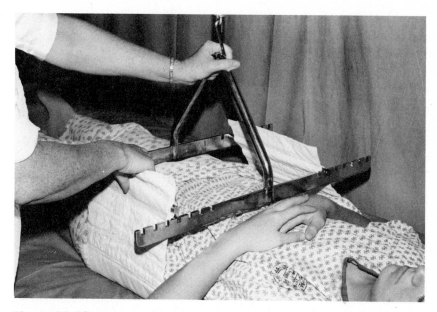

**Figure 11.13** Releasing the pelvic sling by lowering the spreader bar with one hand while releasing the crosspieces. Two persons must reapply the crosspieces simultaneously to maintain the proper position and balance of the sling.

## Additional Materials Needed for Cotrel's Traction

- head halters of various sizes
- pelvic belt

To apply Cotrel's traction:

- Position the patient centered in bed with bed flat.
- Place head halter over patient's head and tighten straps under ears.
- Attach spreader bar to hooks; attach rope to spreader bar; thread rope over pulley and tie to weight holder.
- Place 5–8 lb of weight on holder, as ordered.
- Adjust straps so pull is coming from occipital areas of the halter.
- Place pelvic belt under pelvic area; close straps over abdomen.
- Proceed as for application of pelvic belt on p. 290.
- Recheck patient's position in bed, noting the direction of pull for each of the separate tractions.

## Additional Materials Needed for Head Halter Application

- head halters of various sizes
- additional rope
- one to three pulleys

To apply head halter traction:

- Slide the head halter under the patient's head, and put the chin and occipital areas in their appropriate places in the halter.
- Close the lateral straps snugly.
- Put the halter hooks into the spreader bar, or tie each side hook to a rope to an individual pulley if the patient's face is plump and the halter would exert undue pressure over the facial nerve (see Fig. 11.5b).
- Apply the ordered amount of weight in weight holders to the spreader bar or the individual ropes and hooks.

## Additional Materials Needed for Dunlop's Traction

- Buck's extension materials as given on p. 287 (double sets of materials are needed).

To apply Dunlop's traction:

- Apply Buck's extension to the forearm to facilitate the patient's ability to hold the forearm vertically.
- Apply the second Buck's extension to the injured arm (see Fig 11.8).
- Apply the weights on the weight holders as ordered.
- If requested by the physician, insert 2–4-inch blocks under the bed wheels on the side of the traction. The inclined position may add countertraction from the patient's body to increase the effectiveness of the traction.

With Dunlop's traction, the patient may complain of numbness and tingling of one or more fingers and have decreasing ability to bring the thumb in apposition to the fingers if there is undue pressure on either the radial or ulnar nerves. Removal of the forearm elastic bandage should relieve the symptoms if nerve damage has not occurred.

## SANDBAGS

At times sandbags are used to aid in maintaining an upright position of an extremity in traction. Sandbags against a limb may cause friction, thereby lessening the effectiveness of the traction. If sandbags are used, great care must be taken to prevent pressure over superficial nerves, especially the peroneal nerve over the head of the fibula (see Fig. 11.14). Such pressure could lead to foot drop from weakness or damage to the peroneal nerve. Investigate complaints of numbness, tingling, or inability to perform foot flexion and eversion (see Fig. 11.15).

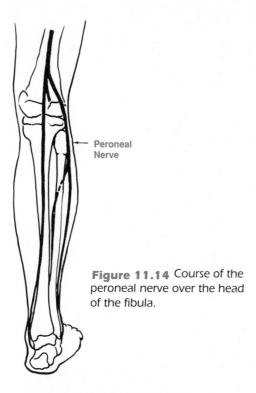

**Figure 11.14** Course of the peroneal nerve over the head of the fibula.

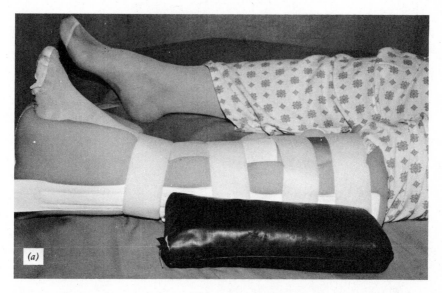

**Figure 11.15** (a) Improper (too high up the leg ) placement of a sandbag, which would cause pressure on the peroneal nerve over the head of the fibula.

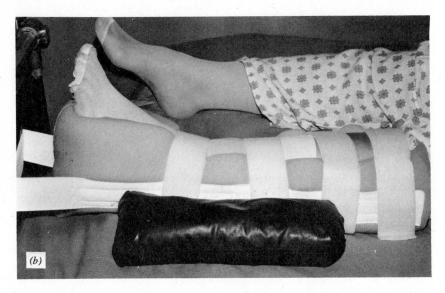

**Figure 11.15** (b) Properly placed sandbag farther down the leg. The sandbag helps maintain the upright position of the leg.

## NURSING CONSIDERATIONS FOLLOWING APPLICATION OF SKIN TRACTION

### NURSING DIAGNOSIS

*ALTERATION IN COMFORT RELATED TO MUSCLE SPASMS OR ACUTE PAIN*

#### Assessment

1. Assess for complaints of muscle spasms, pain presence, type, severity as given on p. 262.
2. Observe or listen for evidence of pain, such as moaning, writhing, crying, and wincing.

#### Expected Outcomes

The patient will:

- be relieved of muscle spasms.
- have relief of acute pain.

## Nursing Interventions

1. Explain the "reasons" for the muscle spasms and acute pain, according to the patient's specific pathology.

2. Check the patient's position every 1–2 hours initially after being placed in traction to note increase or decrease in symptoms of soreness or pain; presence, frequency, or severity of muscle spasms; and other signs of adverse response to the specific traction.

3. *If permitted by the specific traction and the patient's injury,* turn the patient to the side to relieve muscle soreness, spasms, or pain. Adjust the pulleys as required when on the side. *Note:* Persons in head halter, Russell's, Cotrel's, and Dunlop's traction should remain in back-lying positions at all times for the traction to be effective. Persons in Buck's extension can be turned for brief periods to the unaffected side with a pillow placed under the affected limb. The traction pulley should be raised if necessary to maintain proper pull on the affected leg while the patient is in the side-lying position. A pillow placed to the patient's back aids maintaining the desired position.

4. If permitted by the patient's condition, physician's orders and institutional policies, remove the weights and release the person from the traction for brief periods to ease muscle spasms, then reapply the traction. *Note:* Orders may read "in 2 hours, out 2 hours, and out at night" for patients in head halter and pelvic belt traction. Persons in these two types of traction cannot sleep in traction because the muscles would not be able to relax and the traction would exert too much pull on resting muscles, thereby disrupting rest and sleep.

5. Administer ordered medications to relieve muscle spasms and pain. Medications include nonsteroidal anti-inflammatories, muscle relaxants, narcotic or nonnarcotic analgesics, and sedatives.

6. Offer back massage and adjust the patient's position with "mini" adjustments of small pillows or soft blankets to ease discomfort and pain (see Fig. 11.16).

## Evaluation

The patient:

- verbalized relief of muscle spasms and acute pain.
- had no episodes of wincing, moaning, crying, or other evidences of pain.
- was removed from the traction permanently.

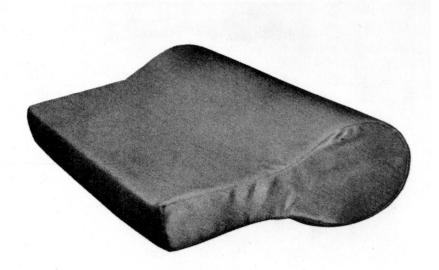

**Figure 11.16** Small pillow, which may be used under the head of a patient in or out of cervical head halter traction.

## NURSING DIAGNOSIS

### IMPAIRED PHYSICAL MOBILITY RELATED TO THE PRESENCE OF THE TRACTION

#### Assessment

1.  Assess for patient's abilities and restrictions because of the specific traction position.
2.  Assess patient's ROM of unaffected muscles.

#### Expected Outcomes

The patient will:

- maintain usual ROM of unaffected tissues while in traction.
- perform ROM and muscle-setting exercises to retain strength while in traction.

## Nursing Interventions

1. Clarify purposes of traction for treatment of specific pathology.
2. Teach ROM and muscle-setting exercise regimens.
3. Assist the patient with movements in bed as needed, to ease stiff muscles and joints (see Fig. 11.17).
4. Secure consultations with physical and occupational therapists to maintain integrity of unaffected musculoskeletal tissues, and to assist with regaining integrity of affected tissues.
5. Assist the patient with ambulation and being up in a chair if allowed up.
6. Have the patient do ROM exercises every 2–4 hours as needed.
7. Have the patient do "quad" setting, gluteal settings, or biceps and triceps strengthening exercises every 2–4 hours as scheduled.

## Evaluation

The patient:

- performed ROM and muscle-setting exercises as scheduled.
- maintained muscle strength while in traction.
- ambulated without soreness or limitation.

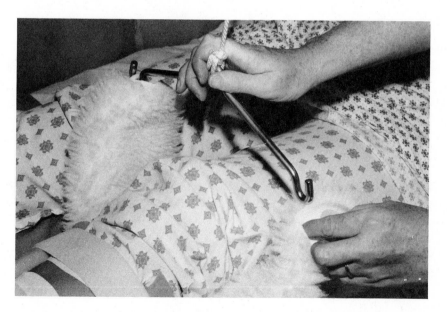

**Figure 11.17** Releasing the knee sling for skin care or neurovascular checks. The spreader bar is lowered by pulling downward and releasing the sling. The spreader bar can be held by the patient to free both hands of the nurse for care.

# NURSING DIAGNOSIS

## *ACTUAL INJURY TO THE MUSCULOSKELETAL TISSUES AND POTENTIAL INJURY RELATED TO NEUROVASCULAR COMPROMISE*

## Assessment

1. Assess neurovascular status: edema, color changes, capillary refill, pain, motor and sensory functions.

2. Assess patient's complaints of numbness, tingling, pins and needles, increased pain.

## Expected Outcomes

The patient will have:

- adequate neurovascular functions.

- no permanent neurovascular compromise or complications.

## Nursing Interventions

1. Do all eight parts of neurovascular checks as ordered, noting changes over time (see p. 255 for checks). *Note*: If a change is noted in one or more part(s) of the checks, repeat the entire check in 15–30 minutes; if the untoward change(s) persists, notify appropriate nursing personnel or supervisor and notify medical personnel as appropriate. Record all findings on neurovascular flow sheet with date and time (see Fig. 11.18 for flow sheet).

2. Apply ice bags to injured tissues as ordered for 48–72 hours.

3. *If ordered and there is no acute injury or bleeding,* after 48–72 hours, apply heat with warm compresses to the sore area (heat may be used in arthritic conditions). Avoid heat in bruises, crush injuries, and fractures to avoid possibility of increasing bleeding.

4. Maintain continuous traction *if* a fracture is present and the patient is in Buck's extension, Russell's, or Dunlop's. A head halter may be used prior to insertion of skeletal tongs for treatment of cervical fractures.

5. Check the entire traction setup every shift: are ropes over pulleys, weights hanging freely, knots all secured? Check patient's overall position and alignment.

| Date | 10/1 | | | | | | | | | | | | | | | Comments | Nurse's signature |
|---|---|---|---|---|---|---|---|---|---|---|---|---|---|---|---|---|---|
| Time | 1 PM | 2 | 3 | 4 | 5 | 6 | 7 | 8 | 9 | 10 | 11 | 12 | | | | | |
| Neurovascular checks | | | | | | | | | | | | | | | | | |
| A. COLOR OF TISSUES<br>Pink (normal) = 1<br>Pale = 2<br>Blue = 3<br>Mottled = 4 | 1 | | | | | | | | | | | | | | | | |
| B. TEMPERATURE OF TISSUES<br>Warm (normal) = 1<br>Cool = 2<br>Cold = 3<br>Hot = 4 | 2 | | | | | | | | | | | | | | | | |
| C. EDEMA<br>None = 0<br>Slight = 1<br>Moderate = 2<br>Marked = 3<br>Pitting = 4 | 2 | | | | | | | | | | | | | | | | |
| D. PAIN<br>None = 0<br>Slight = 1<br>Moderate amount = 2<br>Severe = 3<br>Radiating = 4 | 2 | | | | | | | | | | | | | | | | |
| E. CAPILLARY REFILL<br>2-4 seconds (normal) = 2<br>4-6 seconds = 2<br>longer than 6 sec. = 3 | 2 | | | | | | | | | | | | | | | | |
| F. MOTOR FUNCTIONS<br>Active ROM all joints = 1<br>involved<br>Passive only<br>Weak = 3<br>Paralyzed = 4 | 1 | | | | | | | | | | | | | | | | |
| G. SENSORY FUNCTIONS<br>Discriminates sharp/dull = 1<br>Decreased sensation = 2<br>Pins and needles = 3<br>Numb = 4 | 2 | | | | | | | | | | | | | | | | |
| H. COMPARED WITH LIKE TISSUES<br>Same = 1<br>Different = 2 (also place letter of check that differs) | D.E.G<br>2 | | | | | | | | | | | | | | | Dr. Taylor informed at 1:15 pm, orders given - see order book | S. Smith RN |

**Figure 11.18** Flow sheet for neurovascular checks.

## Evaluation

The patient:

- had temporary (due to acute trauma) but no permanent neurovascular compromise.
- regained normal motor and sensory functions following treatment, if possible.

# NURSING DIAGNOSIS

## *SELF-CARE DEFICIT IN HYGIENE AND GROOMING RELATED TO PATHOLOGY, BED POSITION, AND TRACTION*

### Assessment

1. Assess ability to do own ADL.
2. Assess needs for additional care.

### Expected Outcomes

The patient will:

- do own self-care.
- do own ADL after treatment.

## Nursing Interventions

1. Assist with bathing, hygienic care, and grooming as patient's condition requires.
2. Encourage self-care as the patient's condition permits and functions are regained.
3. Encourage use of cosmetics, shaving, and hair care to improve self-esteem.

## Evaluation

The patient:

- participated routinely in self-care hygiene and grooming.
- used own materials for personal care daily.
- did own ADL by discharge.

## NURSING DIAGNOSIS

## HIGH RISK FOR IMPAIRED SKIN INTEGRITY RELATED TO IMPOSED OR PROLONGED BED REST

## Assessment

1. Assess all skin surfaces and bony prominences.
2. Listen for patient's complaints of soreness, pain, numbness in dependent body areas.

## Expected Outcomes

The patient will:

- retain intact skin surfaces without decubitus development.
- assist with decubitus prevention by adjusting body positions within physical limitations of pathology and traction.

## Nursing Interventions

1. Explain purposes of positioning, lifting, and turning (if permitted) to aid circulation.
2. Check all skin surfaces for signs of pressure or impaired circulation.
3. Check for all pulses under elastic bandages; if pulse is not palpable, remove bandage immediately and palpate for return of pulse. If pulse

returns, reapply elastic bandage more loosely; if pulse does not return, notify physician.

4. Massage around skin pressure areas frequently, being careful not to massage directly over reddened areas (indicates beginning inflammation and disruption of capillaries—rubbing could cause further disruption).

5. Keep bed linens dry, wrinkle-free, and tightened.

6. Apply lotions to keep skin softened, and use lotions in bathwater to provide skin lubrication.

## Evaluation

The patient:

- retained all intact skin surfaces and circulation.
- developed no decubiti.

## NURSING DIAGNOSIS

### POTENTIAL FOR IMPAIRED GAS EXCHANGE RELATED TO IMPOSED BED REST

## Assessment

1. Assess bed position every 2–3 hours.
2. Assess respiratory rates, depth, breath sounds, cough, or chest pain every 2–4 hours.

## Expected Outcomes

The patient will:

- maintain adequate pulmonary perfusion and oxygenation.
- maintain optimal bed positions to aid pulmonary functions.
- use a respiratory aid every 2–3 hours.

## Nursing Interventions

1. Teach the patient about optimal bed positions, deep breathing exercises, and use of respiratory aid to facilitate pulmonary functions. Optimal position is Fowler's position, if not contraindicated, with the patient pulled up in bed, not down toward the foot of the bed.

2. Assist with deep breathing and coughing exercises every 4 hours.

3. Observe vital signs to pick up signs of inflammation or infection, such as tachypnea, tachycardia, fever, or productive cough.

4. Encourage use of respiratory aid or incentive spirometer every 4 hours to maintain pulmonary expansion.

5. Assist with ambulation when patient is allowed up to facilitate respiratory functions.

## Evaluation

The patient:

- maintained optimal bed position as permitted.
- maintained adequate pulmonary perfusion and oxygenation with normal hemoglobin levels.
- developed no pulmonary complications.
- used respiratory aid every 4 hours.

## NURSING DIAGNOSIS

### INADEQUATE NUTRITIONAL INTAKE, LESS THAN BODY REQUIREMENTS RELATED TO ANOREXIA AND INACTIVITY

## Assessment

1. Assess 24-hour intake.
2. Assess patient's food likes and dislikes.

## Expected Outcomes

The patient will:

- have sufficient intake of foods to maintain body requirements and normal weight.
- have activity and exercise regimens to increase appetite and retain weight.

## Nursing Interventions

1. Teach the patient about food groups, vitamins, and minerals for proper nutrition.
2. Assist the patient with menu selections of high biologic value foods, which contain essential amino acids for protein synthesis.

3.  Encourage intake of calories and foods from all food groups to maintain optimal weight, because bed rest leads to weight loss and negative nitrogen balance.

4.  Encourage intake of foods and fluids of patient's likes to maintain optimal systemic circulation and elimination.

5.  Check skin tissues for evidence of hydration; dryness, flaking, tenting are evidence of inadequate hydration.

6.  Check fluid intake every shift to note whether or not it is sufficient. Should have intake of 2500—3000 ml/24 hours.

7.  Encourage the patient to exercise muscles actively to stimulate appetite and lessen anorexia.

8.  Secure an order for nutritional supplements if weight loss, anorexia, or inadequate intake continues for longer than 2 weeks. Weight loss may continue even after appetite and intake markedly increase (related to lack of muscle activity, exercise, and bed rest).

## Evaluation

The patient:

*   regained appetite to achieve intake of foods and calories sufficient to begin regaining toward normal weight levels.
*   actively chose foods daily from the food groups for proper nutrition.
*   remained well-hydrated with normal output.

## NURSING DIAGNOSIS

*POTENTIAL IMPAIRED BOWEL ELIMINATION, CONSTIPATION AND IMPAIRED URINARY ELIMINATION, DECREASED URINARY OUTPUT, RELATED TO BED REST AND DECREASED FOOD INTAKE, BULK, OR FIBER OR DECREASED FLUID INTAKE*

## Assessment

1.  Assess fluid intake and output every shift.
2.  Assess 24-hour food intake.
3.  Assess menu selections.

## Expected Outcomes

The patient will:

- have a soft, formed stool at least every other day.
- select foods with bulk and fiber.
- have fluid intake to achieve urinary output of 30–50 ml/hour.

## Nursing Interventions

1. Assist patient with menu selections for bulk and fiber.
2. Measure intake and output every shift, and total for 24 hours. Intake should be 2500–3000 ml/24 hours to provide a 30–55 ml/hour urinary output.
3. Observe characteristics of urine for signs of infection, such as cloudy, malodorous urine, burning, urgency, or frequency.
4. Check bowel elimination for character and frequency of bowel movements, pain, diarrhea, or constipation.
5. Encourage increase in fluid and fiber intake if indicated by daily totals.
6. Encourage an acid ash diet (see Table 11.1) and foods lower in calcium and oxalate if indicated to decrease possibility of renal calculi. Bed rest and immobility cause calcium to be lost from bones, with possible subsequent development of renal calculi. Calcium intake must be sufficient to facilitate fracture healing if that is reason for traction and bed rest.

**Table 11.1** Foods High in Calcium and Oxalates, and Foods That Produce an Acid Ash

| Food | Amount | Calcium (mg) |
|---|---|---|
| Foods High in Calcium | | |
| Milk, whole (cow's) | 1 cup (8 oz) | 288 |
| Milk, skim (cow's) | 1 cup | 296 |
| Yogurt (whole milk) | 1 cup | 251 |
| Cottage cheese (creamed) | 1 oz. | 27 |
| Cheddar cheese | 1 oz. | 213 |
| Ice cream (10% fat) | 1 cup | 194 |
| Sardines (canned with bones) | 3 oz. | 372 |
| Kale (cooked) | 1 cup | 206 |
| Broccoli (cooked) | 1 cup | 136 |

**Table 11.1** (Continued)

| Food | Amount | Calcium (mg) |
|---|---|---|
| *Foods High in Oxalic Acid (Oxalates)* | | |
| Chocolate | | |
| Dandelions | | |
| Mustard greens | | |
| Rhubarb | | |
| Spinach | | |
| Swiss chard | | |
| *Foods That Produce an Acid Ash* | | |
| Red meats | | |
| Whole grains | | |
| Cranberries and cranberry juice | | |
| Plums | | |
| Prunes and prune juice | | |
| Eggs | | |
| Cheese | | |

## Evaluation

The patient:

- selected foods high in bulk and fiber.
- had a soft, formed stool at least every other day.
- had 30–50 ml/hour urinary output.
- had no urinary tract infections.
- developed no renal calculi.

## NURSING DIAGNOSIS

### POTENTIAL DEFICIT IN DIVERSIONAL ACTIVITY RELATED TO BED REST AND CONFINED SITUATION

## Assessment

1. Assess patient's physical abilities or limitations.
2. Assess patient's concerns about being in traction.

## Expected Outcomes

The patient will:

- actively participate in diversional activities two to three times daily.
- pursue hobbies and personal interests.
- interact actively with relatives, friends, visitors, and others.

## Nursing Interventions

1. Provide active diversional activities to maintain muscle strength and joint functions.

2. Secure physical or occupational therapy consultation for additional exercises and diversional activities.

3. Encourage the patient to work with hobbies, personal interests, and meaningful activities related to employment.

4. Encourage the patient to interact with other patients and participate in games and other activities as able.

5. Encourage visits from family and friends to lessen feelings of isolation or confinement.

## Evaluation

The patient:

- actively pursued hobbies, personal interests, and meaningful activities two to three times daily.
- actively interacted with family, friends, and others.

## NURSING DIAGNOSIS

*ALTERATION IN BODY IMAGE, SELF-ESTEEM, ROLE PER-FORMANCE, AND SOCIALIZATION RELATED TO INJURY AND TRACTION*

## Assessment

1. Assess for patient's reactions or statements about being ill, in traction, or unable to do usual daily activities or employment.

2. Assess for feelings of sadness, depression, anxiety, or concerns about being able to walk again.

## Expected Outcomes

The patient will:

- regain a positive outlook, body image, and self-esteem following treatment.

## Nursing Interventions

1. Listen to the patient's expression of concerns regarding ability to return to customary roles, family expectations, employment, or health as evidence of outward or positive outlook.
2. Allow privacy to the patient and family for expression of concerns, feelings, and sexuality as evidence of esteem and human responses.
3. Offer praise for the patient's attempts to regain mobility and function as healing progresses and pain and muscle spasms are relieved to increase the patient's self-esteem.
4. Assist with participation of family members in patient's self-care, ambulation, and recovery activities.
5. Teach self-care techniques and provide home-care instructions to patient and family to increase confidence, safety and competence in self-care.

## Evaluation

The patient:

- regained a positive body image and self-esteem.
- became ambulatory and outward-looking following treatment.
- was able to do own self-care competently.

## COMPLICATIONS OF SKIN TRACTION

Generally, use of a specific kind of skin traction should lessen the patient's complaints and aid in the patient's return to health. However, at times traction may lead to some temporary "complications" or disabilities, including increased pain, muscle spasms, numbness, tingling, headache, decreased muscle strength, joint laxity and decreased ROM, and skin redness or irritation. With release or adjustment of the traction, each of the above symptoms should be relieved, and no long-term damage should result.

Longer-term complications include development of decubiti, posttraumatic arthritis, and permanent joint or muscle limitation of movements, which would require additional medical follow-up.

## SKELETAL TRACTION

The use of skeletal traction for long-term treatment of orthopaedic injuries has decreased in recent years because of changes in medical care, shorter hospitalizations, and reimbursement policies. Skeletal traction, once initiated, must be maintained over long periods to provide effective relief of muscle spasms and bone realignment and healing. Because of reimbursement policies brought about by diagnostic related groups (DRGs), the long-term hospitalization required for some types of skeletal traction is no longer feasible when other forms of treatment are available. However, some patients are still placed in balanced suspension skeletal traction because of the severity of their injuries; therefore nurses must understand that specific traction setup and functioning, plus other types of skeletal traction for safe care. Other types of skeletal traction include the use of skull tongs and skeletal Dunlop's. The use of tongs and associated nursing care is covered in neurological and neurosurgical texts and will not be incorporated in this text.

The principles of skeletal traction involve the fact that the traction, once instituted, must always be maintained continuously. Weights cannot be lifted or removed, as severe muscle contractions could occur. Such sudden release of weight and the resulting muscle contractions could increase the displacement of the fracture fragments and could also cause rupture or trauma to contiguous nerves, arteries, or veins. Skeletal traction also requires heavier weights to overcome the muscle spasms in the injured tissues. The heavier weight can be used because skeletal traction is applied directly to the involved bone, by means of a strong nail or pin, and not just to the skin, as in types of skin traction. Finally, skeletal traction usually remains in place for periods longer than with skin traction because of the severity of the injury and the amount of muscle spasm, displacement, or other conditions necessitating its use.

The types of skeletal traction included in this chapter are balanced suspension to the femur and skeletal Dunlop's. Discussion of the care of patients in external fixators is also included in this chapter.

## Procedures

## APPLICATION OF SKELETAL TRACTION

### Materials Needed for All Types of Skeletal Traction

- bed with additional metallic frame and side bars
- rope on a roll
- pulleys

- weights and weight holders (have 1, 2, and 5 lb weights available)
- sterile tray with equipment for insertion of particular kind of skeletal pin or wire (tray has towels, syringes, needles, local anesthetic, skin prep materials, knife with blade, and pins or nails of several sizes)
- razor—if area is excessively hairy

In addition to the materials given above, also needed for balanced suspension skeletal traction:

- splint—a Thomas, Harris, or other, covered with sheepskin or stockinette enclosing felt pads to support the thigh (Fig. 11.19)
- Pearson attachment, also with covered felt pads
- foot support—to be applied to Pearson attachment

Some types of skeletal traction may be applied in the operating suite during surgical reduction. Special trays contain the materials needed for initiation of skeletal traction when applied in surgery or on the nursing unit. External fixation devices are applied in the operating suite.

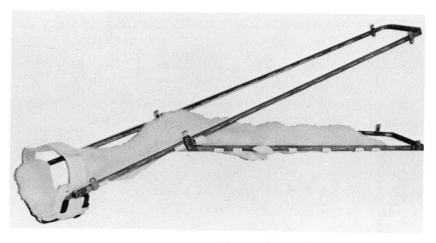

**Figure 11.19** *Thomas splint and Pearson attachment.*

## Procedures

### *APPLICATION OF KIRSCHNER WIRE OR STEINMANN PIN FOR BALANCED SUSPENSION SKELETAL TRACTION (BSST)*

(May be done in operating suite or on nursing unit. See Fig. 11.20 for comparison of wire and pin.)

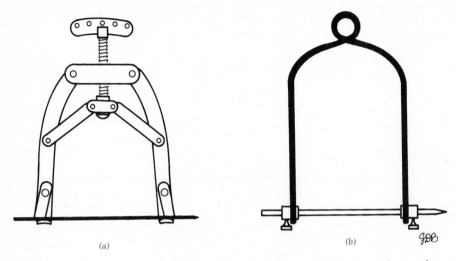

*(a)*          *(b)*

**Figure 11.20** (a) Kirschner wire and spreader. (b) Steinmann pin and spreader.

The physician (and assistants):

- prepares the skin surfaces for pin insertion by thorough cleansing with antiseptic solutions.
- covers the prepared sites with sterile drapes and places sterile drapes on the bed surface for sterile supplies.
- infiltrates pin insertion and exit sites with local anesthetic.
- makes small skin incision for easier wire (pin) insertion.
- inserts the desired pin or wire into and through the bone, usually the upper tibia, and out the exit site. The pin is inserted by drilling through the bone slowly to avoid excessive loss of bone cells. Heat of drilling also causes some loss of bone cells and necrosis.
- attaches the appropriate spreader bar or Kirschner attachment to the protruding ends of the pin or wire and tightens it.
- applies small amount of antiseptic or antibiotic ointment to the pin's entrance and exit sites. The sites may then be left uncovered or a small, sterile dressing may be applied.
- places the limbs in the Harris or Thomas splint and Pearson attachment.
- secures one end of the rope tightly to the Kirschner spreader (or similar spreader), then threads the rope over a pulley on the bed frame, and ties the opposite end to a weight holder.
- ties rope pieces to the ends of the Pearson attachment then to the end of the Harris or Thomas splint, threads the rope over another pulley at the end of the bed, and ties the end of the rope to another weight holder.

- slowly applies desired weights to the weight holder attached to the rope of the traction spreader bar.

- applies weights to the holder attached to the splint and Pearson attachment to suspend the thigh and leg.

For countertraction:

- Attach more rope to the upper portions of the Harris or Thomas splint at the groin area, then thread the rope through a separate pulley, and to another weight holder with weight to equal the weight used for the thigh/leg suspension. Countertraction "balances" the suspension, thus the name.

The skeletal traction is now established. The patient's position is adjusted as needed for comfort and traction requirements. The head of the bed may be raised approximately 30–45° only to assist the patient's efforts to maintain the optimal position in bed (see Fig. 11.21).

Insertion of the wire or pin for skeletal Dunlop's is also done aseptically and is also similar to those previously described (see Fig. 11.22).

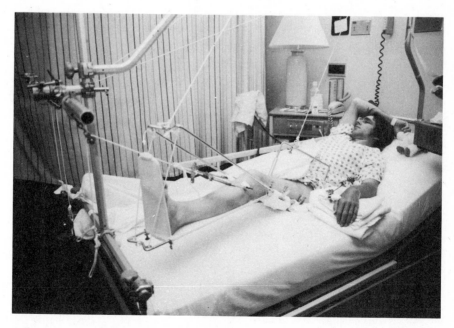

**Figure 11.21** *Balanced suspension skeletal traction to the femur. This patient also has an external fixation device to the left forearm.*

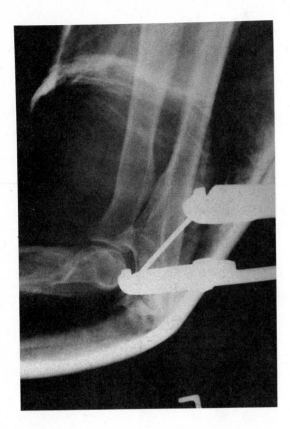

**Figure 11.22** Skeletal Dunlop's to the distal humerus.

Skeletal traction can be applied to many bones of the body including skull, facial, jaw, rib, pelvic, and upper and lower extremities. The patient's specific injury usually dictates which type and weights to apply.

## APPLICATION OF EXTERNAL FIXATION DEVICES

Figs.11.23 and 11.24 show the Hoffman apparatus external fixation device. This apparatus has various sizes and numbers of pins inserted into and through the bone to the fixator frames on both sides of the limb. Insertion of the pins is done aseptically and similarly to either a Kirschner wire or Steinmann pin. Figs. 11.25 and 11.26 show other external fixators.

Nursing observations and care of persons in skeletal traction or an external fixator must include those nursing diagnoses and interventions presented in the section on skin traction in this chapter (see pp. 296–309 for the major nursing considerations). However, additional nursing measures must be performed for the care of patients in skeletal traction or in an external fixator.

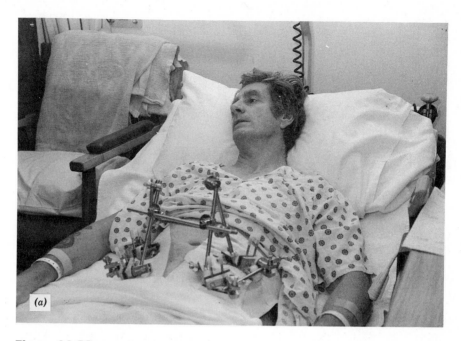

**Figure 11.23** (a) Multiple Hoffman external fixation devices to immobilize bilateral fractures of the pelvis.

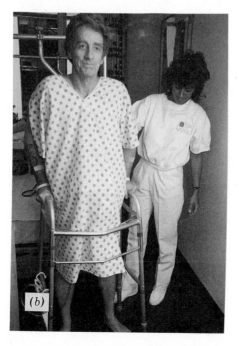

**Figure 11.23** (b) Same patient ambulating the day after application of the device.

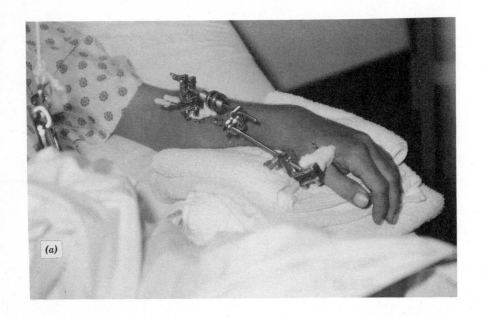

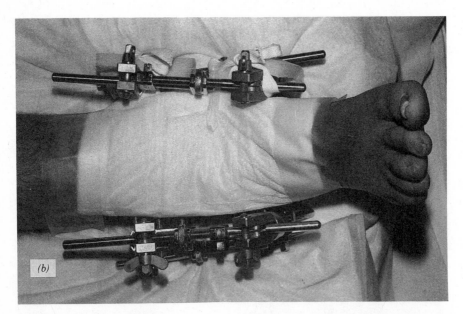

**Figure 11.24** (a) Hoffman external fixation device to the forearm, and (b) to the tibia and fibula.

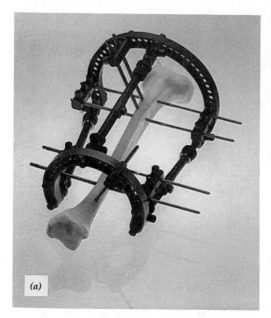

(a)

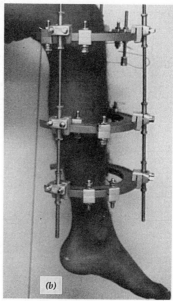

(b)

**Figure 11.25** (a) Ace-Fischer external fixator. (b) Monticelli-Spinelli external fixator.

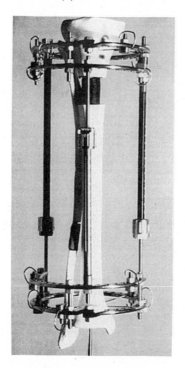

**Figure 11.26** Ilizarov external fixator.

## NURSING CONSIDERATIONS FOLLOWING APPLICATION OF SKELETAL TRACTION

### NURSING DIAGNOSIS

*ACTUAL INJURY TO MUSCULOSKELETAL TISSUES RELATED TO TRAUMA AND SKELETAL TRACTION*

#### Assessment

1. Assess the patient's overall health state and health history.
2. Assess vital signs.
3. Assess specific tissues to be placed in traction for presence of soft tissue trauma, open areas, edema, bruises, rash, bleeding sites, color, amount of hair at site, and for bone fragments in open fractures.
4. Assess patient's knowledge or understanding of the traction and compliance requirements.
5. Assess the patient's current laboratory data.

#### Expected Outcomes

The patient will:
- be relieved of pain, muscle spasms, and local trauma by the skeletal traction.
- achieve bone union at the fracture site(s).
- regain musculoskeletal functions with minimal discomfort or limitation of movement(s).
- maintain adequate functions of unaffected tissues.
- regain full mobility over time.
- experience no complications from the use of skeletal traction.
- return to usual family, social, and community roles and responsibilities.

#### Nursing Interventions

1. Do neurovascular checks as ordered (usually, order is for every hour for 8–24 hours, then every 2 hours, depending on findings). When doing checks, note severity of edema, bruises, ecchymosis, complaints of increasing pain, numbness, or tingling, which may indicate developing compartment syndrome discussed on p. 470.

2.  Measure thighs and legs (or upper arms and forearms) for amount of and increasing edema (a 1-inch increase in circumference indicates loss of one unit of blood into the tissues).

3.  Apply ice bags to lateral surfaces of injured tissues—avoid placing ice bags over arterial areas, which could lessen arterial flow from the pressure of the bag.

4.  Assist with ankle movements, including dorsiflexion, plantarflexion (see Fig. 11.27), inversion, and eversion, plus (when trauma subsides) encourage "quad" setting exercises to relieve inflammatory conditions. Similar exercises should be done for the upper extremities. Exercises should be performed bilaterally every 2–4 hours when the patient is able to do the exercises.

## Evaluation

The patient:

*   regained satisfactory neurovascular functions.
*   had resolution of the inflammatory effects of the trauma.
*   performed ROM and muscle-setting exercises every 2–4 hours.
*   did not develop infection or compartment syndrome.

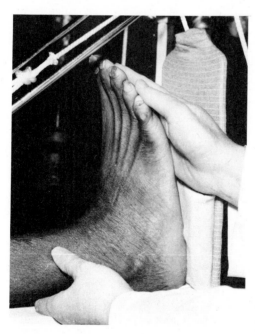

**Figure 11.27** *Assisting a patient with dorsiflexion and plantarflexion exercises.*

# NURSING DIAGNOSIS

## POTENTIAL INJURY RELATED TO THE PRESENCE OF SKELETAL PINS AND TRACTION

### Assessment

1. Assess pin entrance and exit sites twice daily.
2. Assess skin areas contiguous to pin entrance and exit sites.

### Expected Outcomes

The patient will:

1. experience no pin necrosis or infection.
2. have only minimal serous drainage from pin sites.

### Nursing Interventions

1. Monitor pin entrance and exit sites for type, amount, and increase in drainage as signs of resolution or increase in inflammation, infection, or pin necrosis. Pin necrosis is the loss of bone cells caused by the heat and process of drilling through the bone as the skeletal pin or wire is inserted. Some scant serosanguineous drainage is normal in the first 5–7 days following insertion of the wire; occasionally, there may be scant serous drainage for the time the pin or pins are in place (see Fig. 11.28a, b, c.)

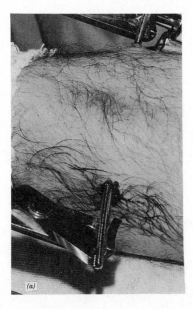

(a)

**Figure 11.28** (a) Serosanguineous drainage from a skeletal pin site.

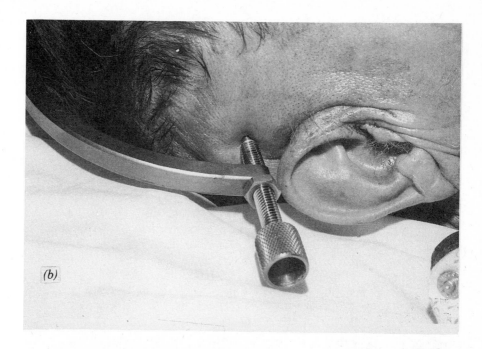

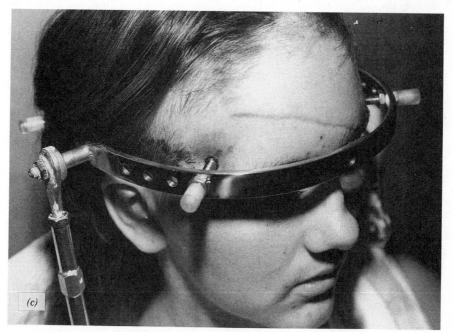

**Figure 11.28** (b) Clean pin site with no drainage. (c) Serosanguineous drainage from a halo pin site.

2. Perform pin site care according to physician's orders and institutional policies. Care of the site varies, but may include several of the following steps:

   a. Cleansing the skin openings around the pin sites with hydrogen peroxide, or mixture of equal amounts of hydrogen peroxide and normal saline, on sterile applicators either once or twice daily.

   b. Allowing the secretions to loosen for 15–20 minutes.

   c. Cleansing and removing the peroxide and secretions with other sterile applicators. Gentle, rolling motions when cleansing avoids traumatizing the epithelium at the sites.

   d. Drying the skin areas gently but thoroughly. No other care may be required.

   Additionally, policies or orders may require that nursing personnel:

   e. Apply a small amount of an antiseptic ointment to the skin around the pin. Commonly used ointments are povidone-iodine and bacitracin-neomycin. Avoid putting ointment into skin-pin openings which would prevent cell "breathing" and could block drainage. Also avoid getting povidone-iodine ointment on the pin or wire itself, because this may cause corrosion and weakening of some kinds of skeletal pins.

   f. Apply a small, dry, sterile dressing at the pin sites if ordered. Most pin sites are routinely left undressed except for the ointment.

   g. Another kind of pin-site care involves cleansing the pin site after insertion of the pins, then wrapping the sites with sterile Kerlex (stretch cling) gauze snugly to prevent movement of the skin on the pins. Sites are unwrapped every three days, checked, and rewrapped. Usually no further cleansing is required (see Fig. 11.29).

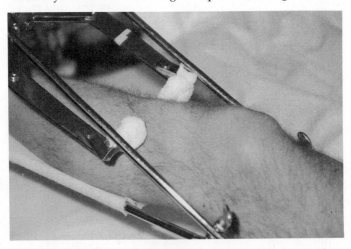

**Figure 11.29** Pin sites covered with stretch gauze for pin site care. The gauze pads are changed every three days. No other pin site care is given.

h. Repeat the pin site care every 4 hours initially (if large amount of drainage is present) or twice daily as required. *All* pin sites must be included in care, especially when multiple pins are present.

## Evaluation

The patient:

- developed no pin site infections.
- had minimal serous drainage from pin sites.

## NURSING DIAGNOSIS

### ALTERATION IN COMFORT RELATED TO ACUTE PAIN, INJURY, OR MUSCLE SPASMS

## Assessment

1. Assess the type, amount, and severity of the patient's pain.
2. Assess the frequency and severity of muscle spasms.

## Expected Outcomes

The patient will:

- experience pain relief with narcotics, muscle relaxants and analgesic administration.
- have relief of muscle spasms in one to three days.

## Nursing Interventions

1. Administer narcotic analgesics with or without potentiator medication (hydroxyzine [Vistaril] is commonly used as a narcotic potentiator) every 3–4 hours "around the clock" during first week of traction. Administering narcotics on an as-needed basis only may allow pain to become so severe that it is not sufficiently relieved by the as-needed medication. Having set times for administering narcotic analgesics relieves the patient of the "clock watching" necessity and conserves energy for the recovery processes.

2. Encourage the patient to use the trapeze and the "post" position to shift self to more comfortable positions to relieve pressure on posterior tissues. The post position involves placing the uninjured foot firmly on the bed with the knee bent, then grasping the trapeze and lifting the body upward. The traction is not disturbed when the patient lifts self.

3. Instruct the patient and family members to avoid rubbing the injured tissues to ease muscle spasms. Rubbing could dislodge clots and could possibly increase trauma in the injury site.

4. As the inflammation of the injured tissues resolves and the patient's comfort increases, administer muscle relaxant and nonnarcotic analgesics to relieve pain and discomfort. Dosages of aspirin, 600–1000 mg, are commonly given every 4 hours during the day as an analgesic, anti-inflammatory, and anticoagulant medication. Aspirin can also be administered early in the injury period between narcotic administrations to enhance pain relief, lessen inflammation, and lessen possibility of emboli.

## Evaluation

The patient had:

- relief of acute pain with medications.

- muscle spasms reduced, then absent, following medications and traction.

- bone realignment and was progressing toward bone union following treatment.

## NURSING DIAGNOSIS

## POTENTIAL FOR IMPAIRED GAS EXCHANGE RELATED TO PULMONARY OR FAT EMBOLI

## Assessment

1. Assess respiratory rate and depth, breath sounds, cough, and sputum production.

2. Assess skin color changes.

3. Assess for presence of petechial rash.

4. Assess for pain in posterior part of calf.

5. Assess for Homan's sign.

## Expected Outcomes

The patient will:

- have adequate pulmonary functions, perfusion, and oxygenation.

- not experience fat or pulmonary embolization.

## Nursing Interventions

1. Monitor the patient carefully in the initial 24–72 hours postinjury for respiratory and other changes the could signify fat embolization. Symptoms include changes in respiratory rates and depth, pain in the chest, changes in the sensorium, feelings of anxiety or danger, blood pressure and pulse changes (pressure drops and pulse increases). A fine petechial rash over the upper chest, neck, and eyelids or conjunctivativae is pathognomonic of fat embolism (see Table 11.2 for treatments).

2. Monitor the patient for sudden chest pain, dyspnea, tachycardia, and blood pressure drops that may follow pain in the calf (usually occurring 10–14 days after the trauma), which may signify pulmonary embolism secondary to thrombophlebitis. Treatments are given in Table 11.2.

**Table 11.2** Comparisons of Fat and Pulmonary Emboli

|  | **Fat Emboli** | **Pulmonary Emboli** |
|---|---|---|
| Pathophysiology | Emboli develop as a result of release of fat molecules from marrow of fractured long bones into bloodstream or from chemical changes in the blood following trauma. There may be multiple microemboli or large emboli that obstruct pulmonary circulation and circulation in other organs. | Emboli develop secondary to thrombophlebitis. They become dislodged, travel in the bloodstream through the heart, and become lodged in the pulmonary circulation, causing obstruction. |
| Occurrence | Most frequently 1–3 days after a long-bone fracture but can also occur at later periods. | Frequently 7–10 days after trauma or development of thrombophlebitis, though can occur weeks or months later. |
| Signs/Symptoms | Sudden development of shortness of breath and dyspnea, changes in mental alertness, confusion, sense of danger, tachycardia, tachypnea, chest pain, drop in blood pressure and appearance of fine, | Same as for fat emboli, except for rash. |

(continued)

**Table 11.2** (Continued)

| | Fat Emboli | Pulmonary Emboli |
|---|---|---|
| Signs/Symptoms (continued) | petechial rash from nipple line on chest, up to neck, and on eyelids or conjunctivae, pallor or cyanosis. | |
| Diagnosis | History of long bone fracture; physical examination with presence of petechiae over chest, neck, and conjunctivae; chest x-ray; arterial blood gases (pa $O_2$ below 60 mm Hg). | History of thrombophlebitis; physical examination; arterial blood gases; complete blood count with differential; ventilation and perfusion scans; chest x-ray; pulmonary angiography. |
| Treatments | Bed rest; $O_2$ therapy; mechanical ventilation, if needed; external hypothermia, if hyperpyrexic; administration of steroids; heparin therapy; intravenous alcohol; administration of antibiotics; intravenous albumin; intravenous hypertonic glucose with insulin coverage. | Bed rest; $O_2$ therapy; intravenous heparin therapy; antibiotic administration; long-term administration of anticoagulant medications. |

3. Assist the patient with deep breathing exercises every 4 hours, plus using respiratory aid every 4 hours.

4. Monitor the patient's temperature readings for possible pulmonary complications; note color and increase in sputum as evidence of pulmonary infections.

5. Help the patient to maintain head of bed in low or flat positions to allow greatest lung expansion and peripheral circulation. Low lying positions do not alter the traction's effectiveness and aid in countertraction.

6. Assist the patient to dorsiflex and plantarflex the feet and ankles to increase venous flow and lessen stasis.

7. Check for presence of Homan's sign (see p. 389 for explanation).

## Evaluation

The patient:

- developed no fat or pulmonary emboli.
- maintained adequate perfusion, oxygenation, and normal skin color.
- performed ankle and foot exercises every 4 hours.

## NURSING DIAGNOSIS

### IMPAIRED PHYSICAL MOBILITY RELATED TO THE SKELETAL TRACTION AND BED REST

### Assessment

1. Assess the patient's muscle strength or limitations.
2. Assess the patient's skin surfaces for condition, breaks, redness, or pressure areas.

### Expected Outcomes

The patient will:

- regain preinjury musculoskeletal functions following treatment.
- regain mobility and ambulation following fracture healing.

### Nursing Interventions

1. Consult occupational and physical therapy for activities to maintain the patient's functions in unaffected tissues.
2. Assist the patient with *active* exercises, rather than passive activities to help maintain body weight and strength. Weight loss of 10 lb or more can occur if skeletal traction is in place for extended periods.
3. Maintain the patient's bed position and the skeletal traction in optimal functioning to lesson length of time for healing. Traction may be required for as long as 4–8 weeks or, currently, for lesser periods prior to surgical repair of the fractured bones.
4. Help the patient with ROM exercises to all joints to maintain strength and mobility.
5. Apply thromboembolic hose to leg(s) not in traction, if the patient is on bed rest, to prevent thrombophlebitis.

## Evaluation

The patient:

- regained muscle strength with exercises and therapy.
- regained mobility with an ambulatory aid until full healing occurred.
- performed ROM exercises every 4 hours.

## NURSING DIAGNOSIS

*SELF-CARE DEFICIT IN HYGIENE AND GROOMING; RISK OF IMPAIRED SKIN INTEGRITY RELATED TO IMPOSED BED REST AND SKELETAL TRACTION*

## Assessment

1. Assess the patient's ability or limitations in self-care.
2. Assess all skin surfaces and bony prominences.

## Expected Outcomes

The patient will:

- perform own self-care hygiene and grooming before discharge.
- maintain intact skin surfaces.

## Nursing Interventions

1. Assist the patient with bath and hygiene as needed.
2. Wash the patient's back and buttocks carefully and thoroughly; examine skin tissues for indications of pressure such as tender, sore areas, changes in skin color, reddened areas, and skin excoriation.
3. Massage the patient's back and buttocks several times daily to increase circulation to those tissues.
4. Apply moisturizing lotions to the patient's elbows and heels to prevent excoriation and pressure areas. Use protective padding as necessary under heels, elbows, and buttocks.
5. Assist the patient with oral hygiene and other grooming activities; teach self-care within limitations.
6. Cleanse the patient's perineal area and check the groin areas and genitalia for evidence of pressure from the Harris or Thomas splint.
7. Apply talcum powder or cornstarch to the back and buttocks to lessen friction when moving the patient up in bed.

8. Assist the patient to lift self off mattress every 1–2 hours to lessen pressure on tissues from the treatment-imposed back-lying position.

9. Change bed linens when damp, and keep linens free of crumbs and wrinkles.

10. Gently assist the patient's efforts to move self up in bed to avoid shearing forces that could disrupt skin surfaces and cause capillary rupture. High Fowler's position increases shearing force, because this position causes the patient to slide down in bed more often.

11. Apply "egg crate," lamb's wool pads, and other padding under bed linens or under the patient to lessen pressure on bony prominences.

12. Secure the side rails in up position to prevent accidental injury to the patient from loss of balance or fall from bed.

### Evaluation

The patient:

• performed own self-care and grooming by time of discharge.

• developed no skin lesions or decubiti.

All the previously mentioned nursing care of patients in various types of skin traction for maintenance of nutrition, elimination, rest and sleep, body image and self-esteem, and diversion also apply to the care of patient in a particular type of skeletal traction.

## Procedures

### CHECKING SKELETAL TRACTION

Maintenance of properly functioning skeletal traction requires that the nurse makes regular "rounds" to:

• Check all ropes, knots, pulleys, freedom of movement, and intactness.

• Check the weights to note that they are free-hanging and not in danger of being "caught" during position changes.

• Make certain that weights are not "lifted" during care. Lifting the weights would release the traction and could cause muscles to contract suddenly. The subsequent shortening would cause disruption of the fragments of the fractured bone. When in skeletal traction, patients should be pulled up to have position changes without the weights being lifted or released.

• Take care not to bump the weights, which could cause pain to the patient by the unnecessary movement of the rope reflected back to the pin.

- Check the entire traction setup, pin site, and all suspension apparatus for tightness or signs of loosening.

- Check all skin surfaces for signs of tolerance or beginning pressure areas.

- Provide for psychological comfort, as well as physical comfort, including answering questions honestly (or having them answered by appropriate person), answering the call light promptly, providing prompt and thorough care, encouraging self-participation as possible, providing diversionary activities, and preparing the patient and family for discharge through discharge planning and teaching.

## COMPLICATIONS OF SKELETAL TRACTION

Infection is an ever-present risk of patients in skeletal traction or external fixators, because of the multiple skin openings. Infection may delay or at times prevent the patient's regaining full recovery. Infection can be superficial or extend to the bone with the ultimate development of osteomyelitis.

Nonunion is also a possibility with skeletal traction and may result from local tissue factors having nothing to do with the treatment. Excessive weight, leading to distraction (separation) of the fracture fragments, also could cause nonunion. Delayed or malunion are also possibilities.

Other complications include posttraumatic arthritis, muscle or nerve weakness, and development of decubiti. Complications that may be secondary to the injury or the imposed bed rest include thrombophlebitis, pulmonary and/or fat embolism, and pneumonia. Hemorrhage and even exsanguination can occur with some severe or multiple fractures. Many major complications are discussed in Chapter 14.

## DISCHARGE PLANNING AND TEACHING

Patients in most forms of skeletal traction must remain hospitalized while the traction is in place. Several exceptions to that situation include those persons with external fixators, those with two Steinmann pins or Kirschner wires through an extremity held in place with a cast, and those in a halo or four-poster traction.

Patients who are discharged in skeletal traction or an external fixator must have oral and written instructions for self-care at home. Also, a family member or significant other should receive the instructions and teaching. Specific instructions on lifting or handling the part or parts in an external fixator should also be given in writing, and practiced by care givers when possible.

Included in the instructions and teaching should be procedures for pin-site care if pin openings are exposed or not encased in a cast. Site care should be done according to the particular physician's orders. The patient should also have written lists of signs or symptoms to report to the physician, including such things as loosening of the pins or wires; loosening of clamps holding pins; movement of one or more pins; beginning or increase in drainage, redness, soreness, or pain; elevated temperature at site of pin(s), or systemic fever; edema; malaise; anorexia; or other unexplainable symptoms. Instructions should also be given concerning diet, analgesic or antibiotic administration schedules, if ordered, exercises, and activities permitted. Prescriptions should be explained, including probable side effects of the medications. If pertinent, instructions for use of sedatives for sleep and laxatives should be discussed. The patient should have a card with the time and date of the next physician's visit if known. Any questions of the patient or relatives should be clarified before discharge. The patient should have a phone number of the physician or the nursing unit to contact if necessary. A continuity-of-care referral should be completed, with the community nurse notified of the patient's conditions and care needs.

## BIBLIOGRAPHY

Behrens, F. (1989). General theory and principles of external fixation. *Clinical Orthopaedics, 241*,15–23.

Ilizarov, G.A. (1989). The tension-stress on the genesis and growth of tissues. *Clinical Orthopaedics, 239*,263–285.

Katz, K., Maor, P., Mizrahi, J., Ross, S., & Seelenfreund, M. (1986). Constant inclined pelvic traction for treatment of low back pain. *Orthopaedic Review, 15*(8),540–545.

Kim, M.J., McFarland, G.K., & McLane, A.M. (1991). *Pocket guide to nursing diagnoses* (3rd ed.). St. Louis: Mosby-Yearbook.

Mears, D.C., & Rubash, H.E. (1986). *Pelvis and acetabular fractures.* Thorofare, NJ: Slack.

Mourad, L. (1991). *Orthopedic disorders.* St. Louis: Mosby-Yearbook.

Rand, J.A. (1987). Failed total knee arthroplasty treated by arthrodesis of the knee using the Ace-Fischer apparatus. *Journal of Bone & Joint Surgery, 69A*(1),39–45.

Rang, M., Moseley, C.F., Roberts, J.M., Wenger, D.R., & Wilkins, K.E. (1989). Management of displaced supracondylar fractures of the humerus (Symposium). *Contemporary Orthopaedics,18*(4),497–535.

Renshaw, T.S. (1986). *Pediatric orthopedics.* Philadelphia: Saunders.

Rockwood, C.A., Jr., & Grun, D.P. (1984). *Fractures in adults* (Vols. 1, 2) (2nd ed.). Philadelphia: Lippincott.

# 12

# NURSING PROCESS FOR PATIENTS HAVING ORTHOPAEDIC SURGERY

Great strides have been made in orthopaedics since its development as a specialty in 1922; many advances were in surgery. Medical, engineering, and pharmaceutical discoveries have all contributed to these advancements. Some of these include the use of the Smith-Peterson nail for hip fractures in 1929, the discovery of penicillin in 1929, the perfection of vitallium and stainless steel nonreactive metals for internal use in 1929, and the introduction and use of sulfonamide drugs such as Prontosil and Neoprontosil in 1930. Other developments such as knee and hip bracing, improved products for wound care, including therapeutic beds, and the use of external fixators which give access to wounds have all made important contributions to healing orthopaedic problems. The length of stay in hospitals has decreased in many cases to 3 to 6 days from 2 to 3 weeks because of the above improvements as well as the greater technical skills of orthopaedic surgeons.

Surgical advances that have influenced orthopaedic surgical techniques include the use of artificial (synthetic) suture materials that are absorbent and cause less inflammation; refinements in anesthetic agents and techniques of administration to decrease the shock of surgery; development of "bloodless" tourniquet techniques; development of respiratory therapy regimens to lessen postoperative pulmonary complications; development of newer antibiotics; development of immunotherapy to permit use of homologous and cadaver bones for bone allografts; and transfusions.

Orthopaedic health care procedures have changed in the last five years because of the technologic advancements just mentioned. The emergence and spread of the acquired immunodeficiency syndrome disease (AIDS) has also caused great changes in health care precautions and promotion of surgical techniques, such as use of the "scope" to minimize invasion of the tissue and therefore minimize blood loss, and development of alternatives to homologous banked blood transfusions. These alternatives to using banked blood include new devices and methods to collect and reinfuse blood intraoperatively, autologous blood transfusion, hypotensive anesthesia, hemodilution, and use of plasma expanders. AIDS, as well as hepatitis non-A and non-B, has also caused hospitals and health care workers to adopt guidelines of universal precautions to prevent further spread. (See appendix for universal precautions as given by the Centers for Disease Control in Atlanta.).

Although blood banks have minimized the risk of receiving HIV-infected blood, the occurrence is 1 in 100,000 and the risk, however small, still exists. To eliminate this risk, the patient now is advised to collect one or more units of his/her own blood prior to surgery. This is called autologous blood donation. Autologous red blood cells may be stored with an additive solution such as Kt at 4°C for 42 days. Therefore the patient should donate blood at least two weeks before surgery to allow sufficient time for recuperation of red blood cells. The patient may also take an iron preparation to increase the formation of red cells prior to surgery. The red blood cells can also be preserved through freezing for months or years. However, the process of freezing and thawing can destroy many of the red blood cells and can be costly.

A patient may also ask a significant other to donate blood; this is called directed donation. However, the patient is most safe when donating his own blood. This autologous blood is then transported to the surgery center and given to the patient, if needed, intra- or postoperatively.

Procedures such as hip and knee arthroplasty and spine surgery in which a patient may lose 2 or more units of blood have also increased the use of blood saving and reinfusion devices. There are several different types of devices on the market that aid the patient by collecting blood intraoperatively, washing cells, then filtering and transfusing this blood back to the patient. These Cell Savers are very useful in surgeries that require 3 or more units of blood replacement. The main disadvantages to using the Cell Savers are expensive setup charges, especially if the hospital does not have the machinery and independent companies are contracted for these services, and the possible damage or loss of coagulation factors and platelets through the filtration process. Other systems collect postoperative blood in a closed drainage system and this blood is then filtered and reinfused.

Autotransfusion is a system used for reinfusion of collected blood (see Fig. 12.1). Such a system uses a wound drain connected to a collection canister by a Y connector. The drainage tube also has a one-way antireflux valve and micron prefilter. Postoperative blood drainage is collected in a sterile, disposable 500-cc bag encased in a rigid canister. The blood bag is kept open by a vacuum inside the rigid plastic shell. Nursing care of this bag includes positioning of the bag below the level of the wound and recording the beginning of collection on the bag. The nurse should also observe the tubing

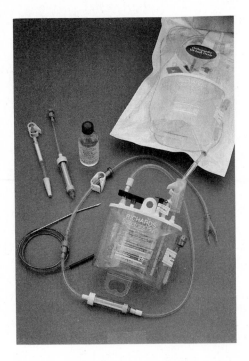

**Figure 12.1** Solcotrans plus orthopaedic drainage/reinfusion system. (Courtesy of Solco Basle Inc.)

for continued drainage or clotting occurring within the tube. The system also has an injection port available for injection of the anticoagulant ACD-A (Anticoagulant Citrate Dextrose, HIH formula A). If this is to be injected, it will be ordered by the physician. Some physicians find that injection of this substance is not necessary if drainage is moderate to heavy. Following collection, the drainage canister is inverted and the blood reinfused through standard blood infusion administration tubing. Directions for use of this or any other reinfusion device should be thoroughly understood before using and manufacturer recommendations and precautions followed. Universal precautions should also be used when working with the blood and blood collection systems.

The blood collected for reinfusion was assessed by Gray and Valerit for viability and function of red blood cells. The blood was collected intraoperatively on dogs and reinfused. The survival rate of red blood cells was 90% of normal and the lifespan and oxygen-transport function of the red blood cells were normal. In addition, hemolysis was minimal.

Side effects or complications of reinfusion devices are minimal but can include fat embolism, sepsis, and febrile reactions; however, the risk of hepatitis and AIDS is eliminated. To reduce the possibility of febrile reactions a study by Faris and Ritter recommends reinfusion of blood within 6 hours or less. The study determined that there was only 2% reaction if reinfusion occurred within 6 hours compared to 22% after 6 hours.

It is reasonable to expect that blood-saving devices and reinfusion will continue, especially for hip and knee arthroplasties and spine surgery. These devices will continue to play an important part in the care of the orthopaedic patient.

Orthopaedic surgery can provide many benefits for the patient including the repair of injured tissues, the restoration of musculoskeletal anatomy, the removal of products of inflammation or infection, increase in joint motion, decrease in pain secondary to surgical repair, and the resection and removal of nonfunctional or harmful tissues such as tumors or cysts. Orthopaedic surgery does carry some inherent risks, such as inadvertent fracturing of bones, hemorrhage, shock, and infection. Fat or pulmonary embolization and, at times, death can also follow orthopaedic surgical procedures. Benefits and risks are discussed with the patient during the preoperative "informed consent" session. Considerations are also given and discussed, comparing the proposed surgery with nonsurgical methods to treat the patient's condition when feasible. Results of diagnostic examinations are also discussed with the patient and family, because the findings influence the choice of treatment options.

Surgical advances have contributed to a high degree of knowledge and complexity of treatment of various disorders. This has led to specialization of orthopaedic surgeons into subspecialties such as hand surgery, joint replacement, and spinal surgery. These subspecialists then concentrate their knowledge and technical skills on problems or disorders of limited body areas.

## PREOPERATIVE ASSESSMENT, PATIENT PREPARATION, AND EDUCATION

### Assessment

Physiologic data are obtained, including vital signs and weight (if it can be obtained without harm to the patient), and neurovascular assessments of the extremities. Pain, its type, duration, and quality are assessed, as is its radiation to other body areas. Pain with ambulation or bed rest is assessed, as are methods used to relieve the pain and the success of these methods. When there are complaints of numbness and tingling, the specific tissues and areas involved are assessed. Physiological reactions to the stress from trauma, hospitalization, or upcoming surgery are assessed, and psychological and personality characteristics are noted. Reactions indicative of anxiety include increased irritability, lack of concentration, lack of eye contact, inappropriate speech, and severe nervousness. Of course this behavior may differ according to cultural background.

The presence or absence of family supports are noted as they influence the patient's reactions and responses. Positive, supportive relationships help to stabilize the patient.

Preoperatively, the patient may express concerns about the effects of the surgery on his/her usual roles, employment, impact on family and friends, or other personal concerns such as sexuality, lifestyle impact, and body image. These concerns may foster feelings of loss or lack of control in the patient and markedly increase the patient's anxiety.

## Preoperative Relaxation Training

Assessment should also include determining the patient's need for preoperative relaxation training. Relaxation procedures assist in reducing the patient's stress reactions, lessen pain, and increase circulation and lung expansion, thereby increasing central and peripheral oxygenation. Relaxation techniques, once learned, help the patient feel more in control. Teaching the techniques to the patient need not take much nursing time, and the nurse does not need to be an expert in relaxation training, but does need the desire to help the patient learn to relax.

Relaxation techniques use principles of awareness and attention to one's internal cues or signs of stress as they influence the person's external responses. Becoming aware of and attending to the internal cues permit the person to choose responses that are not only more externally acceptable and effective, but also are less internally destructive. Therefore, relaxation techniques aid in adapting the person's response(s) to the immediate stressor, the threat, to make it become more manageable and acceptable. Learning to listen to one's internal cues can then enable one to become self-directed after initial teaching sessions.

Relaxation techniques are effective if they reduce the patient's tension and lessen the patient's pain. Concentrating on the relaxation steps—plus the additional oxygenation and perfusion—removes the noxious or painful stimuli to effect relaxation and pain relief. Thus, relaxation techniques reduce signs of tension, such as facial grimacing, rigid muscles in arms or legs, clenched fists, stiffening of the trunk, voice shrillness or tenseness, and rolling the head from side to side.

To begin relaxation training the nurse should close the patient's door for privacy and partially close the curtains if the room is very bright. Speaking in a calm, modulated voice, the nurse asks the patient to close the eyes and think of a past experience in which he or she felt the most relaxed, such as floating in water, lying in a field of grass, lying on a quiet beach, listening to soft music, or hearing leaves rustling gently or waves lapping on the shore. Some patients find it easier to keep the eyes open and concentrate on an object directly in front of the eyes (a focal point); and others may leave the mind blank, instead. The nurse asks the patient to breathe slowly and deeply and continue that breathing pattern.

The nurse then asks the patient to begin at the toes and feet and move up the body, relaxing each part consciously and completely before proceeding upward to the next part, thus, first the toes, feet, calves, thighs, and so on, to the spine. Suggest that the patient "sink into the bed" or "let your body ooze to the bed." Suggestions are continued to the chest, shoulders, arms, hands, and head, suggesting to open the fist, smooth forehead and facial wrinkles, let cheeks droop, let eyelids feel heavy or close, relax the mouth and lips, and let ears drop or relax. By now the nurse should be able to see a calmer, less tense person, and the patient should be able to express feeling more at ease, calmer, and in less pain.

The entire relaxation session takes no more than 5–10 minutes, yet the benefits last for hours or longer. The patient may need reassessment and reminding during subsequent nursing shifts.

Besides relaxation techniques, the nurse also teaches the patient deep breathing and coughing techniques to clear the lungs, and ankle plantarflexion and dorsiflexion to lessen venous stasis. Also preoperatively, the nurse clarifies the patient's understanding of the upcoming surgery; the postoperative recovery procedures; rehabilitation exercises; possible tubes, drains, or intravenous tubings; and the care of the surgical wound.

Additional preparations prior to surgery may include administering nothing by mouth, asking if the patient has had a bowel movement (a small enema or a suppository may be needed to assure emptying of the rectum), having the patient void, removing the patient's jewelry, and checking the vital signs and laboratory data. Some orthopaedic patients will have preoperative antibiotics administered intravenously and might receive preoperative medication to aid muscle relaxation and ease pain. The hair in the operative area may be removed prior to transfer into the operating room, and the patient's skin is thoroughly cleansed with a long-acting antiseptic prior to surgical draping for the operation.

## SPINAL SURGERY

The main indications for spinal surgery are:

- neurological impairment such as loss of bowel or bladder control
- loss of motor function
- progressive deformity impairing loss of function
- severe, intractable pain inhibiting the quality of life
- instability
- invasive tumors.

There are also bone conditions such as fractures, malalignment, and displacement that may cause sufficient problems to warrant spinal surgery. The type of procedure performed—whether it be resection, stabilization with instrumentation or bony fusion, or distraction with or without realignment and use of instrumentation—depends on the disorder or problem, life-style of the patient, patient age and medical condition, and physician preference (see Fig. 12.2a, b).

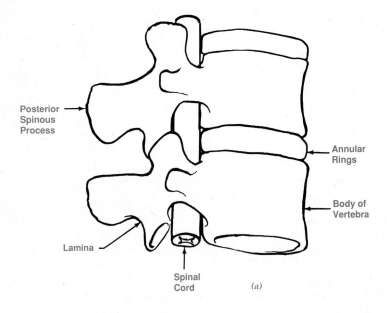

Posterior
Spinous
Process

Annular
Rings

Body of
Vertebra

Lamina

Spinal
Cord

*(a)*

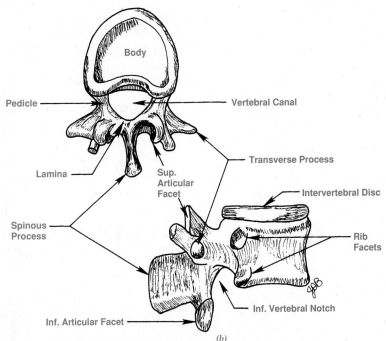

Body

Pedicle

Vertebral Canal

Lamina

Transverse Process

Sup.
Articular
Facet

Intervertebral Disc

Spinous
Process

Rib
Facets

Inf. Articular Facet

Inf. Vertebral Notch

*(b)*

**Figure 12.2** (a) Vertebrae showing annular rings between bodies of the vertebrae. Nuclear pulposus is inside annular rings. (b) Views of vertebrae showing vertebral processes, lamina, and canal for passage of spinal cord.

## Spinal Fusion with or without Instrumentation

Spinal fusion involves the fusing of two or more vertebrae to create a firm, unbending bond. Fusion may be performed using autogenous bone chips or metallic rods, screws, hooks, or plates to hold contiguous bones. Autogenous bone chips may be secured from the anterior or posterior iliac crests or from the tibia. These sites are chosen because the bones have a cancellous, spongy composition that is rich in blood cells, which provide the initial hematoma needed for healing, granulation, and calcium deposition.

The bone chips are placed between the spinous and transverse processes and along the laminar areas posteriorly or may be placed between the vertebral bodies and between the pedicles and transverse process when an anterior fusion is performed. The blood cells in the chips combine with the tissue fluids to form a hematoma. Fibrin then forms, and by way of the processes of healing, granulation, and calcification, the chips become fused with and to their vertebral surfaces, forming a stable bond.

Spinal fusions of the lumbar area may be performed by exposing the operative area from the anterior or posterior routes. Cervical fusions are usually performed anteriorly, however.

Metallic fusions may be created using rods, pedicle screws, or hooks, which are placed over the lamina or plates. The use of this instrumentation provides stability while the bony fusion heals, thereby permitting early ambulation and avoidance of the lengthy bed rest that normally accompanies a fusion without use of instrumentation. However, the use of metal may predispose to infection and loosening from bone resorption (see Figs. 12.3a, b).

Instrumentation is constantly being perfected with new approaches. One of the first developed was the Harrington rod, which was placed on either side of the spinous processes. The rods have hooks at the ends which are placed over the lamina (see Fig. 12.4). Occasionally they become dislodged, requiring further surgery to repair. To prevent or minimize dislodgement, Harrington rods are sometimes wired at each level of vertebra at the spinous process using Drummond or Wisconsin wires, which creates a combination of Harrington and Luque technique. The Luque system was developed in Mexico and provides more rigid fixation through use of sublaminar wires which are placed at each vertebral level and attached to a rod.

Cotrel-Dubousset (CD) (see Fig. 12.5) is a third-generation system of segmental instrumentation which allows manipulation at many levels to permit stability with maintenance of the normal curves, if desired. This system was introduced in 1985 in the United States following use in France. The main advantage of the CD is that the patient does not require postoperative immobilization. The placement of the CD rods, however, is time-consuming and the patient is exposed to a lengthy anesthesia time.

Revisions of the CD led to the development of the Texas Scottish Rite Hospital (TSRH) instrumentation system. TSRH rods are used with horizontal

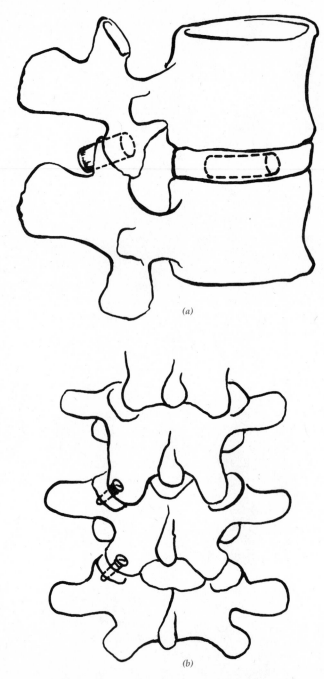

(a)

(b)

**Figure 12.3** (a) Bone grafts (dowels) used as spinal fusion materials. (b) Screws to fuse vertebrae together.

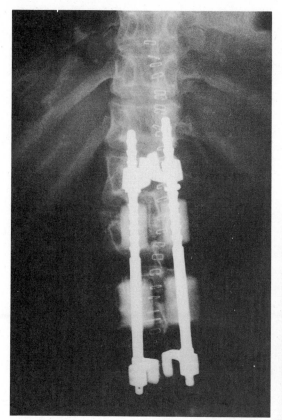

**Figure 12.4** Harrington rods with Edward's sleeves to align and immobilize the vertebrae following a burst fracture of the body of a lumbar vertebra.

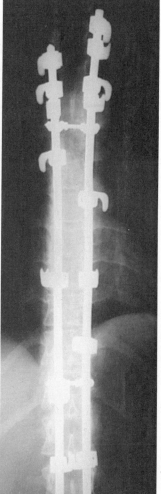

**Figure 12.5** Cotrel-Dubousset rods for scoliosis.

crosslink plates with eyebolt/lock nut rod attachment of hooks. The system is proposed to take less operative time and thereby reduces the lengthy anesthesia while providing a stronger fusion. Its greatest contribution is that it can be added to or changed if needed for spinal revisions.

Another method of fixation is the use of pedicle plates and screws (see Figs. 12.6a, b), which rigidly hold the problem areas of the spine during healing of the bone fusion. Without this rigidity the patient would be required to remain immobile until the fusion heals and the rate of pseudoarthrosis is considerably higher due to difficulty in maintaining bone immobility. This stability maintains alignment of the lumbar spine in fractures, tumors, multiple-level laminectomies, and spondylolisthesis. This has allowed early ambulation for the patient and increased the probability of fusion healing.

## Fractures

Spinal fusion with or without instrumentation may be done for spinal fractures. There are four major types of fractures of the spine: compression, burst, flexion-distraction, and fracture dislocation. The diagnosis of the type of fracture begins with a descriptive history of the mechanism of injury. The mechanism of injury usually proposes which type of fracture the patient may have suffered.

A burst fracture occurs from axial loading on the vertebral disc causing it to shatter into several pieces. Displacement of the bony fragments is usually anterior with the posterior column normally remaining intact. The mechanism of injury involves stress from the head or feet such as falling from a ladder and landing on the feet or a tremendous blow to the head.

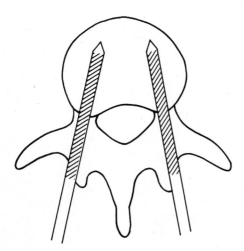

**Figure 12.6** (a) Pedicular screw fixation showing screws through the pedicle into the vertebral body.

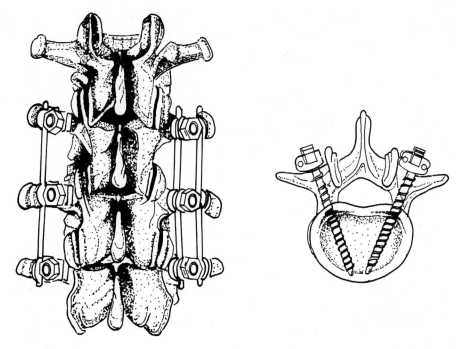

**Figure 12.6** (b) Wiltse system of pedicular screw fixation with screws placed through transverse processes into the pedicle.

A compression fracture (see Fig. 12.7) may occur from a fall, with the person landing on the buttocks, or a blow to the head. Flexion-distraction is normally caused by a seat-belt-type injury and a fracture dislocation from twisting.

A history is extremely important to not only aid in diagnosis but to also help propose the extent of injury. For example, questions regarding temporary dysthesia may indicate spinal cord compromise. A neurologic exam follows the history and an anterior posterior and lateral x-ray of the spine and spine CT is advised.

Treatment may be conservative and consist of bed rest for 1–12 weeks depending on the severity of injury. Bracing with a full-body jacket or cast for 3–6 months may be used. These options have risks of immobility that impact all systems such as deep vein thrombosis, pulmonary emboli, pneumonia, decubiti, constipation, and emotional stress, and therefore surgical intervention may be considered.

Surgical intervention goals include decompression of the neural canal and restoration and maintenance of the spinal column, relief of pain, and stability using instrumentation and fusion. Treatment of choice varies according to physician familiarity and preference of product line but may include instrumentation such as Harrington, Cotrel-Dubousset (CD), or the Texas Scottish

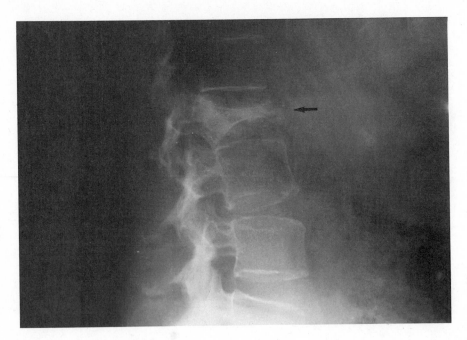

**Figure 12.7** Compression fracture of the spine.

Rite Hospital (TSRH) system. These systems use rods, hooks, and screws to stabilize and prevent further collapse by maintaining distraction. In addition, bone grafting done anteriorly or posteriorly provides spinal fusion.

## Spondylolisthesis

Spinal fusion may also be performed for persons with spondylolisthesis (see Fig. 12.8). "Spondylo" is derived from the Greek words meaning vertebra and "listhesis" means to slip or slide. The vertebra slips forward because of a defect or elongation of the pars articularis or deformity of both of the last lumbar vertebrae or upper part of the sacrum. (The pars is located in the region of the lamina where the lamina and pedicle meet and between the facets above and below the vertebra. See Fig. 12.8b.) This slip of bony structure can impinge upon nerve roots with neurologic symptoms of loss of sensation, weakness, loss or alteration of bowel or bladder function, and pain.

Spondylolisthesis can be identified on x-ray, with the lateral view being the best. The most common site is L4-5 in 80% of cases. However, the slip can also occur at L3-4 and L5-S1. Symptoms usually occur in the fifth to seventh decade of life and are more common in females. Symptoms include low back, buttock,

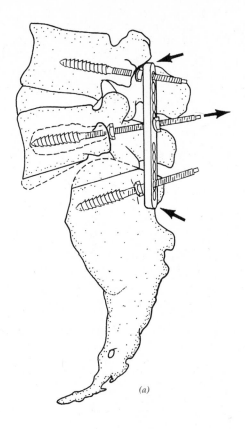

*(a)*

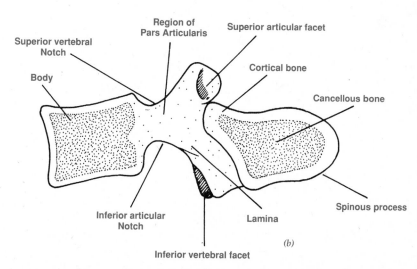

*(b)*

**Figure 12.8** Grade II–III spondylolisthesis of L5 on S1 with pedicular crew fixation.

and thigh pain, bilateral or unilateral radicular pain, and intermittent claudication typical of stenosis. The pain is increased when getting out of a chair or bed, straightening up after bending over, coughing, sneezing, or twisting. On examination there is increased pain to palpation of the facet joints, and the straight leg raise (SLR) may be limited. Also, the patient usually reports weakness and sensory loss along the L5 distribution with relief obtained from flexion, sitting or lying.

Conservative treatment may include bracing, the use of anti-inflammatory medications, physical therapy, and epidural or facet steroid injections. If conservative treatment fails, surgery will involve stabilization using instrumentation and fusion either anteriorly or posteriorly. Instrumentation that may be used includes the use of segmental plates and pedicle screws. This instrumentation is preferred to long rods because it limits the fixation to the area of deformity and provides stability with the pedicle screws. Anterior interbody fusion may also be used to provide increased stability with the posterior instrumentation. Surgery goals will include treatment of the disabling pain, increase of function, and limitation of neurological progression.

## Curve Exaggerations

A spinal fusion may also be done as a treatment for scoliosis (see Figs. 12.9 and 12.10), kyphosis, or severe lordosis. Scoliosis is a lateral curvature of the spine, which, if untreated surgically, may progress to such pronounced curvature and rotation that musculoskeletal, respiratory, cardiac, and circulatory complications may develop and compromise the patient's functioning. A patient with exaggerated curvature of the spine may experience pain, shortness of breath, decreased height or increased deformity, cosmetic deformity, or cardiopulmonary decompression.

A physical exam of a patient with scoliosis typically reveals an S-shaped lateral curvature of the spine, rib hump or exaggerated rib prominence unilaterally, asymmetry of shoulder height with one being higher than the other, particularly evident on bending over, and pelvic obliquity (one side of pelvis higher than other) when standing. The examination then involves curve assessment, the degree of compensation (degree of curvature of bending present in the more distal curvature and how it compares to balance the curvature closest to the head), degree of rib hump, balance, respiratory function, and neurologic findings.

Treatment of abnormal spine curvatures involve close monitoring of the progression of the degree of curvature. A young patient who is not skeletally mature but is in puberty may progress rapidly and therefore should be braced and monitored every few months. An adult usually progresses slowly and should be monitored every 6 months to a year. Treatment of adults also includes bracing, and finally surgery if progression is severe, about 45–50°

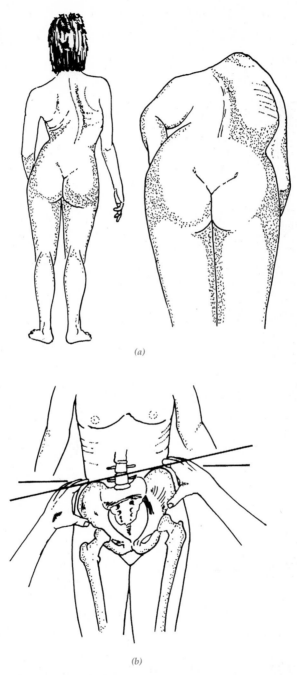

*(a)*

*(b)*

**Figure 12.9** Scoliosis. (a) Lateral S-shaped curve with right rib hump on forward flexion with noticeable shoulder obliquity. (b) Pelvic obliquity in scoliosis.

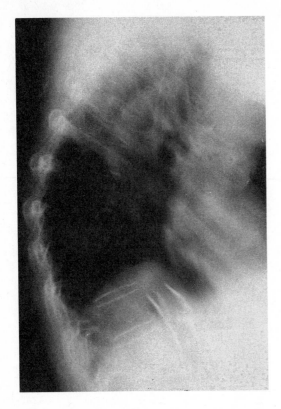

**Figure 12.10** Severe kyphosis in an adult.

with lack of adequate compensation, decompensation or subluxation of vertebra, pulmonary compromise, pain, or neurologic deficit.

Indications for surgery are pain relief, correction of deformity, prevention or treatment of neurologic impairment, treatment of pulmonary compromise, and prevention of further progression of deformity. Surgical treatment may be anterior interbody fusion with use of CD, Dwyer (flexible cable system), Harrington, Zielke (steel rod), or TSRH instrumentation anteriorly or posteriorly. Some experts believe that using anterior bony fusion with posterior instrumentation provides a more stable spine than using anterior or posterior fusion alone.

Kyphosis (see fig. 12.10) is an exaggerated convex curvature of the thoracic spine (hunchback) and lordosis is an exaggerated concave curvature of the lumbar spine (swayback). Abnormal curvatures may also be present such as a thoracic spine that is concave rather than convex, which would then be described as a thoracic lordosis when reporting physical appearance. Each exaggeration in curvature may cause pain, compromise functioning of the patient, and impact their self-esteem.

Another exaggerated curvature of the thoracic spine is Scheuerman's Kyphosis. This curvature causes a gibbus or humpback appearance. It is normally progressive, and females especially have difficulty wearing clothing such as bras due to the convex chest. On x-ray there are 3 contiguous vertebral bodies that are wedged. Vertebral body changes may be noted with Schmorl's nodes present (herniation of disc material into vertebral bodies, seen on x-ray as lucent defects). Surgical correction can be done posteriorly or anteriorly but anterior may give the best results. Harrington or CD instrumentation posteriorly with anterior interbody fusion may be used.

Nursing care of the patient with spinal surgery is explained in nursing diagnoses to follow, but care specific to patients following correction of curves or spinal fusions may include the use of a thoracic lumbar spine orthosis (TLSO). The TLSO will probably be a molded body jacket formed from two bivalved pieces of plastic with velcro straps on the side and possibly shoulder straps as well. This will be worn by the patient whenever up and may be required even when on bed rest, according to physician preference.

Skin integrity should be closely monitored under this TLSO since the plastic predisposes to moisture and skin breakdown. The patient should wear a T-shirt under the jacket to absorb moisture and protect the skin.

Patient care should also include discussion of the cosmetic change in posture following the surgery, which will probably include an increase in patient height. This will impact self-image, length of clothes, relationship to significant other, and proprioception. The change in height can be emotionally disturbing for the female patient if she then becomes taller than her husband or significant other. Also clothes such as pants may need to be altered to a new length.

Spine surgery may also be done for soft tissue disorders such as herniated nucleus pulposus (ruptured disc). This is the herniation of the nucleus through breaks in the annular rings between the vertebrae. The herniation causes an outpouching into the spinal canal and therefore impingement on the nerve roots or spinal cord causing symptoms of back and usually unilateral radicular pain aggravated by sitting, sneezing, and coughing. There may also be neurologic symptoms with muscle weakness and decreased reflexes present. The most common sites for rupture are the interspaces at L4-5, L5-S1 (about 95%). The remaining 5% occur primarily in the cervical spine.

Conservative treatment includes bed rest, anti-inflammatory medication, braces to prevent motion, physical therapy with flexibility and fitness training, aerobic exercise, and weight control. Other modalities include heat and ice therapy, ultrasound, TENS unit, and traction. This treatment may be prescribed for a period of 6 weeks to determine efficacy. If the pain remains refractory to treatment, then the extent of the problem should be determined by the physicians with x-ray, MRI, or myelogram. Following this diagnostic work-up, surgery may be performed.

Surgical removal of a herniated disk is done posteriorly except when the disk is cervical; then the approach is anterior. A laminectomy is done by resecting part of the lamina which affords entry to the area of herniation (see fig. 12.11). The laminectomy is a decompression type of surgery to release pressure on the nerves. The disk rupture may have been anterior, lateral, or posterior toward the spinal cord and care is required by the physician to determine that all the fragments are removed to relieve the pressure. After removal of the herniated material, the wound site is closed and the operation terminated. A spinal fusion may be performed at the time of the laminectomy to strengthen the vertebral column.

Another form of surgical approach for herniated disks is the percutaneous diskectomy (see Fig. 12–12). This is removal of the herniated disk through a small trocar. This procedure is best done on healthy individuals who have not had previous back surgery as this predisposes to scarring, which makes approach difficult; those who do not have disk fragments within the spinal canal; or those individuals with degenerative facet disease, lateral recess stenosis, or ligamentum flavum hypertrophy.

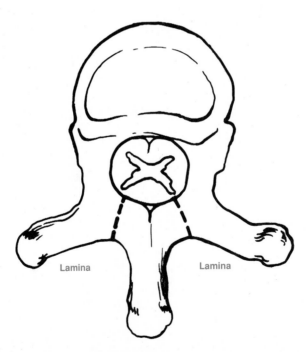

Lamina          Lamina

**Figure 12.11** View showing where lamina are incised and partially removed to gain access to herniated nucleus pulposus.

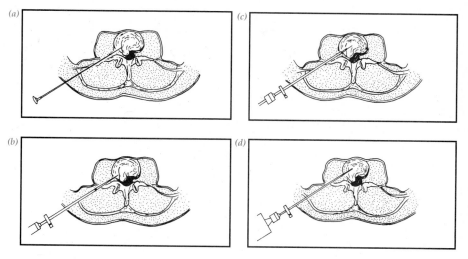

**Figure 12.12** Percutaneous diskectomy: (a) trocar placed posteriorly into the disk; (b) cannula and dilator brought over the trocar into the disk; (c) disk excised with circular trephine; (d) trephine and trocar removed and nucleotome used to aspirate disk.

The surgical procedure is done on an outpatient basis under local anesthesia. The actual surgical time is at least one-half of that required for a laminectomy diskectomy. The patient is placed prone on the operating room table and a 2-mm incision is made approximately 10 cm from the midline. A C-arm fluoroscopy is done to locate the herniated disk and a trocar is advanced to this disk. Using images as a guide, the disk is removed with an aspiration probe (nucleotome) after the annulus has been cut (see Fig. 12–13). The advantage of this type of diskectomy versus laminectomy for removal of the disk is that it is done as an outpatient procedure and the recuperation period is shorter. There is also less trauma to the nerve root.

The main disadvantage of this type of surgery is that it cannot be used in patients who have extruded disks in the spinal canal. The procedure is also more difficult at the L5-S1 level due to the trajectory over the iliac crest that makes approach difficult.

Complications following a percutaneous diskectomy include penetration of the dura, injury to the nerve roots, infection, and incomplete removal resulting in continued pain.

Following the surgical repair, the patient is taken to the recovery room for close monitoring of vital signs, recovery from the anesthesia, return of awareness and alertness, and for early signs of complications. When the patient's condition has stabilized, he/she is returned to the nursing unit and room.

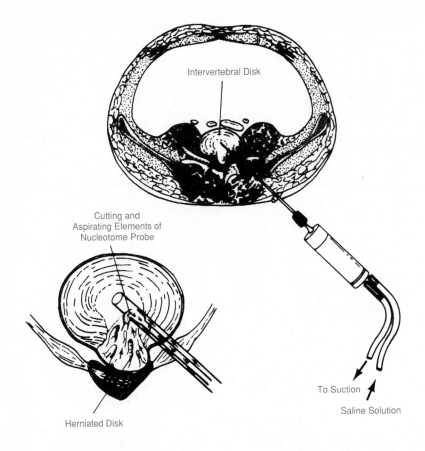

Intervertebral Disk

Cutting and
Aspirating Elements of
Nucleotome Probe

To Suction

Saline Solution

Herniated Disk

**Figure 12.13** Percutaneous diskectomy using nucleotome probe.

## Postoperative Nursing Considerations Following Spinal Surgery

Nursing care for the patient who has had spine surgery differs according to the level of the fusion and the amount of spinal stability that exists following surgery. For example, those patients who have had pedicle plate and screw fixation as well as those with a simple laminectomy may be assisted out of bed the night of surgery. Those patients with fusion without stable instrumentation may require bed rest for several days and then may be dangled (assisted into the sitting position on the side of the bed) with a back brace applied. The patient should be instructed in and demonstrate understanding of the application of this brace. She/he should be able to apply the brace independently. This brace provides some degree of immobility while the spine heals. It does not, however, provide spine support. If the patient has a body jacket cast applied the nursing care must include assessment for superior mesenteric artery syndrome (cast syndrome). (This is included in depth in Chapter 10.)

The use of tubes and drains may include use of an N-G tube, which may be inserted if nausea or vomiting occurs. A urinary drainage catheter may be used either continuously or intermittently to relieve bladder distention for the patient on bed rest or for the patient with bladder dysfunction. A wound drain may also be used to prevent fluid retention and possible infection/abscess formation at the surgical site. These tubes and drains rarely stay in place longer than 2–5 days and the patient is usually discharged within 1 week following surgery.

One important area to address in patient care is sexual activity. Patients who have undergone spinal surgery are usually very apprehensive about this. They should be encouraged to proceed cautiously and avoid twisting, bending, lifting, and jarring of the surgical site, particularly if there has been a fusion, until the site has had time to heal. In addition they should avoid painful positions. Creative positioning to avoid those limitations is possible and the patient can experiment. This return to normal life helps restore feelings of self-worth and reduces anxiety.

Temporary limitations following surgery include no lifting, twisting, bending, or jarring for several weeks as defined by the physician. The patient should rest and maintain an adequate diet. The recovery period may be 6 weeks or longer, depending on the problem and the type of surgical solution. It is not unusual for the patient to continue to experience some pain and decreased sensation for several weeks following surgery or until the edema decreases at the operative site and the nerve memory has decreased.

## Procedures

### LOGROLLING A PATIENT BY TWO PERSONS*

Following a spinal fusion, a patient may be on bed rest for 1 or more days. During this time, the patient is turned by the "logroll" method by personnel.

- Explain the purposes and technique to the patient prior to turning.
- Teach the patient to contract the long muscles of the back to hold the shoulders and pelvis "as a log" while being turned.
- The "near" person (on the side to which the patient is being turned) places a hand on the patient's far shoulder and hip to pull the patient to the side.

---

* Initially patients should be logrolled by two persons to prevent disruption of the hematoma at the operative site. Disruption would delay healing from lack of formation of fibrous tissue. Once the patient has recovered from the initial surgical trauma and is able to hold the shoulders and pelvis "as one," the patient can be taught to turn safely while unattended. However, the patient should not logroll alone or unattended unless the physician permits such independence.

- The second person (on the far side) reaches under the patient's shoulder and hip and gently pushes the patient to the side as the first person pulls the patient to the side.
- The "far" person shifts the patient's hip and shoulder into straight alignment and props pillows to the patient's back and between the legs to support the patient while in the side-lying position (see Figs. 12.14 a,b,c,d).

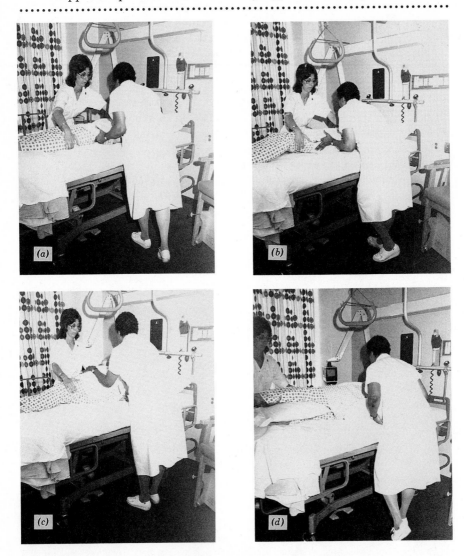

**Figure 12.14** (a) Nurses beginning to logroll a patient. (b) Continuing to logroll the same patient. (c) Patient logrolled to side. (d) Pillows between the legs and to the back to support a patient in the side-lying position.

## NURSING DIAGNOSIS

### POTENTIAL FOR IMPAIRED SKIN INTEGRITY RELATED TO USE OF A BRACE OR BODY CAST

#### Assessment

1. Assess skin for signs of increased pressure.
2. Assess incision for signs of wound breakdown.
3. Assess bony prominences for skin condition.

#### Expected Outcome

The patient will

- maintain healthy, intact skin surfaces without evidence of pressure.
- experience no decubiti or wound infection.

#### Nursing interventions

1. Observe skin and bony prominences for signs of pressure (if a brace is used) including color change or complaints of soreness or numbness. Include all areas that might have pressure, such as over the ribs, sacral areas, shoulders, and axilla. If there is a cast and you are unable to observe the skin, question the patient for any pain, burning, or numbness in these areas.
2. Inspect the skin 2–3 times daily while patient is lying in bed to assess skin integrity. Some physicians permit the brace to be loosened for inspecting the skin.
3. Maintain a shirt or other protective covering between the skin and brace. If a cast is used, when placed on the patient the padding must be sufficient to protect the skin.

#### Evaluation

The patient:

- maintained intact, healthy skin surfaces and bony prominences.
- experienced no decubiti or wound infection.

# NURSING DIAGNOSIS

## POTENTIAL FOR IMPAIRED GAS EXCHANGE RELATED TO ANESTHESIA, IMMOBILITY, OR BED REST

### Assessment

1. Assess for changes in vital signs and temperature elevations.
2. Assess for presence or absence of rales, rhonchi, congestion, or wheezing.
3. Assess for orientation to time, place, and person.
4. Assess skin color and capillary refill.

### Expected Outcomes

The patient will:
- maintain adequate gas exchange and oxygenation.
- not develop atelectasis, pneumonia, or other lung infections.
- attain maximum lung expansion and pulmonary perfusion.

### Nursing Interventions

1. Have the patient deep breathe and cough every 2 hours to prevent atelectasis and pneumonia.
2. Monitor lung sounds for presence of rales, rhonchi, congestion, or wheezing as indications of lung infection or pneumonia.
3. Logroll the patient every 2 hours to aid maximum lung expansion.
4. Assist the patient's use of an incentive spirometer every 2 hours to promote maximum lung expansion.
5. Monitor mental alertness every 4 hours as one indication of adequate oxygenation. Disorientation might indicate inadequate oxygenation.
6. Monitor the patient's skin color and capillary refill as signs of peripheral perfusion.

### Evaluation

The patient:
- remained alert and oriented during the hospital stay.
- maintained lungs free of congestion and did not develop atelectasis or pneumonia.
- regained pink skin color and capillary refill in 2–4 seconds.

# NURSING DIAGNOSIS

## *ALTERATION IN TISSUE PERFUSION RELATED TO SURGICAL TRAUMA AND IMMOBILITY*

### Assessment

1. Assess neurovascular status through neurovascular checks (also referred to as laminectomy checks following spinal surgery).
2. Assess for presence of and changes in type, severity, duration, and site(s) of pain.
3. Assess patient's ability to do prescribed exercises.

### Expected Outcomes

The patient will:

- maintain adequate peripheral perfusion and oxygenation.
- have return of normal neurovascular status.
- not have venous stasis or deep vein thrombosis.

### Nursing Interventions

1. Do neurovascular or laminectomy checks every 1–2 hours for the first 24 hours, then every 4 hours to monitor regression or progression of symptoms (see p. 255 for indications of compromise). Following spinal surgery, the patient may experience initial motor and sensory changes that can be related to either the preoperative condition or the surgical trauma. The patient may complain of numbness, tingling, or (rarely) complete loss of feeling and anesthesia. (However, notify the physician of these changes.) Motor function also may be weaker postoperatively due to anesthesia effects, preoperative pressure on the nerves, or muscle weakness. Both motor and sensory functions should become more normal in 24–48 hours if recovery is proceeding normally and there are no complications. All eight parts of neurovascular checks are important and should be carefully monitored, not only the motor and sensory functions.
2. Have the patient do the dorsiflexion, plantarflexion, and circumduction exercises of the ankles and feet to aid circulation and lessen stasis.
3. Logroll the patient every 2 hours to aid peripheral perfusion and lessen venous stasis.
4. Do Homan's sign check (see p. 489) to assess for thrombophlebitis.

5. Administer medications every 3–4 hours as ordered or use patient-controlled analgesia pump to achieve pain relief from the surgical trauma or repair.

## Evaluation

The patient:

- maintained adequate peripheral perfusion with pink color and capillary refill in 2–4 seconds.
- did not develop deep vein thrombosis or phlebitis.
- maintained pain relief with oral analgesics by the time of discharge.

## NURSING DIAGNOSIS

### POTENTIAL FOR ALTERATION IN BOWEL ELIMINATION RELATED TO ANESTHESIA, IMMOBILITY, BED REST, AND SURGICAL TRAUMA

## Assessment

1. Assess for bowel sounds, abdominal distention, and passage of flatus every 4 hours.
2. Assess for complaints of constipation.
3. Assess for passage of stool.

## Expected Outcomes

The patient will:

- regain bowel sounds with peristaltic movements every 30–45 seconds.
- pass flatus to relieve distention.
- have no constipation or difficult defecation.
- have soft, formed, brown stool at least once every other day or resume the patient's normal pattern by the time of discharge.

## Nursing Interventions

1. Listen for bowel sounds and passing of flatus every 4 hours to indicate return of peristalsis.
2. Measure the abdominal girth every 4 hours to note presence of or increase in girth as an indication of possible ileus; a decrease in girth and passage of flatus are indications of return of peristalsis.

3. Irrigate a nasogastric tube if present (used infrequently) to maintain its patency.

4. Maintain suction of the nasogastric tube if present to remove gastric contents until peristalsis returns.

5. Begin food and fluid intake slowly when ordered by the physician to note the patient's ability to tolerate the oral intake. Nausea and vomiting or increasing gastric or abdominal distention are signs of intolerance or ileus.

6. Administer a suppository or laxative as ordered to aid in the evacuation of stool.

7. Observe the amount, color, and characteristics of the stool; color should be brown with firm mass; the amount will vary with patient's intake and frequency of defecation.

8. Record the bowel movements for safety and continuity of care.

## Evaluation

The patient:

- regained normal peristalsis with bowel sounds, passage of flatus, and evacuation of a brown, formed stool every other day by the time of discharge.

- regained an appetite and had intake of three meals of foods from all food groups daily.

- experienced no paralytic ileus or constipation.

- began to regain lost weight by the time of discharge.

## NURSING DIAGNOSIS

### ALTERATION IN MOBILITY RELATED TO THE SURGICAL INTERVENTION

## Assessment

1. Assess the patient's ability to do ankle and foot dorsiflexion and plantarflexion.

2. Assess the patient's ability to participate in own self-care, hygiene, ADL, within limitations imposed by surgery.

3. Assess the patient's knowledge of future use of an ambulatory aid, such as a walker or cane.

4. Assess patient's ability to apply the back brace if one is ordered.

## Expected Outcomes

The patient will:

- regain the ability to perform ADL activities, such as bathing and dressing.
- learn the use of an ambulatory aid to assist ambulation until able to ambulate independently.

## Nursing Interventions

1. Teach the patient to perform dorsiflexion, plantarflexion, and circumduction exercises to feet and ankles every 2 hours to prevent venous stasis.

2. Teach the patient to logroll and the purpose of logrolling to prevent venous stasis, promote maximum lung expansion, and prevent pressure areas.

3. Assist the patient with bathing, oral hygiene, and dressing, using adaptive equipment, if necessary, such as a long-handled bath sponge.

4. Apply the back brace, if ordered for the patient with a spinal fusion, and teach the patient how to apply.

5. Teach proper body position to avoid bending at the waist and therefore prevent injury to surgical area.

6. Teach proper body mechanics in lifting or stooping to prevent further back injury.

7. Teach the patient to use ambulatory aids, until patient can ambulate independently per physician's order.

## Evaluation

The patient:

- was able to perform ADL activities independently by time of discharge.
- ambulated independently following short-term use of an ambulatory aid.
- was able to apply and remove a back brace.
- had maximum bone healing and/or fusion over time.
- returned to previous life-style.

Complications of spinal surgery include fracture of the vertebra, slippage or breakage of instrumentation, abdominal ileus, pneumonia, atelectasis, deep vein thrombosis, wound infection, loss of bowel or bladder function, neurological impairment with parasthesia of extremities, loss of sexual function, increased back or leg pain, and pseudoarthrosis.

## CHEMONUCLEOLYSIS

Some patients with a herniated nucleus pulposus may be treated with chymopapain, an enzyme which breaks down the collagen fibers in the disk into their basic constituents of amino acids, carbohydrates, and water, which lessens the pressure from the ruptured or swollen disk. Through the processes of inflammation, the disk tissues are replaced with scar tissue. Treatment with chymopapain is referred to as chemonucleolysis; because of some severe and at times life-threatening complications, it is a controversial treatment for a herniated nucleus pulposus.

Chymopapain was initially used in 1964, and was approved by the Food and Drug Administration in 1972. The approval was withdrawn because of controversial research data, but it was reapproved in 1982. It is now used as an alternative to open surgical intervention for intervertebral disk disease.

Because of the possibility of the patient's having an allergic reaction to the chymopapain, the patient is carefully and thoroughly studied prior to the decision to have the procedure. Information is secured about a history of allergic reactions; a pregnancy test is performed on the female patient; and an informed consent is secured by the physician. The informed consent includes the risks of reaction to the local anesthesia used at the site, possible side effects of the chymopapain, including appearance of a rash, hives, or swelling of the lips or eyes, and the possibility of an anaphylactic reaction (reported in 1% of patients). The consent also includes the possibility of posttreatment muscle spasms, continued or unrelieved back pain, stiffness or soreness in the low back area, and, rarely, paralysis.

Chymopapain effectiveness ranges can be as broad as 40% to 90% and therefore leaves doubt as to the actual benefit of this procedure. Also the procedure may not be done if there is herniation of the nucleus pulposus through the annulus.

## Procedures

## PREPARATION FOR CHEMONUCLEOLYSIS

### Responsibilities of the Physician

- Explain the procedure to the patient and family and have the informed consent form signed.
- Ask about and clarify the patient's history of allergies and allergic reactions.

- Explain the effects of chymopapain within the disk space.

- Discuss possible side effects of chymopapain, such as a rash, hives, swelling of the lips or eyes, and the possibility of an anaphylactic reaction, posttreatment muscle spasms, stiffness or soreness in the low back area, continued or unrelieved back pain, and, rarely, paralysis.

- Order laboratory studies, including a complete blood count, bleeding and clotting studies, hematocrit and hemoglobin, urinalysis, electrocardiogram, chest x-ray, and, if the patient is a female, a pregnancy test.

- Schedule the procedure with the operating room personnel.

- Order the medications, including diphenhydramine (Benadryl) 50 mg every 4 hours for 3 doses the evening before the procedure.

- Order that the patient not be given morphine, meperidine, or urecholine in the 24-hour period preceding the procedure.

## Responsibilities of Nursing Personnel

- Admit and orient the patient to the nursing unit and complete the admission papers and procedures.

- Clarify the preoperative events as needed.

- Administer bedtime sedative, if ordered.

- Administer nothing by mouth after midnight.

On the morning of the operative procedure, the nurse will:

- Complete the patient's preoperative preparations and checklist.

- Initiate an intravenous infusion and insert a heparin well in another vein.

Following transportation to the operating suite, the operating room nurse will:

- Administer the ordered methylprednisolone (Solu-medrol) 250 mg I.V. push one hour prior to the surgery.

- Administer the ordered cimetidine (Tagamet) 300 mg I.V. over 30 minutes in the 30 minutes preceding the surgery. The methylprednisolone and cimetidine are given to decrease the possibility of allergic reactions.

- Assist with the operative procedure as required.

## NURSING CONSIDERATIONS FOLLOWING CHEMONUCLEOLYSIS

## NURSING DIAGNOSIS

*IMPAIRED PHYSICAL MOBILITY RELATED TO CONTINUED BACK PAIN OR MUSCLE SPASMS POSTOPERATIVELY*

### Assessment

1. Assess the patient for "position of comfort."
2. Assess for complaints of pain, back pain, or muscle spasms.
3. Assess ability to do self-care.

### Expected Outcomes

The patient will:

- experience relief of back pain and muscle spasms with oral analgesics by time of discharge.
- perform own self-care.

### Nursing Interventions

1. Assist the patient to position of greatest comfort—usually is side-lying, with pillows to back and between legs or on back with head elevated 30–45° and knee gatch elevated 30–45° to relieve muscle spasms and pain.
2. Assist the patient to turn as needed to reduce muscle tension and aid tissue perfusion.
3. Apply ice bags or heating pad to back to relieve spasms. The patient is given the option to use either one or to try both at different times.
4. Administer analgesics and muscle relaxant medications every 4 hours to aid relaxation and pain relief.
5. Observe patient for effects of medications and other nursing interventions to evaluate results.
6. Teach patient positioning and transfer procedures when ambulatory for safe care and patient comfort.

## Evaluation

The patient:

- experienced relief of pain and muscle spasms with use of oral analgesics by the time of discharge.
- participated in self-care and ambulation.

## NURSING DIAGNOSIS

### POTENTIAL FOR INJURY RELATED TO THE EFFECTS OF ANESTHESIA OR CHYMOPAPAIN

## Assessment

1. Assess vital signs.
2. Assess bowel sounds and abdominal distention.
3. Assess urinary output.
4. Assess breath sounds.
5. Assess for rash, hives, periorbital edema.

## Expected Outcomes

The patient will:

- regain usual vital signs.
- regain bowel sounds in all quadrants.
- have equal fluid intake and output.
- experience no anaphylactic reaction.

## Nursing Interventions.

1. Monitor vital signs every hour for 24 hours, then every 2 hours for 8 hours, then every 4 hours until stable.
2. Listen to bowel sounds every 4 hours and check abdominal girth to note return of peristalsis.
3. Ask patient if flatus has been expelled as evidence of return of motility.
4. Measure intake and output every 8 hours to note fluid balance.
5. Begin oral intake slowly after bowel sounds are active and the patient is passing flatus.
6. Listen to breath sounds to note adequacy of pulmonary perfusion.

7. Observe the patient's skin and face for rash, hives, or edema indicative of allergic reaction. Report findings of any one of these to the physician immediately, and have emergency medications ready—such as epinephrine, aminophylline, diphenhydramine, hydrocortisone, and sodium bicarbonate.

8. Record and report patient's relief of symptoms and recovery to note progression or resolution of symptoms.

For some patients, chemonucleolysis has been very beneficial and has completely resolved their back pain. For others, their pain has persisted, and laminectomy with open surgical disk removal has been required. Therefore, the controversy persists about this treatment of herniated nucleus pulposus.

## SURGICAL TREATMENT OF FRACTURES

Treatment of a fracture must involve consideration of the risks and benefits of surgical versus nonsurgical care. While conservative, nonsurgical treatment may involve a longer period of immobility, require compliance with restricted weight bearing, and delay the patient's return to employment, surgical treatment presents the risks of anesthesia, hemorrhage, and superficial or deep wound infections. The physician, patient, and family should discuss the various options in terms of their success rates, healing patterns, and possible outcomes to arrive at mutually agreeable decisions for the treatment of the specific fracture. Nonsurgical treatments of fractures were discussed in Chapters 4, 10, and 11.

Many metallic devices may be used in the surgical treatment of a fractured bone or bones. Use of a specific device is determined by the configuration of the patient's fractured bones, the amount of stability required, the weight-bearing nature of the fractured bone, the device's known characteristics and reliability, and the preference of the physician.

Some of the metallic devices used to fix or repair fractures internally include pins, wires, plates, screws, compression screws, nails, and intramedullary rods (see Fig. 12.15). Plates are used on the sides of the fractured bone (see Fig. 12.16), and are held in place with screws or nails. A screw can be used alone to attach a small fragment of bone to a larger portion, such as in a displaced tibial plateau fracture. An intramedullary rod may be used in the medullary canals of the femur, humerus, radius, ulna, or tibia. This type of rod may be placed percutaneously through a small skin incision to lessen the chance of infection or may be placed through a larger surgical opening during open surgery (see Fig. 12.17). Compression screws are used for proximal femoral fractures and consist of a side plate with a screw in the proximal portion of the plate, which compresses during weight bearing. The screw extends up the femoral neck into the head (see Fig. 12.18).

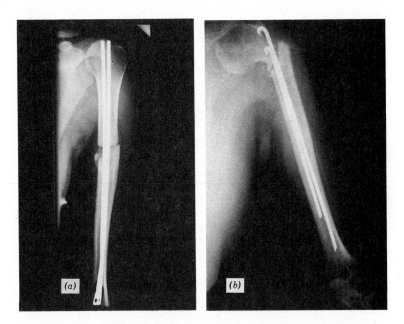

**Figure 12.15** (a) Intramedullary rods used to immobilize a midshaft fracture of the humerus. Note that bone grafts are also present. Patient had a nonunion of the fracture site prior to these treatments. (b) Rush pins used as intramedullary rods to treat a fracture of the neck of the humerus.

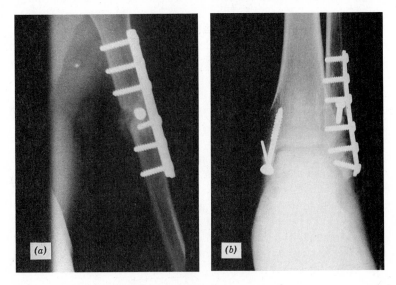

**Figure 12.16** (a) Compression plate and screws used to treat a comminuted fracture of the humerus. (b) Compression plate with screws plus a screw and nail used to treat bimalleolar ankle fractures.

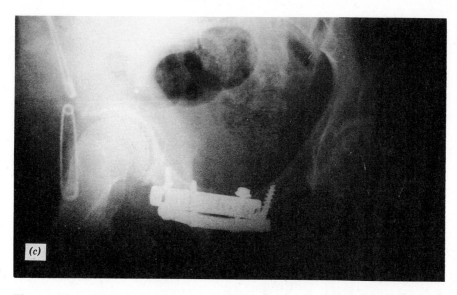

**Figure 12.16** (c) Plate with screws used to treat a separated symphysis pubis area. The plates are at right angles to one another. Patient healed well.

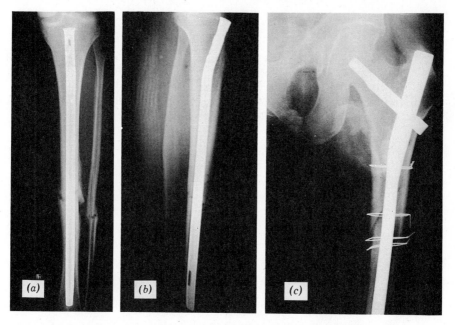

**Figure 12.17** (a) Another type of intramedullary rod for tibial fracture. (Note associated fracture of the fibula.) (b) Same type of rod for treatment of a midshaft fracture of the femur. (c) Same rod with transfixing screw and circlage wires to treat a comminuted fracture of the femur.

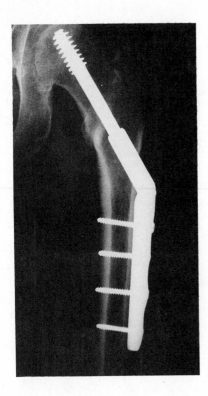

**Figure 12.18** Sliding compression screw and side plate to treat a fracture of the femoral neck.

Several internal fixation devices may be used for treatment of different types of fractures of the hip. Fractures of the femoral head and neck, generally referred to as intracapsular fractures, because they are within the hip capsule (see Fig. 12.19), may be treated by removal of the head and neck and insertion of a metallic prosthesis as shown in Fig. 12.20. Replacement of the head and neck is done to avoid the necessity for a reoperation if the fracture were treated with a hip nail. Reoperation might be required because of the high incidence of development of avascular necrosis that is common with intracapsular fractures because of the loss of some of the blood supply to the head of the femur from disruption of the ligamentum teres at the time of the injury. The ligamentum teres supplies 30% or more of the nutrition to the head of the femur, and loss of that nutrition may lead to avascular necrosis.

Fractures of the hip that are intertrochanteric and also extracapsular are commonly treated with various hip nails with or without a side plate or with one or more of a variety of long pins (see Figs. 12.21 and 12.22). Intertrochanteric fractures generally heal well with pins or nails, because the blood supply to the head is usually not disrupted at the time of injury. The blood supply to the intertrochanteric areas of the femur come from the circumflex artery and other smaller arteries in the area, and bone union can be achieved with the hip nail or multiple pins.

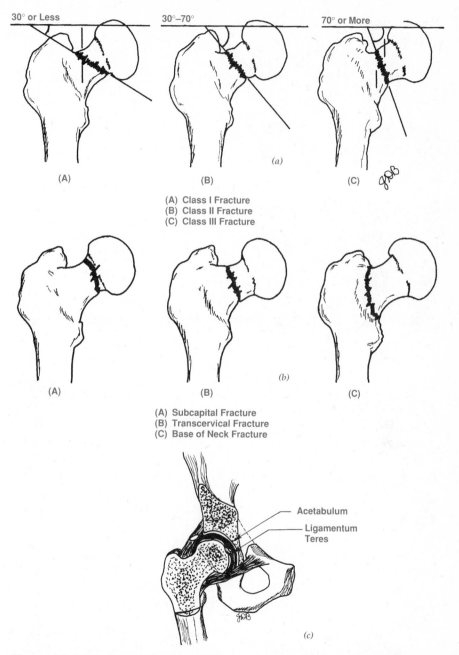

**Figure 12.19** (a, b) Classifications of intracapsular fractures of the femur. (c) Capsule of the hip showing ligamentum teres, which nourishes the head of the femur with arterial blood. It is frequently torn and disrupted in intracapsular fractures of the femoral head and neck.

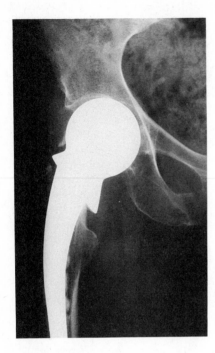

**Figure 12.20** Prosthesis to replace the femoral head and neck.

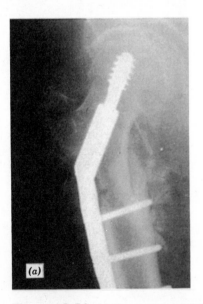

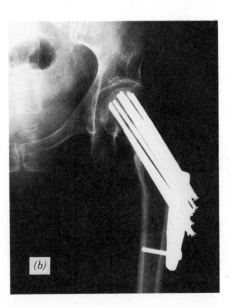

**Figure 12.21** (a) Compression (sliding) nail used for intertrochanteric or extracapsular fractures of the proximal femur. (b) Multiple pins with plate used to treat the fracture in (c).

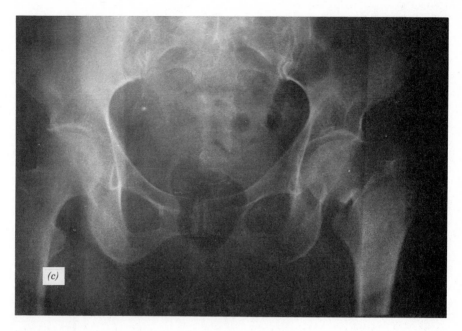

**Figure 12.21** (c) Fracture of the intertrochanteric region of femur (right side of picture).

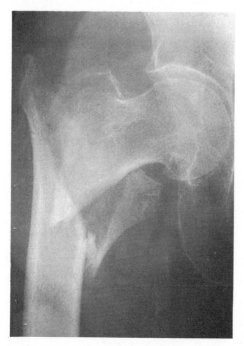

**Figure 12.22** Comminuted intertrochanteric (extracapsular) fracture of the proximal femur.

It is vital following an open reduction with internal fixation (ORIF) that the nurse read and follow the physician's orders for the nature and amount of weight bearing and motion allowed, both of which are determined by the stability of the fractured bones and the nature of the device used.

### Nursing Considerations Following Open Reduction with Internal Fixation of Fractured Bones

The nursing diagnoses and their nursing interventions are the same as discussed above under spinal fusion, and the reader is referred to those pages. These nursing diagnoses are potential for impaired gas exchange related to anesthesia and immobility; potential for impaired tissue perfusion related to immobility and the specific injury; and impaired physical mobility related to the fracture and surgery. Another nursing diagnosis that is vital for safe care and must be discussed following open reduction with internal fixation is alteration in comfort related to acute pain, surgical trauma, and edema.

## NURSING DIAGNOSIS

### ALTERATION IN COMFORT RELATED TO ACUTE PAIN, SURGICAL TRAUMA, AND EDEMA

#### Assessment

1. Assess for presence, type, site, duration, and characteristics of pain.
2. Assess neurovascular status of tissues.
3. Assess limb alignment.
4. Assess elevation of extremity.
5. Assess operative site for edema, drainage, or other signs of inflammation or infection.
6. Assess cast (if present) for dampness, drying, and rough edges.

#### Expected Outcomes

The patient will:

- regain pain relief with narcotics and analgesics.
- have relief of edema and other signs of inflammation.
- experience wound healing without infection.
- maintain desired elevation of extremity.

## Nursing Interventions

1. Do neurovascular checks every 2 hours for 24 hours, then every 4 hours to monitor recovery or development of untoward symptoms (see Fig. 11.18). Check for numbness in the web space between the fingers and thumb as one indication of developing compartment syndrome (see p. 470).

2. Elevate the limb to heart level to minimize edema by increasing venous return.

3. Apply ice bags to the operative site to aid vasoconstriction and lessen bleeding and edema formation.

4. Administer analgesics or narcotics every 3–4 hours for pain. Pain is acute and requires a therapeutic blood level of medication for effective pain relief.

5. Monitor and record the results of medications to relieve the patient's pain, and note absence of pain indicators (moaning, wincing, crying).

6. Monitor the wound site during dressing changes for signs of wound healing or for signs of infection, including increased redness, pain, edema, and drainage.

7. Assist the patient to change positions every 2–3 hours to increase comfort by relieving pressure.

8. Assist the patient to do ROM exercises to increase circulation, lessen pain or muscle soreness, lessen edema and maintain muscle/joint strength. With hand fractures obtain doctor's order before ROM.

9. Check cast tightness, drying state, and edges for roughness (care of patients in casts is discussed in Chapter 10).

## Evaluation

The patient:

- experienced relief of acute pain by use of oral analgesics by the time of discharge.
- had resolution of edema and other signs of inflammation by the time of discharge.
- had primary wound healing.

Following an open reduction with internal fixation of a fracture, the patient remains hospitalized for 3–5 days to permit close monitoring of pain relief, wound healing, and ambulation. The patient is then discharged, after being taught wound care, ambulation with weight-bearing restrictions, cast care, dietary considerations, fluid intake, and bowel elimination techniques; these aspects of care were discussed in Chapters 4 and 10. Also, if a sling is needed to maintain elevation or immobility of an upper extremity, its application is taught and practiced by the patient and family.

Complications following open reduction with internal fixation include hemorrhage, superficial or deep wound infection, malunion, nonunion, fat or pulmonary embolism, deep vein thrombosis, and neurovascular impairment, all of which are discussed in Chapter 14.

## JOINT ARTHROPLASTY

An arthroplasty is an operation to repair a joint. Arthritis and degenerative joint disease have high incidence rates throughout the world. Sooner or later many of those persons afflicted with arthritis and degenerative joint disease will undergo one or more arthroplastic repairs to decrease pain and increase mobility.

An arthroplasty may involve one or both joint surfaces and one or more of the joint tissues: muscles, ligaments, tendons, cartilage, bones, membranes, nerves, and blood vessels. Surgical procedures involving joints are always difficult because of the many different joint tissues that are involved.

Three types of arthroplasties performed commonly are called resectional, interpositional, or replacement arthroplasty.

*Resectional arthroplasty* involves removal of portions of bone from one or both bone surfaces of the joint, creating a gap of 2 cm, which eventually fills with scar (fibrous) tissue. Resectional arthroplasty restores motion and relieves pain, but diminishes the joint stability. Examples of this type of arthroplasty include the Keller bunionectomy procedure and the Girdlestone operation (see Fig. 12.23).

*Interpositional arthroplasty* involves insertion of a substance between the two reconstructed joint surfaces. Substances used include metals, plastic, skin, or fascia. The Smith-Peterson cup arthroplasty is the most common example of this type, though now it is less frequently performed as a cup arthroplasty alone (see Fig. 12.24). In cup arthroplasty, a metallic cup is placed over the head of the femur to provide a smooth surface for articulation with the acetabulum. The cup replaces the worn or degenerated cartilage over the head of the femur. The cup is held in place by a pointed projection on its inner surface, which is pounded into the femoral head as the cup is put in place.

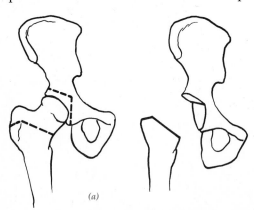

*(a)*

**Figure 12.23** (a) Area of bone removed in a Girdlestone operation.

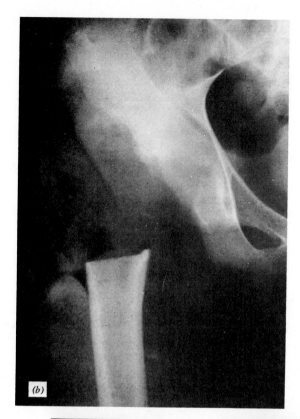

**Figure 12.23** (b) Patient with Girdlestone operation to remove infected total hip prosthetic materials. This operation creates a "flail" hip.

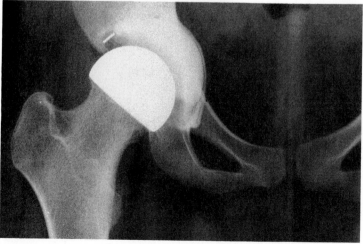

**Figure 12.24** "Conservative" hip replacement that replaces the acetabulum, but conserves the head of the femur by covering it with a metallic cup.

*Replacement arthroplasty* usually involves the replacement of one or both of the joint surfaces with metallic or plastic prosthetic parts. Earliest joint replacements involved the removal of the femoral head and insertion of a femoral prosthesis into the shaft of the femur. Austin Moore was one proponent in this type of arthroplasty. Many modified types of femoral shaft prostheses are now used for this operation, depending on the size and shape of the femur and acetabulum. Use of the femoral shaft prosthesis is common following subcapital fractures or fractures of the femoral neck that result in loss of blood supply to the femoral head, because of the possibility of the development of avascular necrosis.

*Total joint replacement arthroplasty* involves replacement of both joint surfaces—one surface with a metallic prosthesis and the opposing surface with a high-density polyethylene (plastic or ceramic) component. The components might be cemented into their respective bones with a compound called methyl methacrylate, or they might be placed in the joints uncemented, but held in by bone chips; by the porous, coated components; and by the joint muscles, bones, and ligaments themselves. The decision to use the cemented versus uncemented components varies with the specific patient's joint condition and the physician's preference, although it appears that one reason uncemented replacements are being performed is related to the problem of loosening occurring with cemented prostheses, which often require reoperation in approximately 10 years.

Total joint operations are done commonly on the hip, shoulder, knee, elbow, and ankle. Joints of fingers or toes may have silicone (silastic) used for their replacements.

## Procedures

### GENERAL PREOPERATIVE PATIENT PREPARATION

### Responsibilities of the Physician

- Perform a thorough physical examination.
- Order laboratory hematologic studies, such as a complete blood count, electrolytes, prothrombin time, partial thromboplastin time, platelets, type and cross-match (number of units of blood is also ordered); liver function tests such as serum glutamic oxaloacetic transaminase (SGOT), serum glutamic pyruvic transaminase (SGPT), lactic dehydrogenase (LDH), and alkaline phosphatase.
- Order x-rays, CT, or MRI scans of the affected joint(s) or limb.
- Order urinalysis.

- Order electrocardiogram and chest x-ray.

- Order medications for pain management, sedatives, and laxatives or enema as needed.

- Order antibiotics and intravenous solutions.

- Explain the upcoming operative procedure and secure the patient's signature on the informed consent form.

## Responsibilities of Nursing Personnel

- Orient the patient to the nursing unit

- Clarify and prepare the patient physically and emotionally for the operation.

- Perform neurovascular assessments.

- Teach the patient to do antiseptic cleansing of the operative site.

- Clarify the events on the preoperative evening.

- Administer an enema, if ordered, to empty the lower bowel.

- Clarify the events and prepare the patient on the morning of surgery, including hygienic care, insertion of an indwelling bladder catheter, initiation of an intravenous infusion, administering preoperative medications and antibiotics as ordered.

- Complete the preoperative checklist and charting.

- Send to the operating room if ordered: a knee immobilizer or a passive motion machine for a patient having a total knee replacement, an abduction pillow for the patient having a total hip replacement, and a sling and swathe for the patient having a total shoulder replacement.

- Prepare the room for the patient's postoperative care.

## Total Hip Replacement

This operation is most often performed because of degenerative joint disease from osteoarthritis (see Fig. 12.25), but it may also be done to treat avascular necrosis (see Fig. 12.26) of the head of the femur secondary to use of steroids. The operation involves replacing the acetabulum and the head and neck of the femur (see box—"Anatomy of the Hip"). The acetabular component is a high-density polyethylene material that may be metal-backed, and the femoral component is metallic. There may also be a third piece between the first two components made of polyethylene or ceramic material; therefore the total joint

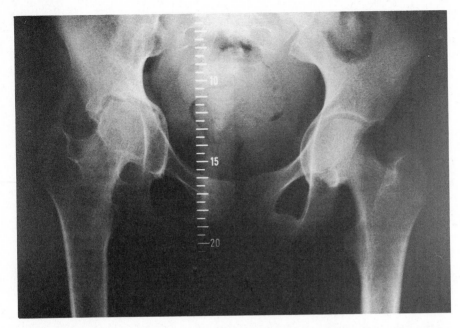

**Figure 12.25** Osteoarthritis of right hip (left side of picture) from degenerative joint disease.

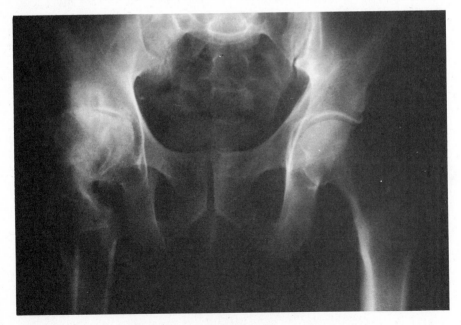

**Figure 12.26** Avascular necrosis of the head of the femur secondary to steroid therapy in a patient following a renal transplant.

## ANATOMY OF THE HIP

The hip joint, designed for weight bearing, is the largest ball-and-socket joint in the body (see Fig. 12.27). The spherical head of the femur articulates with the acetabulum within the innominate bone of the pelvis. The articular surfaces of the bones are covered with cartilage, which is lubricated by synovial fluid produced by the synovium lining the inner aspects of the joint. The bones are held snugly in approximation by a capsule that completely surrounds the joint. The capsule is composed of three main ligaments: the iliofemoral, pubofemoral, and ischiofemoral ligaments. The iliofemoral ligament is the strongest ligament in the body and helps one maintain an erect posture.

The blood supply to the head of the femur comes from the ligamentum teres, a tough band of fibrous tissue extending from a notch in the central portion of the femoral head to the central acetabular notch. Additional blood supply to the hip joint comes from branches of the internal and external iliac arteries, terminating in the circumflex artery within the hip capsule ligaments. The nerves that supply the hip area come through branches of the sciatic, obturator, and femoral nerves.

Hip joint movements include flexion, extension, adduction, abduction, rotation, and circumduction. Movements are limited by the depth of the acetabulum, the size and position of the femoral head within the acetabulum and its labrum (rims), and the strength of the muscles.

replacement may be two or three prostheses. As was stated above, the acetabular and femoral prostheses may be cemented into the bones with methyl methacrylate or may be uncemented, porous coated prostheses. When left uncemented, the porous coating provides rough surfaces for bony ingrowth. Uncemented prostheses must fit tightly into their respective bones for the ingrowth to occur. The porous coating was designed to avoid prosthetic loosening. However, because of the bony ingrowth, removal of the noncemented prosthesis is very difficult if it should need to be removed for any reason (see Fig. 12.28).

New developments in total hip implants now include computer generation of the charts of the patient's femur and acetabulum with construction of the total hip implant to fit that anatomy. This technology is now on site in a few major implant centers. While the patient is in the operating room the implant is made from a mold of the patient's femur taken during surgery. This implant is made in a nearby on-site laboratory in about half an hour and delivered to the surgical suite for implantation. These chrome cobalt hip components are porous coated and are press fit without the use of methyl methacrylate, thus are cementless.

**Figure 12.27** Hip capsule showing the ligaments and muscles plus the hip trochanteric and iliopsoas bursae.

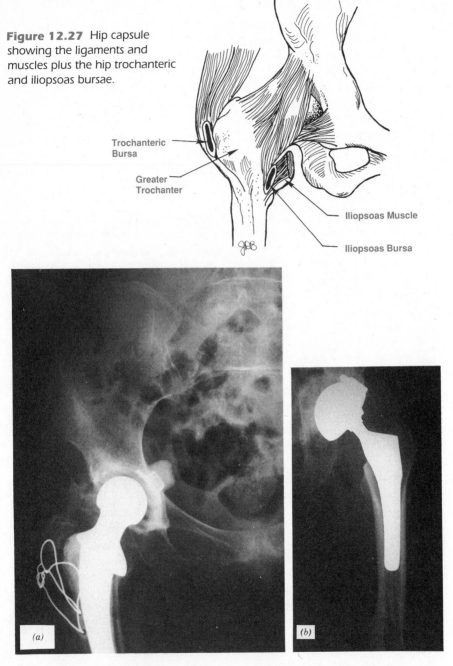

Trochanteric Bursa

Greater Trochanter

Iliopsoas Muscle

Iliopsoas Bursa

(a)

(b)

**Figure 12.28** (a) Cemented total joint replacement with extrusion of cement into pelvis. (b) Noncemented total hip replacement.

The main advantage of this hip implant is the custom fitting. But waiting for the custom-generated prosthesis adds at least 30 minutes to the operative time, which is of concern especially to elderly patients because of extending anesthesia time. Another disadvantage is that the patient is required to use crutches with WBAT (weight bearing as tolerated) for 6 weeks until the prosthesis is stable and the area healed.

The preoperative preparation of the patient for a total hip replacement follows that given above as general preparation. In addition, this patient will discuss with the physician the type of prostheses that are likely to be used, whether these will be cemented into the sites or uncemented, porous coated prostheses, and the usual postoperative course. Benefits and risks are included in the discussion.

Preoperative teaching is done to prepare the patient for the postoperative presence of the abduction pillow, a urinary catheter, and for the need to do frequent deep breathing and coughing procedures, foot and leg exercises, and turning. Methods for pain management are also included in preoperative teaching, as are ambulation and weight-bearing restrictions.

The patient is transported to the operating suite in his/her bed so that postoperative transfers are minimized. The operation is conducted in a laminar flow operating room, with access kept to an absolute minimum. Operating room personnel and the surgical team wear nearly occlusive wraps and gowns to minimize the possibility of wound contamination. The length of the operative procedure varies from 1–3 hours and is somewhat dependent upon the patient's joint pathology, the operative technique, and the ease or difficulty of fitting and "seating" the various prostheses in their proper positions. The physician makes every effort to have the limbs be of equal length postoperatively, although a length discrepancy of 1/8 – 1/4 inch can be treated with a heel or shoe lift.

## Postoperative Nursing Considerations Following Total Hip Replacement

One of the primary concerns postoperatively involves helping the patient maintain the limb in correct alignment to prevent dislocation or subluxation. Proper positioning is especially vital for noncemented prostheses, which might be more easily dislocated than the cemented ones. The usual requirements postoperatively for each type of prosthesis is to maintain the operative limb abducted with the hip extended or not flexed. Placing an abduction pillow (see Fig. 12.29) between the patient's legs helps to maintain the desired position.

The self-adherent straps attached to the pillow fit around the patient's legs to hold the pillow and legs in the proper position. (If the abduction pillow is not available, it can be substituted for by propping two or more pillows between the patient's legs so they form an *A* with the acute angle of the *A* at the

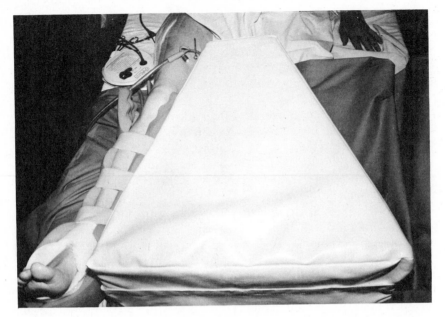

**Figure 12.29** Abduction pillow used following a total joint replacement. The patient's catheter is clamped prior to removal.

groin.) The straps on the abduction pillow should be checked several times per shift for tightness or loosening to be sure they neither constrict circulation, produce pressure areas, or come undone. A knee immobilizer can also be used to prevent hip flexion by restricting knee motion.

The second concern following total hip replacement involves proper turning techniques and schedules. Physicians' orders vary, but whatever the preference, the order must be written concerning turning to either side; only to the operative side or only to the nonoperative side. Some physicians think that turning the patient to the operative side helps apply pressure to minimize blood loss and maintain the femoral prosthesis within the acetabulum. Other physicians want the turning to be to the nonoperative side, because it is less painful and the elevation of the uppermost leg helps maintain the prostheses in the joints.

## Procedures

### TURNING TECHNIQUES FOLLOWING TOTAL HIP REPLACEMENT

When turning the patient to the nonoperative side, the nurse should:
- Place the abduction pillow between the patient's legs and secure the pressure-sensitive straps.

- Reach over to the patient's far or operative side, place a hand on the hip and under the operative knee and pull the patient with the patient's help to turn the body to the side (a second nurse should help turn the patient in the first few postoperative days until the patient is recovered sufficiently to help a lone nurse with the turning). The nurse(s) must use care to avoid "pulling" the operative leg in front of the body, which could dislodge the prosthesis from the hip joint. The operative leg should be in correct alignment with the body, both during and after the turning is completed.

- Place a pillow to the patient's back to aid in maintaining the side-lying position (see Fig. 12.30).

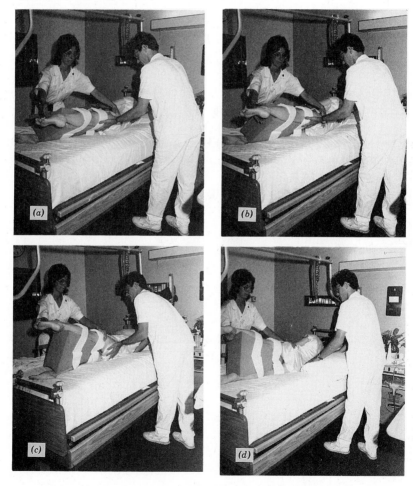

**Figure 12.30** (a) Nurses beginning to turn a patient to the unoperative side with abduction pillow in place. (b, c) Continuing turning process. (d) Turning completed, and a pillow placed to aid the patient while in the side-lying position.

- Raise the side rails to the up position.
- Place the call signal in an accessible position.

When turning the patient to the *operative* side, the nurse should:

- Place the bed in flat position if the head is elevated.
- Remove the abduction pillow from between the legs.
- Reach over to the patient's far side, place hands to assist or pull the patient to the side (a second nurse is needed until the patient can help with the turning), using care to avoid dislocating the prosthesis while shifting the patient to the optimal side-lying position.
- Place a pillow to the patient's back and between the legs for comfort and to aid in maintaining the side-lying position.
- Raise the side rails to up position.
- Place the call signal in an accessible position.

Many nursing diagnoses following total hip replacement are the same as for other surgical patients, including impaired gas exchange related to anesthesia; potential for impaired perfusion related to immobility and bed rest; potential for injury related to wound infection; alteration in food and fluid intake related to anorexia, ileus, or bed rest; and impaired physical mobility. In addition, these patients have potential for injury related to displacement of prostheses, deep vein thrombosis, wound or joint infection; impaired physical mobility related to weight-bearing limitations and use of ambulatory aids; and alteration in urinary elimination related to presence of a urinary catheter and bed rest. Nursing interventions for the first five diagnoses above have been given under spinal fusion in this chapter. The nursing interventions and expected outcomes for the remaining diagnoses follow.

## NURSING DIAGNOSIS

### POTENTIAL FOR INJURY RELATED TO DISPLACEMENT OF A PROSTHESIS

#### Assessment

1. Assess for complaints of increased pain in surgical area of hip.
2. Assess for shortening and external rotation of operative extremity.
3. Assess for deformity in operative hip.
4. Assess for patient's ability to maintain proper position of operative limb.
5. Assess for patient knowledge of proper positioning.

## Expected Outcomes

The patient will:

- maintain proper alignment of the operative limb.
- not experience dislocation or subluxation.
- achieve weight bearing without pain and with the use of an aid until the physician permits unassisted ambulation.

## Nursing Interventions

1. Explain to the patient the importance of maintaining proper positioning and to:

   a. avoid adduction of the legs and not to cross the ankles.

   b. maintain elevation of the head of the bed less than 90° to prevent unsafe hip flexion.

   c. keep operative leg abducted during turning with pillows between legs or with use of an abduction pillow (see Fig. 11.28).

   d. use a knee immobilizer to prevent hip flexion caused by flexion of the knee.

2. Turn the patient as per physician's order to the operative or nonoperative side using two nurses to assist the patient. Keep the operative limb in abduction.

3. Place pillows to the patient's back to help the patient remain in the side-lying position and keep the abduction pillow under the operative leg when turning the patient to the unoperative side.

4. Have the patient use the "post position" when raising or lifting off the mattress. The post position involves having the patient flex the knee of the unaffected leg and firmly planting or "posting" the foot on the bed. The patient then stiffens the vertebral column and pelvis, grasps the trapeze, and lifts the body while pushing up with the posted foot and leg. Using this position helps prevent prosthetic dislocation or subluxation (see Fig. 12.31).

5. Maintain the patient on bed rest for the ordered period, then assist the patient to be out of bed. Bed rest periods vary from 3–5 days for patients with uncemented hip replacements to 1–5 days for those with cemented replacements. When up, the patient is cautioned to avoid 90° flexion of the hip and to avoid *adduction* of the operative extremity.

6. Remind the patient to maintain the ordered weight-bearing restrictions while assisting the patient to ambulate. Restrictions vary by physician and type of replacement, but usually the patient is asked to maintain

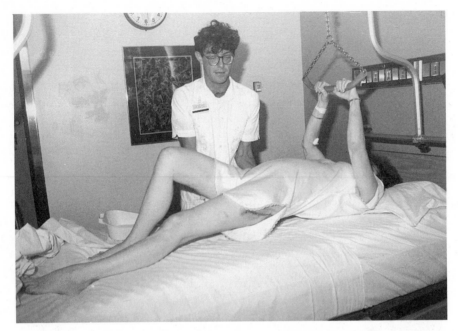

**Figure 12.31** "Post" position to raise the patient's body. Patient plants or "posts" foot and lifts self by pushing down on the planted foot and pulling from trapeze.

partial weight-bearing for 1–3 months, using a walker initially and then crutches. The patient is usually permitted to begin walking in 3–7 days following hip replacement. Variations occur because of concerns for the stability of the prosthetic replacements, joint muscle strength, and physician's preference (see Table 12.1).

7. Assists the patient with the use of a "fracture" bedpan to lessen pressure on the operative site. The smaller bedpan is more comfortable for the patient than a larger bedpan.

8. Provide a toilet riser and "high" seat in chairs when the patient is allowed up in a chair or uses the bathroom facilities to prevent overflexion of the hip, which could dislodge the prosthesis (see Fig. 12.32).

9. Listen to and assess any complaints of increased pain in the operative area. Holding the limb in external or internal rotation, or expressions of "I felt a pop and had a lot of pain in my hip when I turned," can indicate subluxation or dislocation.

## Evaluation

The patient:
- was able to maintain the proper position throughout the recovery period.
- had no dislocation or subluxation.

**Table 12.1** Exercises for Patients Having Total Hip Replacement

Preoperative exercise program. Repeat each exercise 10 times.

- Move ankles up and down, then side to side; then make circles with feet.
- With knee straight, push heel down into bed. Hold 5 sec. Relax muscles. (Do legs separately.)
- With knee straight, tighten kneecap and pull toward head. Hold 5 sec. Relax.
- Pinch buttocks together. Hold 5 sec. Relax.
- With knee straight, make one leg shorter than the other by hiking one hip, then the other.
- Pull knee toward buttocks, lifting knee off bed about 6 in.
- Maintain arm motion and strength by moving and using arms in bed (use trapeze and T-bar).
- Breathe deeply three times. Use respiratory apparatus as instructed.

Postoperative program. Carry out under the direction and in the presence of a physical therapist, nurse, or nursing attendant.

- Basic exercise program is continued. Use of respiratory breathing apparatus is performed at least four times daily.
- Lie flat in bed majority of time daily. Can sit in bed with head elevated for only 30 min at a time.
- Dangle feet over edge of bed, stand at bedside, walk with walker or crutches with weight bearing as prescribed by physician.
- Sit in chair with knee lower than hip. Sit only 30 min at a time. Then lie flat in bed.
- Continue basic exercise program and walking.

Exercise program postoperatively is done in stages (lying, standing, walking, sitting) and in the presence of a health team member up to the time of discharge, usually. Their presence assures patient safety in the event of weakness or overly eager activity.

Additional exercise program following postoperative visit to physician (usually 6–8 wk after replacement).

- Lie flat on back; push shoulders and heels into bed, lifting buttocks off bed. Hold 5 sec. Relax. Repeat five times.
- Lie flat on back; lift operative leg straight off bed about 12 in. Hold 5 sec. Relax. Repeat five times.
- Sit with feet on floor; lift knee of operative leg straight up off chair about 4 in. Hold 5 sec. Relax. Repeat five times.
- Lie on the unoperated side with a pillow between knees; attempt to lift operated leg straight up off pillow, holding it up 5 sec. Relax. Repeat five times.

Individual programs for use of a cane (used in hand opposite operative hip), stair climbing, riding in a car, etc., are reiterated during office visits.

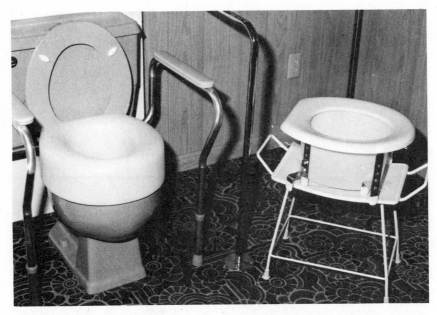

**Figure 12.32** Raised toilets to prevent overflexion of the hip following a total joint replacement.

- walked with the use of a walker or crutches when permitted, within the ordered weight-bearing restrictions.
- achieved pain-free ambulation by the time of discharge.

## NURSING DIAGNOSIS

### POTENTIAL FOR INJURY RELATED TO DEVELOPMENT OF DEEP VEIN THROMBOSIS

#### Assessment

1. Assess neurovascular status every 2 hours.
2. Assess for positive Homan's sign.
3. Assess for complaints of calf soreness.

#### Expected Outcomes

The patient will:

- maintain unobstructed peripheral circulation.
- experience no deep vein thrombosis.

## Nursing Interventions

1. Do neurovascular checks every 2 hours. Note or listen to patient's complaints of calf pain, soreness, edema, or redness along venous pathways.

2. Check Homan's sign by dorsiflexing the patient's foot. If the patient complains of pain "deep inside" the calf, Homan's sign is said to be positive; however, false-positive Homan's signs may be related to operative positioning or musculoskeletal soreness.

3. Assist the patient to perform foot and ankle exercises of dorsiflexion and plantarflexion to prevent venous stasis.

4. Apply antiembolism hose to increase venous return and lessen venous stasis.

5. Administer aspirin, coumadin, or low-dose heparin (3000–5000 u., s.q., b.i.d.) to decrease the possibility of deep vein thrombosis. If the patient is receiving one of these medications:

   a. Monitor the bleeding and clotting values as ordered. (A prothrombin time is ordered when the patient is taking coumadin, and a partial thromboplastin time is done for patients on heparin. Each test is done serially every 6–12 hours or daily.)

   b. Notify the physician if the values indicate need for a change in the ordered dosages of medications. The desired range of prothrombin time when the patient is on coumadin is $1^1/_2$ times its normal value (normal is 11–12.5 seconds). The antagonist for coumadin overanticoagulation is vitamin K given intramuscularly by physician's order. The desired therapeutic range for the partial thromboplastin is also $1^1/_2$–$2^1/_2$ times normal (normal is 30 seconds), and the heparin dose is adjusted according to the results. The antagonist for overheparinization is protamine sulfate, given per physician's order. Aspirin is given orally once or twice daily when used as an anticoagulant in a dosage of 600–1000 mg.

   c. Monitor the patient for easy bruising, ecchymosis, or frank bleeding.

   d. Perform a guaiac test on all stools, and use a hemastix for urine at least once each shift for presence of blood.

   e. Hold venipuncture sites for 3–5 minutes to aid clot formation or lessen bleeding.

   f. Post a sign above the patient's bed with the above interventions for all caregivers.

   g. Clarify any patient concerns about the need for frequent monitoring, repeated laboratory testing, and the need to inform nursing personnel of signs of bleeding.

## Evaluation

The patient:

- maintained adequate circulation without venous stasis.
- did not experience bleeding episodes related to anticoagulation therapy.
- did not experience deep vein thrombosis.

## NURSING DIAGNOSIS

### POTENTIAL FOR INJURY RELATED TO WOUND OR JOINT INFECTION

## Assessment

1. Assess wound for signs of infection (see below).
2. Assess for complaints of increased pain in incisional area.
3. Assess for temperature elevations.

## Expected Outcomes

The patient will:

- regain an intact incisional area with well-approximated wound edges.
- experience no superficial or deep wound or joint infection.

## Nursing Interventions

1. Do wound dressing changes with strict aseptic techniques to avoid transfer of pathogens.
2. Empty wound drainage tubing or container every 4–8 hours to avoid overfilling, which could cause stasis and cause the organisms to remain in the wound area. Careful aseptic technique while emptying the container prevents external contamination of the container and tubing, with infection ascending into the wound.
3. Monitor the patient's temperature and other vital signs for signs of infection, such as elevated temperatures for prolonged periods, temperature spikes, tachycardia, and tachypnea.
4. Observe the wound area for redness, edema, purulent drainage, or development of an abscess as signs of a wound infection.
5. Regard complaints of dull, aching pain in the hip area on weight bearing as one possible indication of joint infection.

## Evaluation

The patient:

- had a well-healed, well-approximated wound by the time of discharge.
- regained normal temperature ranges by discharge.
- experienced no joint pain on weight bearing.

## NURSING DIAGNOSIS

### IMPAIRED PHYSICAL MOBILITY RELATED TO WEIGHT-BEARING LIMITATIONS AND USE OF AMBULATORY AIDS

### Assessment

1. Assess for complaints of pain on weight bearing in the operative limb.
2. Assess for patient's knowledge of the proper amount of weight to be borne on the operative limb.
3. Assess patient's knowledge of the proper use of ambulatory aids, such as crutches, walker, or cane.
4. Assess the patient's ability to maintain proper position of the operative limb.
5. Assess patient's physical ability to use the ambulatory aid when ambulating.

### Expected Outcomes

The patient will:

- learn proper use of ambulatory aids.
- maintain proper positioning of operative extremity during ambulation.
- achieve desired weight bearing during ambulation.
- achieve correct and safe ambulation without injury.

### Nursing Interventions

1. Assist the patient to maintain the desired position of the operative joint and limb. Avoid 90° flexion or adduction past neutral.
2. Assist the patient with ambulation and weight-bearing restrictions according to the physician's orders.
   a. The patient is usually allowed out of bed within the first 3 days with partial to nonweight bearing on the operative extremity while using a walker. The patient then progresses to the use of crutches or a cane.
   b. Teach the patient use of the proper aid to limit weight bearing.

3. Assist the patient up and down stairs using crutches while maintaining weight-bearing restrictions.

4. Use the ambulatory aid most useful to the patient to maintain weight-bearing limitations; that is, use platform crutches or a walker for the patient with rheumatoid arthritis or fractures of the radius or ulna, who is unable to bear weight on the hands or wrists.

5. Adjust the height of the ambulatory aid to fit the patient—see correct crutch adjustment in Chapter 13.

## Evaluation

The patient:

- regained mobility in 1–3 postoperative days with restricted weight bearing as required.

- used ambulatory aids correctly to maintain restricted weight bearing.

- maintained correct alignment of the operative limb during ambulation.

## NURSING DIAGNOSIS

*ALTERATION IN URINARY ELIMINATION RELATED TO THE PRESENCE OF A URINARY CATHETER AND BED REST*

## Assessment

1. Assess for patency of the urinary catheter.

2. Assess for adequate oral or venous intake of fluids and output of urine.

3. Assess for complaints of urgency or pain in the bladder area, which may be due to a urinary tract infection, renal colic, or a nonpatent catheter.

4. Assess vital signs for temperature elevation or tachycardia.

## Expected Outcomes

The patient will:

- maintain adequate fluid intake.

- maintain adequate urinary output.

- remain free of a urinary tract infection.

- maintain a patent urinary catheter and drainage system.

## Nursing Interventions

1. Monitor daily intake and output and record as required.
2. Check urinary catheter for patency by observing urine flow. Flow should be at least 30 cc per hour for an adult.
3. Follow hospital policy for irrigation of the urinary catheter. The system is usually not interrupted for irrigations unless the catheter is not patent, in order to maintain a closed system to lessen the chance of infection. If doing a catheter irrigation, avoid excess force by using a sterile bulb syringe or 60-cc piston syringe and sterile solution.
4. Turn the patient every 2 hours to facilitate proper urinary drainage.
5. Force fluids if patient's condition permits to aid in maintaining patency of the catheter and urinary drainage.
6. Wash the perineal area with warm water and mild soap twice daily to help prevent ascending infection.
7. Keep the drainage tubing above the collection bag to avoid stasis of the urine in the drainage tubing, which could lead to bacterial growth and infection.
8. Monitor vital signs and report increased temperature or tachycardia as possible signs of urinary tract infection.
9. Observe the patient for signs of flank pain or lower abdominal pain as indicative of renal involvement or a nonpatent catheter.
10. Remove the urinary catheter as early as feasible to lessen the chance of urinary infection.

## Evaluation

The patient:
- maintained adequate intake and output during hospitalization.
- remained free of urinary tract infection.
- was able to void satisfactorily following removal of the urinary catheter.

In addition to displacement of the prostheses, vein thrombosis, or wound or joint infection, other complications can occur following total hip joint replacement. These include uneven limb lengths, intraoperative femoral fracture, perforation of the ilium bone, nerve injury from surgical trauma or prolonged pressure on the sciatic nerve, hemorrhage, and stress fractures around the prosthetic components. Despite these complications, the benefits far outweigh the risks; a successful total hip replacement helps the patient regain pain-free mobility with improved joint ROM.

## Total Knee Replacement

Prosthetic replacement of the femoral and tibial condylar surfaces within the knee joint is done for traumatic, arthritic (rheumatoid arthritis), and degenerative conditions, including osteoarthritis (see Fig. 6.1c, d, and box "Anatomy of the Knee") or the degenerative condition secondary to repeated hemorrhages into the joint experienced by persons with hemophilia.

Nursing considerations following total knee, shoulder, ankle, wrist, and elbow replacements will be grouped together to avoid repetition and redundancy. Care that is specific for a particular joint will be clearly stated.

---

## ANATOMY OF THE KNEE

The knee joint is a composite of hinge and gliding types of joints formed by the articulations of the femur with the condyles of the tibia and the posterior portion of the patella, the kneecap (Fig. 12.33). The capsule of the knee only partially surrounds the joint, being replaced in the anterior surfaces by the patellar ligament (ligamentum patellae) and the quadriceps expansions on each side of the ligament. The collateral and oblique ligaments attached to the posterior and lateral tibial, fibular, and femoral bones add additional stability to the knee joint. The joint is lined by synovial membrane, which is the most extensive synovium in the body, extending from the femoral condyles forward to the posterior surfaces of the patella and distally to the tibial cartilages. Structures within the knee joint are the anterior and posterior cruciate ligaments and the two semilunar cartilages (menisci). The cruciate ligaments cross one another as they pass from their tibial origins to their insertions in the femur. The semilunar cartilages—so named because they resemble a crescent moon—end in the anterior and posterior horns. The transverse ligament of the knee joint connects the anterior horns of the semilunar cartilages. The cruciate ligaments prevent the tibia from being forced too far backward or forward. The semilunar cartilages provide gliding joint movements and are partial shock absorbers within the joint (see Fig. 12.34).

Other structures within the knee include the bursae. The clinically significant bursae include the prepatellar, located directly on top of the patella; the superficial infrapatellar and deep infrapatellar, located above and below the patellar tendon (the patellar tendon inserts into the tibial tubercle from the inferior border of the patella); and the pes anserine bursa, located on the upper medial aspect of the tibia below the pes anserine between the tendons of the sartorius, gracilis, and semitendinosus muscles (see Fig. 2.12a).

Branches of the femoral and popliteal arteries supply the blood to the knee joint. Branches of the obturator, femoral, tibial, and common peroneal nerves provide the innervation. Because the obturator and femoral nerves also supply part of the innervation to the hip area, pain from hip diseases may be referred to the knee.

Movements of the knee joint include flexion, extension, and axial rotation during the first few degrees of flexion and the last few degrees of extension.

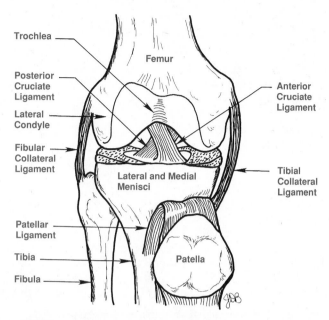

**Figure 12.33** Normal anatomy of the knee. Note menisci and ligaments.

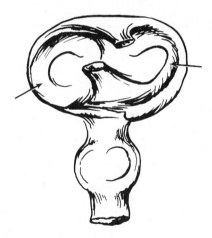

**Figure 12.34** Semilunar cartilages, the menisci, of the knee (arrows).

## Total Shoulder Replacement

A total shoulder replacement is done for avascular necrosis of the humeral head, crush injury to the humerus, tumor resection of the humerus, and for rheumatoid arthritis and osteoarthrosis. (See box, "Anatomy and Physiology of the Shoulder Joint.")

The shoulder is a ball-and-socket joint like the hip joint; thus, shoulder joint replacement has similar concerns and operative techniques to those of the hip joint. The polyethylene glenoid prosthesis corresponds to the acetabular component. A metallic prosthesis extends down the humeral shaft. Both components are cemented in place with methyl methacrylate, or a porous coated prosthesis can be used without cement for the humeral shaft.

Because of the muscles in and around the shoulder joint, replacement is technically somewhat difficult. Postoperatively, the prostheses require strong muscle action for satisfactory joint strength.

## ANATOMY AND PHYSIOLOGY OF THE SHOULDER JOINT

The shoulder is a ball-and-socket joint formed by the articulation of the spherical head of the humerus with the glenoid cavity of the scapula. The joint has a loose capsule that permits freedom of movement but makes it subject to dislocations. Coracohumeral and three glenohumeral ligaments reinforce the joint anteriorly and superiorly. The capsule is lined with synovial membrane. Nerve supply comes from the suprascapular, axillary, and lateral pectoral nerves and the blood supply from the axillary and brachial arteries. Movements of the shoulder joint include flexion, extension, abduction, adduction, circumduction, and rotation. The muscles of the shoulder girdle elevate and depress the shoulder joint and move it forward and backward (see Figs. 12.35 and 12.36).

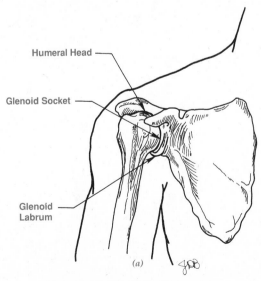

Humeral Head

Glenoid Socket

Glenoid Labrum

(a)

**Figure 12.35** (a) Posterior view

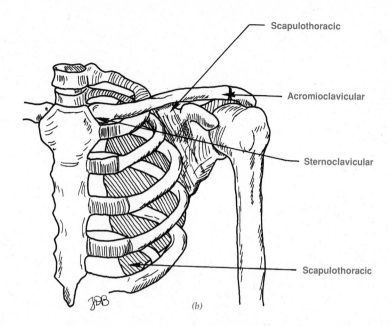

**Figure 12.35** (b) anterior view of shoulder girdle.

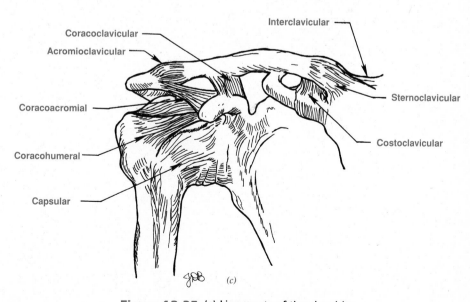

**Figure 12.35** (c) Ligaments of the shoulder.

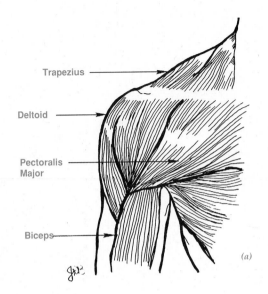

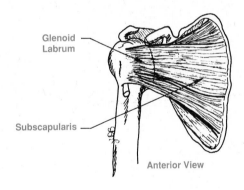

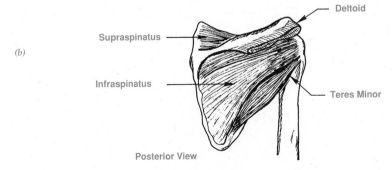

**Figure 12.36** (a) Muscles of the shoulder. (b) Rotator cuff muscles of the shoulder.

## Total Replacement of the Ankle, Elbow, and Wrist

Replacement of each of these joints is done for degenerative joint disease or traumatic conditions that destroy the cartilage and joint surfaces (see Figs. 12.37, 12.38, and 12.39). Several types of replacement prostheses are available for ankle, elbow, and wrist replacements.

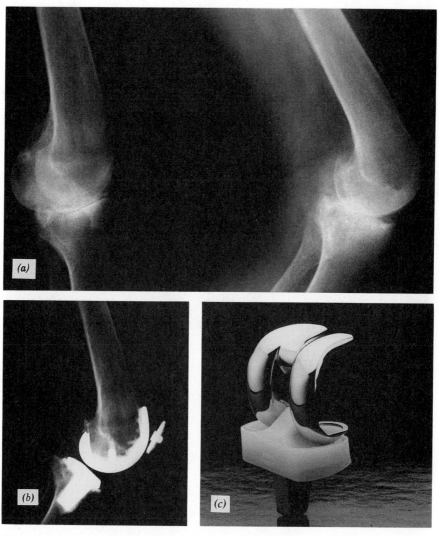

**Figure 12.37** (a) Osteoarthritis, degenerative joint disease, of the knee. (b) Total knee replacement with patellar cap. (c) Insall/Burstein knee components for total knee replacement (Courtesy of Zimmer, Warsaw, IN.)

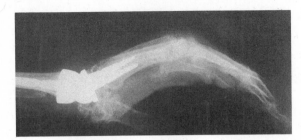

**Figure 12.38** Total wrist replacement.

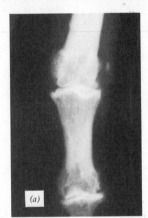

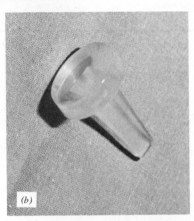

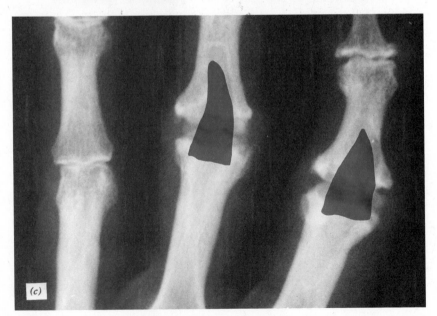

**Figure 12.39** (a) Rheumatoid arthritis of interphalangeal joints of fingers. (b) Silicone implant for interphalangeal joints. (c) Implants in place in interphalangeal joints.

## Nursing Considerations Following Total Replacement of the Knee, Shoulder, Ankle, Elbow, or Wrist

## NURSING DIAGNOSIS

### POTENTIAL FOR IMPAIRED GAS EXCHANGE RELATED TO IMMOBILITY

#### Assessment

1. Assess lungs every 4 hours for breath sounds and presence of rales, rhonchi, or wheezes.
2. Assess vital signs every 2–4 hours.
3. Assess respirations for dyspnea, tachypnea, or orthopnea.
4. Assess for productive cough.

#### Expected Outcomes

The patient will:
- regain maximal lung expansion and perfusion.
- regain normal gas exchange.
- not experience pulmonary complications.

#### Nursing Interventions

1. Assist the patient to deep breathe and cough every 2 hours to prevent atelectasis and pneumonia.
2. Listen to the lung sounds every 4 hours, noting presence of rales, rhonchi, or decreased breath sounds as indications of decreased exchange and possible atelectasis or pneumonia.
3. Turn the patient every 2 hours to promote maximal lung expansion. Patients with total ankle, wrist, or knee joint replacements can be turned to either side. A knee immobilizer may be used for the patient with a total knee replacement, and a sling or swathe for the patient with a total shoulder replacement to maintain the desired joint positions.
4. Assist the patient to use the incentive spirometer every 2 hours to facilitate maximal lung expansion.
5. Observe the position of the "airplane" splint (if present) following a total shoulder replacement to note adequacy of check expansion.

#### Evaluation

The patient:
- regained maximal lung expansion and perfusion before discharge.
- had normal gas exchange and normal blood gases.

- had no rales, rhonchi, atelectasis, or pneumonia.
- had respiratory rates of 16–20 by discharge, with no dyspnea or orthopnea.

## NURSING DIAGNOSIS

*POTENTIAL ALTERATION IN PERIPHERAL TISSUE PERFUSION RELATED TO SURGICAL INTERVENTION AND IMMOBILITY*

### Assessment

1. Assess neurovascular status every 2–4 hours.
2. Assess skin color.

### Expected Outcomes

The patient will:

- regain satisfactory peripheral perfusion.
- regain normal ranges of neurovascular status.
- experience no peripheral edema or venous stasis.

### Nursing Interventions

1. Do neurovascular checks every 1–2 hours for the first 24 hours, then every 2–4 hours as indicated by the patient's data. Untoward signs include increasing numbness or tingling, inability to move joints, increasing pain, severe edema, and sluggish capillary refill (normal is refill in 2–4 seconds; sluggish is 4–6 seconds, which should be reported).
2. Assist the patient to change positions every 2 hours to maintain peripheral perfusion and to prevent venous stasis.
3. Have the patient move the fingers and wrists and the toes and ankles every 2 hours to maintain joint mobility.
4. Monitor the functioning of the passive motion machine if in use. Passive motion machines aid the patient with joint flexion and aid in passive muscle motion to lessen stiffness and aid venous return. A passive motion machine may be used following total knee, shoulder, wrist, elbow, or ankle replacements, although there is some controversy about its use because of the possibility that it might contribute to loosening of the prostheses and may increase bleeding. If a passive motion machine is to be used after a total knee replacement, it is usually

placed under the knee in the first few postoperative hours with 0–30° flexion of the knee (according to physician's orders). If a passive motion machine is not used, the joint motion may be restricted by the use of a knee immobilizer or a restrictive dressing.

## Evaluation

The patient:

- regained satisfactory peripheral perfusion in 24–48 hours postoperatively.
- regained normal limits of neurovascular status in 48–72 hours or by the time of discharge.
- experienced no peripheral edema or venous stasis by the time of discharge.
- experienced no circulatory complications, such as phlebitis or deep vein thrombosis.

## NURSING DIAGNOSIS

### POTENTIAL FOR IMPAIRED SKIN INTEGRITY (POTENTIAL FOR SKIN BREAKDOWN) RELATED TO EXTENDED BED REST AND PRESENCE OF INCISION

## Assessment

1. Assess skin for signs of increased pressure.
2. Assess incision for signs of wound breakdown.
3. Assess bony prominences for skin condition.

## Expected Outcomes

The patient will:

- maintain healthy, intact skin surfaces without evidences of pressure.
- regain well-healed, well-approximated wound edges.
- experience no decubiti or wound infection or dehiscence.

## Nursing Interventions

1. Observe skin and bony prominences for signs of pressure including color change (could be white, reddened, or bluish), complaints of soreness or numbness, and for excoriated or open areas. Include all areas that might have pressure, such as: under a sling or swathe; behind

the neck; under the arm; under the heel area; in the coccyx or sacral areas; around the shoulder blades, elbows, or iliac crests; under the knee; and on the plantar surface of the foot.

2. Turn the patient every 2 hours to relieve pressure areas.

3. Massage the patient's back and bony prominences every 4 hours to stimulate circulation and to relieve tired muscles. Do *not* massage over reddened areas, which could increase trauma to the site. Reddened surfaces can indicate capillary damage. Massage gently *around* the reddened area only.

4. Change the wound dressing as ordered, using strict aseptic technique to prevent introduction or transfer of organisms into the wound (see Fig. 12.40).

5. Observe the wound healing and suture line for redness, edema, increased warmth, or purulent drainage as signs of infection.

6. Apply mattress pads, sheepskin pads, "egg crate" pads, or other pads to help distribute pressure over larger areas (see Fig. 12.41).

## Evaluation

The patient:
- maintained intact, healthy skin surfaces and bony prominences.
- regained an intact, well-approximated wound incision by the time of discharge.
- experienced no decubiti or wound infection.
- participated in turning to prevent skin breakdown.

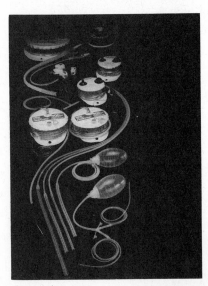

**Figure 12.40** Hemovac (left) and Jackson-Pratt (right, grenade-shaped) drains and drainage tubes.

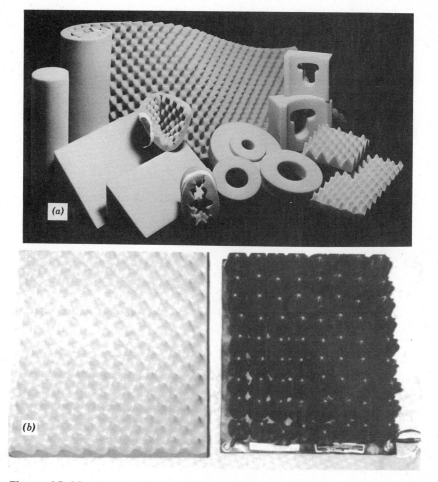

**Figure 12.41** (a) Various sizes and shapes of pads. (b) Foam pad (left) with peaks and valleys to change pressure areas, and (right) inflatable pad to alternate pressure areas.

## NURSING DIAGNOSIS

### *ALTERATION IN PHYSICAL MOBILITY RELATED TO SURGICAL INTERVENTION*

Assessment

1. Assess the patient's knowledge and understanding of the need for bed rest.
2. Assess the patient's ROM of unaffected tissues.
3. Assess the patient's knowledge of the use of the ambulatory aid prescribed (walker, cane, crutches).

## Expected Outcomes

The patient will:

- regain mobility with weight-bearing limitations as required.
- be able to negotiate stairs with crutches.
- be able to do self-care using adaptive aids if necessary.

## Nursing Interventions

1. Assist the patient to maintain the desired position of the operative joint and limb.

   a. After a total shoulder or total elbow replacement, maintain the affected limb adducted and in a sling or swathe.

   b. After a total knee replacement, maintain the knee in extension with the degree of flexion ordered, with or without a knee immobilizer (see Fig. 12.42 and Tables 12.2 and 12.3).

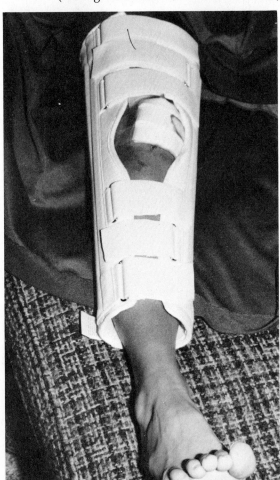

**Figure 12.42** Knee immobilizer.

**Table 12.2** Exercise Program Following Total Knee Replacement

Program is initiated according to individual patient's progress and recovery. It is usually begun on the first postoperative day. Exercises are repeated 10 times.

- Move feet up and down at ankles; make circles with feet and turn feet side to side at ankles.
- With knee straight, push heel down into mattress. Hold 5 sec. Relax. (Do legs separately.)
- With knee straight, pull on kneecap and tighten thigh muscle. Hold 5 sec. Relax.
- Pinch buttocks together. Hold 5 sec. Relax.
- Use arms to maintain muscle strength and arm motion while in bed.
- Breathe deeply three times. Use breathing apparatus as instructed.
- With operative knee straight and opposite knee bent, lift operative leg straight off bed.

Later stages of postoperative activity program. Therapist will be present during performance of activity.

### Stage 1

- Continue exercise program above.
- Use deep breaths and breathing apparatus to keep lungs expanded.
- Sit with head elevated in bed for 30 min only at any one time; then lie flat in bed.

### Stage 2

- Continue basic program above.
- Sit in chair at bedside for 30 min at a time.
- Knee bending will be started by therapist once bulky dressing is removed.* Instructions for use of knee sling in bed will be given.

### Stage 3

- Continue basic program above.
- Stand at bedside and walk using walker or crutches with 9–14 kg (20–30 lbs) weight on operated leg.
- Maintain activity only 30 min at any one time; then lie flat in bed.

*Knee range of motion is determined by physician. Some physicians have the patient begin exercises immediately postoperatively and others have the patient wait 2–3 weeks before doing active exercises.

**Table 12.3** Home Program of Exercises Following Total Knee Replacement

Program is to be repeated three times daily for 20–30 min each time.

- Lie on back with a towel roll under the ankle; push knee down into mattress. Hold 5 sec. Relax. Repeat six times. (Do legs separately.)
- Lie on back with towel roll under the ankle; push heel down into mattress. Hold 5 sec. Relax. Repeat six times.
- Lie on back; slide the heel on the bed back toward buttocks (bend the knee). Pull, hold 5 sec. Relax. Repeat six times.
- Lie on back; with right knee bent and foot on bed, lift left leg straight off bed, 6–12 in. Hold to count of 10. Relax. Repeat six times. Then repeat with opposite leg.
- Sit in chair: slide foot back under chair as far as you can. Keeping foot beneath you, bend over touching both hands to ankles. Then sit up straight and using your leg muscles, pull your foot back another inch; then bend over touching ankles. Do exercise five times per leg.

Following total knee replacement patients maintain 9–14 kg (20–30 lbs) weight bearing for first 6–8 wk after surgery. They may use crutches or a walker. They should limit sitting time to less than one hour daily, using a high chair with a firm seat and arms. The foot of the operative leg is kept out in front when sitting or rising. Patients are usually cautioned not to ride in cars. They are encouraged to be up, to go outside and take brief walks, and to maintain rest periods. Antiemboli hose are worn until first office visit.

    c. After a total ankle replacement, maintain the operative ankle in a neutral position.

2. Turn the patient every 2 hours to relieve tired muscles and increase circulation.

3. Secure physician's order for consultation with physical therapists for assistance with postoperative exercises and ambulation.

4. Assist the patient with ambulation and weight-bearing restrictions according to the physician' orders.

    a. After a total shoulder or elbow replacement, the patient is usually allowed out of bed on the first postoperative day, with the operative arm in a sling and swathe, or for an ankle replacement, restricted weight bearing and the use of a walker or crutches.

    b. After a total knee replacement, the patient is usually allowed out of bed on the second or third postoperative day with the use of crutches or a walker.

5. Assist the patient up and down stairs with crutches following a total knee or ankle replacement.
6. Secure physician's order for consultation with occupational therapists for adaptive equipment for:
   a. Patients following total knee replacement: reachers, sock pullers, long-handled bath sponge, bedside commode, walker, or crutches.
   b. Patients following total shoulder replacement: long-handled bath sponge.

## Evaluation

The patient:

* regained mobility in 1–3 postoperative days with restricted weight bearing as required.
* walked up and down stairs safely several times prior to discharge.
* used adaptive devices to aid in doing own self-care.

## NURSING DIAGNOSIS

### ALTERATION IN COMFORT AND ACUTE PAIN RELATED TO SURGICAL INTERVENTION

## Assessment

1. Assess the patient's complaints of pain—its type, location, severity, and duration.
2. Assess the patient for signs of pain.
3. Assess effects of analgesics.
4. Assess patient's ability to do relaxation techniques.

## Expected Outcomes

The patient will:
* experience pain relief over time during hospitalization.
* have pain controlled by narcotic and nonnarcotic analgesics.
* use relaxation to aid pain relief.

## Nursing Interventions

1. Observe the patient for evidences of pain, such as moaning, crying, wincing, withdrawal, or increased irritability.
2. Reposition the patient to alter pain sensations.

3. Administer narcotics (or use the patient-controlled analgesia pump as ordered) every 3–4 hours to maintain therapeutic blood levels to aid pain relief. A patient may also be treated by epidural analgesia.

4. Teach the patient self-administered analgesia by infusion pump if ordered, to give the patient more control over pain relief and analgesia.

5. Offer massage to relieve tired, sore muscles.

6. Alternate narcotic doses with administration of nonnarcotic analgesics every 4 hours to aid pain relief.

7. Apply ice bags to the operative joint to lessen edema and thereby relieve pain.

8. Check the tightness of the dressing as a contributor to "throbbing" pain. Ace bandages may need to be rewrapped to aid circulation.

9. Have the patient do relaxation techniques to aid pain relief by relieving muscle tension.

## Expected Outcomes

The patient:

- experienced relief of acute pain by the time of discharge or had pain relieved by oral analgesics.
- used several techniques to aid pain relief.
- was pain-free during self-care and ambulation.

Complications associated with total joint replacements include loosening of the prostheses, fracture of the bones (shafts of humerus, femur, or tibia), infection, nerve damage, hemorrhage, and increased pain; all are discussed in Chapter 14.

Many other orthopaedic surgical procedures are done as treatment for various orthopaedic conditions.

## CORE DECOMPRESSION OF THE FEMORAL HEAD

Core decompression, the removal of a core of bone in the femoral head, is done in an attempt to relieve pressure in the femoral head and to slow the process of avascular necrosis and obviate the possible need for a total hip replacement. Some physicians believe that this surgical procedure is useful in the treatment of the early stage of avascular necrosis, but the benefits of core decompression are controversial.

Before the procedure is done, a bone pressure reading is done to determine if the operation is necessary. A cannula is placed in the intertrochanteric areas, under local anesthesia. The baseline pressure is usually 20–30 mm Hg.

If the baseline pressure is normal, 5 ml of normal saline is injected into the bone, and the pressure is recorded 5 minutes postinjection. The "stress test" pressure is usually less than 10 mm Hg above the baseline pressure. If both tests are normal, the cannula is placed in the head of the femur and the test repeated. If there is an abnormally high reading, core decompression is performed.

Preoperative assessment includes a history of hip pain, a history of steroid use, or a previous hip fracture. A bone scan will usually show increased radioisotope uptake in the femoral head. A core decompression will not be effective to relieve symptoms if the avascular necrosis has progressed too far.

Complications following a core decompression include fracture of the hip, a possibility of infection, or progressive degeneration of the head of the femur, necessitating an endoprosthetic replacement.

Postoperatively, the patient is maintained on bed rest for the operative day and is then allowed out of bed with a walker and partial weight-bearing. The remainder of the postoperative care following a core decompression corresponds to that following a hip arthroplasty.

## ARTHRODESIS

Arthrodesis is a surgical procedure to fuse a joint; it is done to relieve pain, halt disease processes, and provide joint stability. The fusion is accomplished by the use of bone grafts and metal devices that stabilize and fuse the joint surfaces.

The operative procedure may be intra-articular, extra-articular, or a combination of both. Intra-articular fusion is done by removing the diseased tissues and then approximating the cancellous bone surfaces. Bone grafts—preferably autogenous from the patient's body—of cancellous bone are used to obtain a more rapid fusion. Extra-articular fusion is done by approximating bone surfaces entirely from outside the joint capsule.

Following an arthrodesis, the operative joint is permanently stiff and without motion. Therefore, the major purpose or benefit of an arthrodesis is to relieve pain by decreasing the joint motion. The major risks are nonunion and infection.

An arthrodesis may be done on joints of the ankle, knee, hip, elbow, shoulder, wrist, hand bones (metacarpal bones), and one or more vertebrae. Immobilization of the operative area is required postoperatively to permit bone healing and union (see Fig. 12.43).

Following arthrodesis (fusion) of the shoulder, the patient may be placed in a shoulder spica cast for as long as 3 months. A patient with an elbow arthrodesis will be immobilized in a cast for 2 months. After wrist or hand

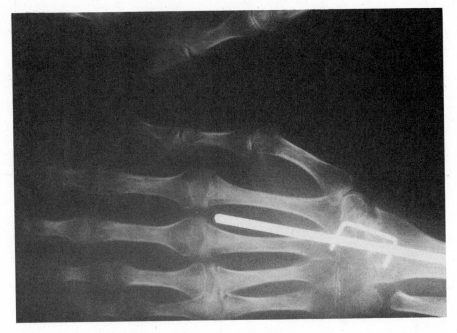

**Figure 12.43** Arthrodesis of the wrist.

arthrodesis, the arthrodesis area is immobilized in a cast, splint, or a bulky, stiff dressing for several weeks.

Nursing considerations will be discussed with those of care of a patient after an osteotomy, because the nursing diagnoses and care are very similar.

## OSTEOTOMY

An osteotomy is a surgical procedure performed to correct varus or valgus deformities (see Fig. 12.44). These deformities concentrate stresses of weight bearing in either medial or lateral areas of the cartilage surfaces of the bones in the joint, causing the cartilage to wear away or deteriorate with weight bearing. Through an osteotomy (bone cutting), the bone having the diseased cartilage is cut, with a wedge-shaped portion of bone removed. The cut bone edges are then approximated and held together with pins, plates, and screws. Through the resulting bone realignment, the joint cartilage has new weight-bearing surfaces; thus, the cartilage wear is decreased or stopped (Fig. 12.45 and 12.46).

The major benefit of an osteotomy is the retention of joint cartilage with corresponding painless weight-bearing. The major risks are nonunion and infection.

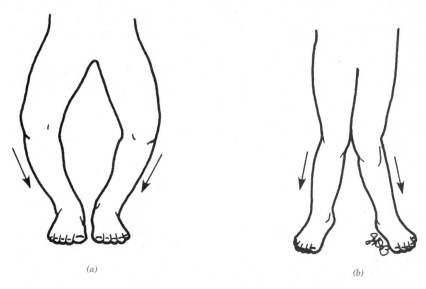

(a)
(b)

**Figure 12.44** (a) Varus (bowlegs) and (b) valgus (knock knees) deformities.

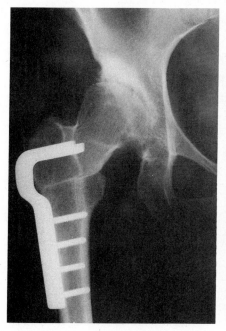

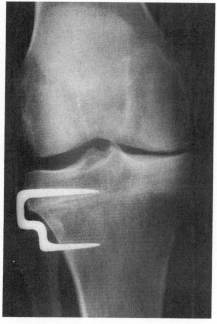

**Figure 12.45** Osteotomy of the proximal femur, with immobilization by blade and screws.

**Figure 12.46** Osteotomy of the proximal tibia held with a step stable.

## NURSING CONSIDERATIONS FOLLOWING AN ARTHRODESIS OR OSTEOTOMY

## NURSING DIAGNOSIS

*ALTERATION IN TISSUE PERFUSION RELATED TO SURGICAL TRAUMA*

### Assessment

1. Assess neurovascular status of operative site.
2. Assess for proper position of operative tissues.
3. Assess for signs of pressure from dressing, cast, or splint.
4. Assess vital signs.

### Expected Outcomes

The patient will:

- retain satisfactory neurovascular functions during the immediate post-operative period.
- regain normal ranges of neurovascular functions following recovery.
- maintain the desired postoperative position of operative area.
- develop no pressure areas or infection.

### Nursing Interventions

1. Elevate the operative extremity or tissues to heart level to increase venous return and to lessen edema.
2. Do neurovascular checks every 1–2 hours for the first 24 hours, then every 4 hours. Signs of neurovascular compromise include a "burning" sensation, increasing numbness or pain, severe edema, and a capillary refill of greater than 4–6 seconds. Notify the physician if any one of those signs develops.
3. Explain the proper position of the operative limb that is to be maintained by the patient and the purposes of maintaining that position, which are to permit bone surface approximation to permit healing and thereby bring about bone union. A neutral position is usually desired, whereas external rotation is undesirable.
4. Apply ice bags to the affected areas to aid vasoconstriction, thereby lessening edema.

5.  Check the skin surfaces near the dressing, splint, or cast for signs of pressure, such as changes in color, temperature, skin indentations, and other neurovascular changes listed under Intervention 2. All bony prominences also should be checked for signs of pressure.

6.  Assist the patient to be up at the bedside, up in a chair, and to ambulate when permitted. The patient should hold an upper extremity in a sling (if it is not in a shoulder spica cast); if the operative limb is the lower extremity, full weight-bearing is restricted for 3–4 months, although partial weight-bearing aids adherence of the bone grafts or cut bone surfaces to aid bone union.

7.  Monitor the patient's vital signs for evidence of hydration or blood volume, physical status, readiness for ambulation, and signs of infection.

8.  Administer antibiotics every 4–6 hours as ordered to maintain therapeutic blood levels.

9.  Check the dressing or cast for any drainage, for the extent of postoperative bleeding or, if the drainage is purulent or malodorous, for infection.

10. Turn or assist the patient to turn every 2 hours to relieve pressure on dependent tissues.

11. Massage the back and around bony prominences to aid circulation and perfusion.

12. When ordered, change dressings using strict aseptic technique to lessen chances of infection. Note healing of wound by approximation of wound edges and absence of drainage or pain.

## Evaluation

The patient:

*   regained satisfactory neurovascular status by the time of discharge.
*   maintained the proper limb positions when in or out of bed.
*   developed no pressure areas, no wound drainage, and no infection.
*   regained intact wound edges with approximation.

## NURSING DIAGNOSIS

### *ALTERATION IN COMFORT WITH ACUTE PAIN RELATED TO THE TRAUMA OF SURGERY*

## Assessment

1.  Assess the patient's complaints of pain, its duration, intensity, location, and quality.
2.  Assess patient for objective signs of pain.

3. Assess need for and effectiveness of analgesics.
4. Assess the patient's relaxation skills.

## Expected Outcomes

The patient will:

- regain a relatively painless operative area.
- experience pain control with analgesics.
- not develop complications associated with severe pain in the operative limb, such as compartment syndrome.

## Nursing Interventions.

1. Monitor patient's complaints of pain—usually pain is sharp, fairly intense, and fairly constant for the first 3–4 postoperative days; then it becomes less intense and intermittent.
2. Reposition the patient to relieve painful or sore tissues.
3. Administer narcotic analgesics every 3–4 hours around the clock to relieve pain and to maintain therapeutic blood levels.
4. Assess pain relief after medicating to note effectiveness of the medications.
5. Teach relaxation techniques to reduce muscle tension and to relieve pain or soreness.
6. Listen to and evaluate a patient's complaints of increasingly severe pain accompanied by numbness and tingling or changes in function of the involved tissues as signs of increasing venous pressure and possible beginning signs of compartment syndrome, especially if the patient's extremity is encased in a cast (see p. 470 for discussion of compartment syndrome).
7. Suggest use of a patient-controlled analgesia pump for persistent pain that is unrelieved by intermittent nurse-administered analgesics. If use of a patient-controlled analgesia pump is decided upon by the physician and patient, the nurse should teach the patient how to administer the analgesic and monitor the results.

## Evaluation

The patient:

- experienced pain controlled by oral analgesics by the time of discharge.
- developed no complications, such as compartment syndrome.
- did not display behaviors associated with pain.
- ambulated with an ambulatory aid without discomfort.

## AMPUTATION

Amputation involves the removal of a body part, either at or through a joint or through the circumference of a part. When the part is removed at the joint, the operation is referred to as a disarticulation and amputation.

Amputation is required when the affected part is necrotic, gangrenous, or severely infected, or when the involved tissues are traumatically crushed or contain a malignant tumor.

The level at which the amputation is done is determined by the absence of infected or damaged tissues; there should be a section of healthy tissue between the level of the amputation and the diseased tissues. An arteriogram may assist the physician in determining the site of amputation by providing indications of circulatory adequacy to help assure wound healing.

### Hemipelvectomy or Hind-quarter Amputation

Hemipelvectomy involves disarticulation of the leg and thigh at the hip level, with resection of the ilium and resection of the pelvis from the pubic and ischial rami to the ischial tuberosity. This very radical amputation is performed to remove a malignant tumor and the surrounding tissues, hopefully to effect a curative situation. The operation is being done less frequently because of the great morbidity that accompanies it, the improved resectional techniques for limb salvage, and the availability of chemotherapeutic agents to treat local or systemic malignant cells (see Fig. 12.47).

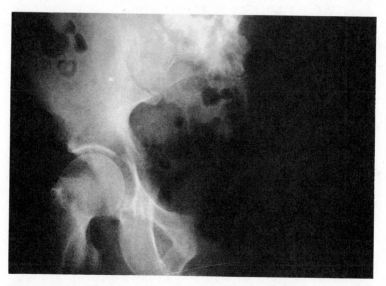

**Figure 12.47** Hemipelvectomy for treatment of osteogenic sarcoma of the femur.

## Fore-quarter Amputation

Fore-quarter amputation involves disarticulation of the humerus and forearm from the shoulder joint, with resection of the clavicle, scapula, and ribs. The operation is done for malignant tumors, but, like hemipelvectomy, is being done less frequently for the same reasons: better resectional limb salvage techniques and the availability of chemotherapeutic agents.

## Preoperative Patient Preparation and Education

Many of the preparations are the same as those stated for other surgeries—securing the patient's history, physical examination, obtaining hematologic, urinary, and radiologic studies; electrocardiogram, blood type and crossmatch, and bleeding/clotting data. Neurovascular assessments are done every 1–2 hours. The patient with a tumor will also undergo vascular studies (arteriogram), scans—including a CT scan, MRI, or bone scan—and may have a biopsy, although the biopsy is usually done at the time of definitive surgery.

Patient education is very necessary, and a thorough understanding of the proposed surgery is vital so the patient can express his concerns preoperatively, receive some answers or assurances of the probable nature of surgery, and expectations for postoperative recovery patterns and activities. When it is feasible and possible, having a well-rehabilitated person with a similar amputation visit the patient might provide some assurance and help to calm the patient's fears. The patient has to be given sufficient time to adjust to the upcoming surgery to enable physiologic and psychologic adjustment and to aid the patient's postoperative adaptation. Family members must be included in the preoperative discussions to help support the patient during this trying period. Of course, the time for patient preparation and education is greatly condensed or shortened when the patient has a life-threatening, severely crushed extremity that requires immediate, emergency surgical removal to lessen the dangers from hemorrhage, shock, and infection.

Other preoperative physical and psychological preparations are the same as have been discussed above: food and fluid restrictions, skin preparations, and teaching for postoperative events and care.

## NURSING CONSIDERATIONS FOLLOWING AN AMPUTATION

## NURSING DIAGNOSIS

*DISTURBANCE IN BODY IMAGE AND SELF-CONCEPT RELATED TO LOSS OF ALL OR PART OF AN EXTREMITY*

### Assessment

1. Assess patient's physical and emotional reactions and responses to the loss of the limb.

2. Assess the patient's willingness and ability to participate in self-care and ADL.

3. Assess the patient's grieving processes.

## Expected Outcomes

The patient will:

- resume usual life-style within limitations after rehabilitation.
- develop a positive, realistic body image and self-concept following the amputation.

## Nursing Interventions

1. After an upper-extremity amputation, assist and teach the patient to do hygiene, self-care, and other ADL that are difficult to do with only one upper extremity to lessen feelings of helplessness or frustration and to increase the patient's abilities for self-care.

2. Listen to the patient and family or significant others express fears, anxieties, and grief about loss of the body part to aid them toward a healthy adaptation.

3. Consult occupational therapists for one-handed training for an upper extremity amputation and for adaptive devices to aid self-care and adaptation (long-handled bath sponges, sock pullers, and curved-sided bowls).

4. Execute physician's order for an orthotist to measure the patient for a prosthesis, to explain its use, and to discuss the upcoming rehabilitative processes to provide the patient with some assurance.

5. Schedule a postoperative visit with a well-rehabilitated person with an amputation similar to the patient's, if the physician and patient are agreeable.

6. Consult, with the physician's order, mental health personnel if the patient's grief and adjustment are prolonged or markedly debilitating.

## Evaluation

The patient:

- was adjusting and adapting to the amputation by the time of discharge.
- was able to express a positive outlook toward the future.
- was able to do own self-care and ADL with use of adaptive devices.
- verbalized eagerness to return to usual activities and life-style.

## NURSING DIAGNOSIS

*ALTERATION IN COMFORT RELATED TO ACUTE SURGICAL TRAUMA OR PHANTOM PAIN*

### Assessment

1. Assess for patient's expressions of acute incisional-area pain.
2. Assess for patient's expressions of pain in toes or fingers of amputated limb (phantom pain).
3. Assess the patient's ability and willingness to participate in self-care and ADL.
4. Assess the patient's ability to relax and to use imagery techniques.

### Expected Outcomes

The patient will:

- experience mild-to-moderate incisional pain controlled by analgesics.
- experience decreasing episodes of phantom pain, relieved over time by resolution of inflammation at the operative site.
- use relaxation and imagery techniques to aid pain relief.
- not develop a neuroma.

### Nursing Interventions

1. Listen to the patient's expressions of incisional pain.
2. Listen to the patient's statements such as "my fingers (or toes) feel cramped and hurt," indicative of phantom pain. Phantom pain is a sensation of soreness, stiffness, cramping, or pain in the missing tissues as if they were still present.
3. Explain the "reasons" for phantom pain (inflammation of the nerves in the operative site, or pressure on the nerve endings from operative edema) and that it is usually experienced in the early postoperative period.
4. Administer analgesic medications every 3–4 hours to maintain a therapeutic blood level; or the patient may use a patient-controlled analgesia (PCA) pump for self-administered analgesics for prolonged pain.
5. Teach and assist the patient to use relaxation and imagery techniques to help with pain relief.

6. Reposition the patient to aid perfusion and lessen pain or tiredness in sore muscles or joints.

7. Massage the patient's back to aid in relaxation and relieve tired muscles.

8. Consult with pharmacists, if necessary, for assistance with patients experiencing intractable or uncontrollable pain. It is vital to control this pain early in the postoperative period to prevent imprinting of phantom pain. Most patients who undergo an amputation for trauma or tumor and who have not had prior preoperative pathology or long-standing pain usually have less severe or prolonged phantom pain than do those patients with long-standing preoperative pathology.

## Evaluation

The patient:

- experienced relief of incisional pain with healing and resolution of inflammation.
- experienced phantom pain episodes with less frequency by the time of discharge.
- expressed understanding of reasons for phantom pain.
- had remaining pain controlled by oral analgesics.
- used relaxation and imagery techniques successfully to relive pain.

## NURSING DIAGNOSIS

### ALTERATION IN SKIN INTEGRITY RELATED TO SURGICAL INCISION

## Assessment

1. Assess wound for signs of inflammation.
2. Assess vital signs.
3. Assess wound healing.
4. Assess patient's interest and ability to participate in wound care and wrapping.

## Expected Outcomes

The patient will:
- have wound healing by primary intention.
- understand and verbalize principles of aseptic wound care.
- change wound dressings aseptically.

- develop a well-approximated scar without excessive scar formation.
- not experience wound bleeding or hemorrhage.

## Nursing Interventions

1. Do wound care and dressing changes using strict aseptic technique to avoid causing wound infection. Infection results in delayed wound healing and excessive scar formation. Excessive scar tissue may cause problems with wearing or walking with a lower-extremity prosthesis. Scar tissue is avascular, and pressure areas develop easily and heal slowly when on a weight-bearing surface.

2. Observe the wound for evidence of healing or signs of infection.

3. Teach aseptic principles and wound care techniques to the patient and significant others for self-care and home care.

4. Teach the patient signs or symptoms of wound infection or pressure areas in the stump tissues.

5. Keep a tourniquet at the bedside in the event of arterial bleeding to lessen blood loss. If arterial bleeding should occur, the tourniquet should be applied above the stump end and tightened to stop the bleeding. The physician should be called immediately, because the artery will have to be closed either by suturing or application of a caustic substance, such as silver nitrate stick. The tourniquet should be removed every 15 minutes to allow tissue perfusion and can be removed permanently when the artery is resutured or closed. A tourniquet must be applied gently to avoid tissue trauma and loosely enough that arterial vasospasm will not occur.

6. Teach stump wrapping techniques for proper compression and shaping the stump (see Fig. 12.48).

7. Administer ordered antibiotics to lessen the possibility of wound infection and to aid healing by primary intention.

8. For patients with a hemipelvectomy:
   a. Monitor the position of the urinary catheter to prevent kinking or obstruction to the urinary drainage to prevent stasis or infection, which could lead to wound infection.
   b. Cleanse the rectal area carefully to prevent spread of organisms to the incisional area.

## Evaluation

The patient:

- experienced wound healing by primary intention and without excessive scar tissue.
- performed own dressing changes aseptically.
- performed stump wrapping correctly.
- experienced no bleeding or hemorrhage.

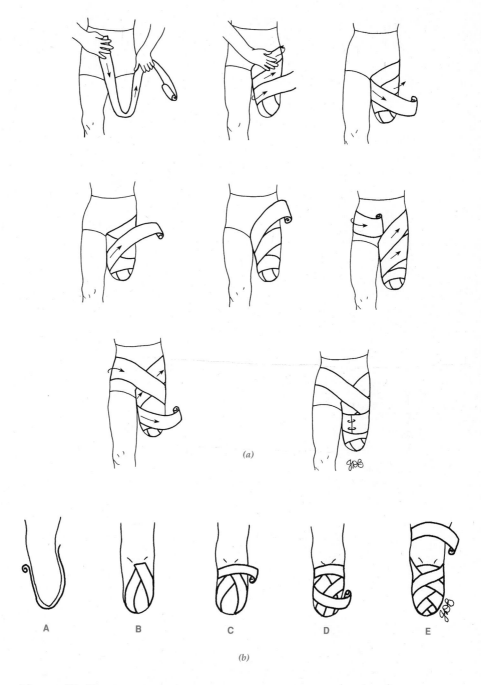

*(a)*

*(b)*

**Figure 12.48** (a) Technique for wrapping a stump following an above-the-knee amputation. (b) Wrapping following a below-the-knee amputation.

# NURSING DIAGNOSIS

## IMPAIRED PHYSICAL MOBILITY RELATED TO THE LOSS OF AN EXTREMITY

### Assessment

1. Assess physical strength and ROM of joints.
2. Assess impact of loss of limb on patient's balance.
3. Assess understanding and knowledge of use of specific ambulatory aid needed.
4. Assess the patient's ability to do own self-care and ADL.

### Expected Outcomes

The patient will:

- ambulate with use of an ambulatory aid.
- maintain posture and balance when ambulating.

### Nursing Interventions

1. Elevate the stump area for only 24 hours postoperatively to lessen edema formation. After 24 hours, the stump should be put flat on the bed to lessen the possibility of development of flexion contractures.
2. Assist the patient to lie prone and flat in the bed following lower extremity amputations to lessen chance of flexion contractures.
3. Teach the patient use of the trapeze to assist in positioning, turning, and transferring from bed to chair.
4. Teach the patient exercises to increase strength and to lessen chances of developing contractures:
   a. Teach and assist the patient to do quadriceps-setting exercises to increase strength for ambulation. Exercises should be done every 4 hours for above- or below-the-knee amputations.
   b. Teach and assist the patient to do biceps- and triceps-strengthening exercises following below-elbow amputation to prevent contractures.
   c. Teach and assist the patient to do straight leg-raising exercises following below-the-knee amputations. The knee must be fully extended during these exercises.

d. Teach and assist the patient to do biceps- and triceps-strengthening exercises in preparation for walking with crutches or a walker.

e. Teach the patient adduction exercises to prevent abduction contractures following an above-the-knee amputation.

5. Secure physician's order to consult physical and occupational therapists to assist patient with exercises, ambulation, self-care, and ADL activities.

6. Assist the patient to ambulate when ordered; note ability, skill, and balance.

## Evaluation

The patient:

- regained physical strength and mobility by the third to fifth postoperative day.
- ambulated with an ambulatory aid as needed.
- performed the muscle-strengthening exercises every 4 hours.
- did not develop contractures.
- did own self-care and ADL within limitations.

The majority of patients experience no complications following amputations for trauma or tumors. However, complications are common after amputations of infected tissues, and include wound dehiscence, wound infection, hemorrhage, or shock. Other complications include abnormal grief and maladaptation to the loss of a body part and development of flexion contractures.

Chapter 14 describes complications following surgery, trauma, sports injuries, and other accidental injuries.

## ILIZAROV METHOD

Professor Gavril Abramovich Ilizarov designed a circular fixator in 1951 in the then Soviet Union, which utilized Kirschner wires for fixation of fractures. Usage of this fixator led to his development of a distraction/compression device of soft tissue and bone known as the Ilizarov method. This method was introduced to North America in 1986 by Dr. Victor Frankel, followed by Dr. Gianfranco Bagnoli.

The Ilizarov method is principally used to promote bone lengthening but can also be used in the treatment of pseudoarthrosis, fractures, and axial dislocations and rotational defects by stimulating bone formation. It is most often used for tibial problems or disorders.

The biological principle is that continuous distraction of the periosteum while keeping the endosteal diaphyseal circulation intact promotes the growth of a fibrous tissue. The fibrous tissue is initially poorly vascularized, then

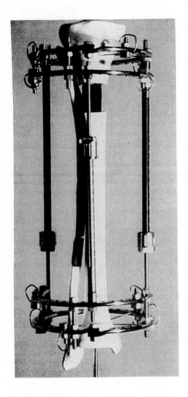

**Figure 12.49** Ilizarov apparatus for limb lengthening and other therapies.

forms a solid mass from which osteogenesis begins in the core. This osteogenesis continues as the distraction is decreased and invades the entire tissue once the desired length is reached and the traction ended. The "regenerated" bone cells, as Ilizarov calls them, are arranged along the lines of the greatest use. Soft tissue stretches and grows to accommodate the bone lengthening (see Fig. 12.49).

Fixation of the Ilizarov is through use of Kirschner wires for traction and Olive or stopper wire with bead for support, which are placed through the bone with fixation on both ends to form internal fixation, and are then connected to the rings or half-rings by a wire fixation bolt, buckle, or slotted washer. Great care is taken during placement of these wires to minimize bone necrosis from drill heat, avoid nerves such as the peroneal, and avoid major blood vessels or disruption of the bone blood supply. These wires are connected to the external fixator, which consists of threaded stainless steel rods, nuts, and rings or half-rings. The rings are connected to each other with rods and nuts. The rods are then distracted or compressed through adjustment of the nuts. One full turn of the nuts is 1mm. Following connection of the rings and rods, the transosseous wires are then attached to the rings and rods and tension applied.

This method provides a stable, elastic fixation which can maintain reduction of a comminuted or oblique fracture and permits early weight bearing and mobility of adjacent joints. Studies show that healing times with this method of fixation are shorter.

Prior to the use of the Ilizarov device a corticotomy (cortex osteotomy) is performed to allow for faster distraction. A corticotomy is done through a 1-cm incision, and 2/3 to 3/4 of the circumference of the bone is cut. The remainder is cut when the rings are turned in opposite directions, thereby fracturing the cortex. This procedure is careful to preserve the medullary blood supply which is necessary for new bone growth.

Distraction of the bone usually begins 2 to 10 days postoperatively and does not usually exceed 1 mm per day. This 1 mm may be accomplished by increments throughout the day, such as a .25-mm turn four times a day, or may be done once a day. Distraction done too quickly can lead to ischemia of the bone and soft tissue and if done too slowly can lead to healing of the bone, preventing timely distraction.

Weight bearing should be encouraged to facilitate healing during the use of this device. Distraction is stopped when the desired result has been obtained but the device is maintained until the bone has healed. Healing is determined by x-ray, lack of pain, no swelling or limp.

Preoperative care includes patient and family teaching about the appearance of the device, since any instrumentation that is seen entering and exiting the body can be a source of anxiety and disturbance in body image. The patient may have fear of not being accepted by their significant other, fear of injury if the device is bumped or touched, and anxiety about the ability to care for the device. Family members or significant others may be fearful of the nursing care involved, or may have difficulty looking at the device or the patient. The best way to allay these emotions is to properly teach the family and patient through pictures and/or illustrations about the Ilizarov device and how to care for it. A hands-on model that allows touching of the device is excellent to quiet fears and anxieties. The family and patient should also be prepared for the curiosity of people when they are out in public. This curiosity is normal and natural and does not mean that the patient is abnormal.

Preoperative care should include early assessment for hospital discharge planning. A home assessment (by the office nurse) as to who will provide care and if there is a need for home health care should be determined prior to hospitalization. Assessment of the neurovascular status of the limb should be determined and recorded for comparison postoperatively.

Postoperative care includes the usual neurovascular assessment as presented throughout the book. Also included is pin tract site care which includes observance of the pin tract site for evidence of infection. Recommended care involves placing of dry sponges at the base of the wire next to the skin, which is initiated 2 or 3 days postoperatively. A rubber stopper can be placed over the sponge to prevent skin motion and friction, decreasing irritation, pin tract infection, and bleeding. (This care is also recommended for all pin tract sites.) There will be some redness and swelling at the site but purulent drainage, increased redness, pain, or swelling should be reported to the physician.

The affected limb will have some swelling and pain in the early postoperative period, but this should decrease after the first 3–7 days. A decrease in the swelling can be assisted with elevation of the limb.

The patient will have expected pain immediately after surgery and should be medicated as needed and prior to ambulation. Pain medications that are frequently used include morphine sulfate, Demorol (meperidine), and Dilaudid (hydromorphone). As pain decreases the patient may be switched to oral pain medications such as Percocet. The patient may continue to feel some continuance of knee pain due to the proximity of the wires to the knee. Continued pain may be managed with relaxation techniques, imagery, and distraction. In addition, wire inspection should be done to assess tension since loss of tension can result in instability and increased pain.

Ambulation is begun approximately 2–5 days postoperatively as prescribed by the physician. Physical therapy will probably assist with crutch or walker ambulation. Partial weight-bearing as tolerated is encouraged but full weight-bearing may disrupt distraction and is therefore usually discouraged. Physical or occupational therapy may also assist with assistive devices for picking up objects off the floor, sock and shoe application, and toe or foot slings to prevent equinus contracture or foot drop. These assistive products help the patient to feel in control of the environment and help establish autonomy. When ambulating, prevention of injury through falls or bumping the device is of major concern to the nursing staff and patient, and care should be taken to clear a path for safe ambulation by moving any furniture in the way.

## NURSING DIAGNOSIS

Diagnoses that apply include:

Alteration in comfort related to acute pain (p. 296); alteration in body image and self-esteem, role performance, and socialization related to injury and traction (p. 00); impaired physical mobility as related to injury or presence of a cast (substitution of Ilizarov device for cast applies); potential for injury related to the presence of wire tract sites and distraction.

### Assessment

1. Assess wire entrance and exit sites twice daily.
2. Assess skin areas contiguous to wire entrance and exit sites.
3. Assess neurovascular status of the affected limb. (Distraction can cause nerve paralysis.)
4. Assess for foot drop daily.

## Expected outcomes

1. The wire sites will remain free of infection as evidenced by lack of purulent drainage, minimal redness, and minimal swelling.
2. The neurovascular status of the affected limb will remain within normal limits as evidenced by capillary refill in less than 3 seconds, warm skin, normal color, normal sensation.
3. The foot will not develop an equinus contracture.

## Nursing Interventions

1. Do wound care of the wire sites as ordered. Usually this will involve changing a sponge 2–3 times daily over the site with application of a rubber stopper over the sponge.
2. Report to the physician any signs of infection of the sites such as purulent drainage, increased redness, swelling, and increased pain.
3. Elevate affected limb to prevent swelling.
4. Post instructions for distraction at the bedside and inform the patient to prevent errors. The nuts or distraction rod should be marked with nail polish or some other medium to delineate amount of turns done. Distraction should only be altered with physician instruction.
5. Instruct the patient and significant others in self-care with the device.
6. Prevent injury during ambulation by clearing a path for ambulation. Assistive devices such as crutches or walker should be adjusted to the patient to provide maximum stability.
7. Administer antibiotics as ordered.

## HAND SURGERY

Hand surgery is done to relieve pain, maintain or restore alignment, and restore function. Indications include resection of disease processes such as tumors or growths impeding function or sensation, realignment of fractures or dislocations, and to improve function or cosmesis (see Fig. 12.50).

### Finger fractures

Kirschner wires may be used percutaneously in the treatment of fractures of the fingers. The wires are placed through the skin and bone fragments to stabilize the fracture. Generally Kirschner wires are used with balls or pieces of cork placed at the wire's end to prevent injury from a sharp wire. Care must be given to avoid bumping or motion of the pin as this may displace the fracture and increase the patient's pain.

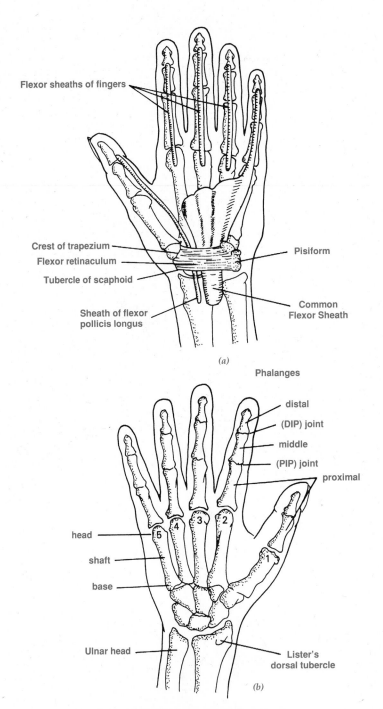

**Figure 12.50** Anatomy of the hand.

Injuries that produce hand fractures may also cause lacerations of tendons. Tendons are cords of condensed collagen having great tensile strength. To permit function of joint motion the tendon must be able to move freely. Extensor tendons are located on the top or dorsum of the hand and provide extension. Flexor tendons are contained in tendon sheaths and are located on the palmar or volar aspect of the hand, and produce flexion. If a flexor tendon is repaired in conjunction with fracture reduction the patient is placed in a dorsal splint and a rubber band attached to the fingernail of the affected finger. This rubber band is then attached to the dressing at the wrist level with the finger flexed. The finger then can move slightly and is controlled to prevent tearing of the repaired tendon and yet allow enough motion to prevent scarring of the tendon within the sheath. Flexor tendons require a much longer immobilization than extensor tendons. Extensor tendons are dressed with a volar splint and the fingers are allowed motion early on. Return to work following flexor tendon injury takes approximately 6 weeks, extensor tendons usually 3 weeks. Finger fractures generally take 3–6 weeks to heal and the patient's ability to return to work is determined by the patient's age, health, and job duties. Nursing care is impacted if the hand fracture is complicated by tendon injury, because usually orthopaedic assessment includes determination of range of motion, but not with tendon injuries. The patient should *not* be asked to move the fingers if the tendon has been lacerated.

Hand surgery is also done to relieve growths or pressure on nerve roots that impede sensation and function, such as with carpal tunnel syndrome. Carpal tunnel syndrome occurs when swelling within the carpal canal results in median nerve entrapment on the volar aspect of the wrist. The median nerve is compressed within the carpal tunnel, which is beneath the transverse carpal ligament. This condition exhibits symptoms of pain and paresthesia of the thumb and index and long fingers, with symptoms worsening at night. The patient often complains of hand weakness and dropping objects. Often there has been some type of repetitive activity such as computer work, where the wrist is bent and there is continuous finger motion, or certain kinds of factory work, where there is constant wrist bending and twisting.

Carpal tunnel release may be performed when there has been an EMG and nerve conduction study confirming the presence of carpal tunnel syndrome and conservative treatment, including use of a resting hand splint, use of NSAIDS, and possible steroid injections, has failed. In addition the patient may have a positive Tinel sign and positive Phalen (see p. 309).

Carpal tunnel release is performed as an outpatient procedure under general or regional anesthesia. The incision usually is placed along a palmar crease to minimize scarring (see p. 65). A cast, splint, or restrictive dressing will be applied for 1–2 weeks according to physician preference. Stitches may be removed within 2 weeks. The patient may return to work 3–6 weeks following the surgery, depending on the type of duties involved. For example, if the patient normally does repetitive wrist-bending tasks such as computer work, then the return may be delayed. The patient should be counseled about the possibility of a return of this syndrome if the job duties have contributed to the diagnosis. The patient may need to consider a job change or retraining. Also, ergonomics, which is adjusting the workplace to help prevent these injuries, may help, such as placing a keyboard at a height that does not require extreme wrist flexion.

Carpal tunnel surgery may also be performed through an arthroscope. This requires 2 small incisions on the volar aspect of the hand. This is a recent development and as yet is not widely used. The main benefit of the use of the scope is that it is less invasive and therefore recovery time is shortened. The patient does not have a cast, splint, or restrictive dressing but rather a light ace wrap. Normal activities may be resumed within the same week of surgery. The main disadvantage is that the technique requires considerable skill.

## BIBLIOGRAPHY

Anderson, L. (1989). Educational approaches to management of low back pain. *Orthopaedic Nursing, 8*(1);43–46.

Arciero, R.A. (1986). Irrigating solutions used in arthroscopy and their effect on articular cartilage: An in vivo study. *Orthopedics, 9*(11),1511–1515.

Arvidsson, I., (1986). Reduction of pain inhibition on voluntary muscle activation by epidural analgesia. *Orthopedics, 9*(1),1415–1424.

Arvidsson, I. & Erickson, E. (1986). Postoperative TENS pain relief after knee surgery: Objective evaluation. *Orthopedics, 9*(10),1346–1351.

Aston, J.W., Jr., & Henley, B.M. (1989). Physical growth arrest of the distal radius treated by the Ilizarov technique. *Orthopaedic Review, 8*(7),813–816.

Bagnoli, G. (1990). *The Ilizarov method.* Philadelphia: B.C. Decker Inc.

Bridwell, K.H., & DeWald, R.L. (1991). *The textbook of spinal surgery* (Vols. 1–2). Philadelphia: Lippincott.

Bridwell, K.H. (1988). Cotrel-Dubousset instrumentation. *Orthopaedic Nursing, 7*(1),11–16.

Brinkley, L.B. (1989). Predeposit autologous blood for elective orthopaedic surgery. *Orthopaedic Nursing, 8*(1),25–28.

Brosman, H., & Berda, P. (1990). Pedicle screw fixation in the lumbar spine. *Orthopaedic Nursing, 9*(6),22–32.

Camp, J.F., & Colwell, C.W. (1986). Core decompression of the femoral head for osteonecrosis. *Journal of Bone and Joint Surgery, 68A*(9),1313–1319.

Ceccio, C.M. (1988). AIDS: Scientific update, treatment, and nursing care. *Orthopaedic Nursing, 7*(5),13–25.

Clay, K.L., & Stirn, M.L. (1986). Documentation of discharge teaching of patients who have had hip surgery. *Orthopaedic Nursing, 5*(5),22–24.

Cole, H.M. (Ed.). (1989). Questions and answers, diagnostic and therapuetic technology assessment (data), chemonucleolysis. *Journal of the American Medical Association, 262*(7),953–956.

Collin, C. (1986). Localized, operable soft tissue sarcoma of the lower extremity. *Archives of Surgery, 121*(12),1425–1434.

Cornell, C., & Ranawat, C.S. (1986). The impact of modern cement techniques on acetabular fixation in cemented total hip replacement. *The Journal of Arthroplasty, 1*(3),197–202.

Crocker, C.G. (1986). Acute postoperative pain: Cause and control. *Orthopaedic Nursing, 5*(2),11–18.

Doheny, M., O'Bryan, M., & Sedlak, C.A. (1987). Body image considerations for the adult scoliosis patients having spinal fusion surgery. *Orthopaedic Nursing, 6*(6),18–22.

Dutka, M. (1986). Elbow and wrist arthroscopy: Perioperative nursing care. *Orthopaedic Nursing, 5*(4),29–34.

Engh, C.A. (1987). Porous-coated hip replacement. *Journal of Bone and Joint Surgery, 69B*(1),45–55.

Esses, S.I., & Bednar, D.A. (1989). The spinal pedicle screw: Techniques and systems. *Orthopaedic Review, 18*(6),676–682.

Faris, P.M., & Ritter, M.A. (1991). Unwashed filtered shed blood collected after knee and hip arthroplasties. *The Journal of Bone and Joint Surgery, 73-A*(8),1169–1178.

Figgie, H.E., (1986). A critical analysis of alignment factors affecting functional outcome in total elbow arthroplasty. *The Journal of Arthroplasty, 1*(3),169–174.

Figgie, H.E. (1986), A critical analysis of alignment factors influencing functional results following trispherical total wrist arthroplasty. *The Journal of Arthroplasty, 1*(3),149–156.

Figgie, H.E., (1986). A critical analysis of mechanical factors correlated with bone remodeling following total elbow arthroplasty. *The Journal of Arthroplasty, 1*(3),175–182.

Frankel, V.H., Gold, S., & Golyakhovsky, V. (1989). The Ilizarov technique. *Orthopaedic Review, 18*(2),46–52.

Fraser, R.D. (1986). Exacerbation of back pain after chemonucleolysis. *Alternatives in Spinal Surgery, 3*(1),5–7.

Frymoyer, J.W. (Ed.). (1991). *The adult spine principles & practice* (Vols. 1–2). New York: Raven Press.

Gannon, D.M., Lombardi, A.V., Jr., & Mallory, T. (1991) An evaluation of the efficacy of postoperative blood salvage after joint arthroplasty. *The Journal of Arthroplasty, 1*(2),109–114.

Goldstein, T.B. (1986). Chemonucleolysis: Still controversial, but worthwhile for skeletal patients. *Journal of Musculoskeletal Medicine, 3*(6),21–35.

Gore, D.R., (1986). Correlations between objective measures of function and a clinical knee rating scale following total knee replacement. *Orthopedics, 9*(10),1363–1367.

Gottschalk, F., (1986). Early fitting of the amputee with a plastic temporary adjustable below-knee prosthesis. *Contemporary Orthopedics, 13*(1),15–21.

Grantham, S.A., & Craig, M. (1986). Open intramedullary nailing of the femoral shaft fracture. *Orthopaedic Review, 15*(7),426–432.

Green, S. (1989). The Ilizarov technique: The first English language course in Siberia. *Surgical Rounds for Orthopaedics, 2,*36–41.

Greenwald, T.A., & Keene, J.S. (1991). Results of Harrington instrumentation in type A & type B burst fracture. *Journal of Spinal Disorders, 4*(2),149–156.

Groh, G., Buchert, P.K., & Allen, W.C. A comparison of transfusion requirements after total knee arthroplasty using the solcotrans autotransfusion system. Abstract from the University of Missouri Health Sciences Center.

Guyer, D.W., & Wiltse, L.L. (1989). Pedicle screw fixation of the lumbar spine. *Surgical Rounds for Orthopaedics, 2,*17–21.

Hallock, G.C. (1986). Severe lower extremity injury, microsurgical reconstruction rationale. *Orthopaedic Review, 15*(7),465–470.

Hammerberg, K.W., Rodts, M.F., & DeWald, R.L. (1988). Zielke instrumentation. *Orthopedics, 11*(10),1365–1371.

Hanley, E.N., Jr., & Eskay, M.L. (1989). Thoracic spine fractures. *Orthopedics, 12*(5),689–696.

Harper, M.C. (1986). Open and closed intramedullary nailing of the femur. *Contemporary Orthopaedics, 13*(3),31–36.

Hunter, S. (1986). Southern hip exposure. *Orthopedics, 9*(10),1425–1428.

Inglis, A.E. (1982). *Total joint replacement of the upper extremity.* St. Louis: Mosby.

Ippolito, E. (1986). Idiopathic condrolysis of the hip: An ultra-structural study of the articular cartilage of the femoral head. *Orthopedics, 9*(10), 1383–1392.

Jauernig, P.R. (1990). Organizing and implementing an Ilizarov program. *Orthopaedic Nursing, 9*(5),47–55.

Johnson, L. (1986). *Arthroscopic surgery* (Vols. 1–2) (3rd ed.). St. Louis: Mosby.

Jorgensen, U. (1987). Long-term follow-up of meniscectomy in atheletes. *Journal of Bone and Joint Surgery, 69B*(1),80–83.

Staff. (1986). Consensus Conference: Prevention of venous thrombosis and pulmonary embolism. *Journal of The American Medical Association, 256*(6),744–749.

Kostuik, J.P. (1988). Anterior Kostuik-Harrington distraction systems. *Orthopedics, 11*(10),1379–1391.

Kraker, D., (1986). Early post-surgical prosthetic fitting with a pre-fabricated plastic limb. *Orthopedics, 9*(7),989–996.

Kricum, M.E. (1988). *Imaging modalities in spinal disorders.* Philadelphia: Saunders.

Levine, A.M., & Edwards, C.C. (1988). Low lumbar burst fractures. *Orthopedics, 11*(10),1427–1432.

Luque, E.R., & Rapp, G.F. (1988). A new semirigid method for interpedicular fixation of the spine. *Orthopedics, 11*(10),1445–1450.

MacArthur, B.J. (1986). Arthroscopy of the shoulder. *Orthopaedic Nursing, 5*(4),26–28.

Maciunas, R.J. & Onofrio, B.M. (1986). The long-term results of chymopapain chemonucleolysis for lumbar disc disease. *Journal of Neurosurgery, 65*(9),1–8.

Magid, D. (1986). A systemic approach to the hip: Computed tomography with multiplanar reconstructions. *Contemporary Orthopaedics, 13*(6),15–23.

Mallory, T.H. (1989) Advances in total hip arthroplasty. *Surgical Rounds for Orthopaedics, 17*–22.

Maroon, J.C., Onik, G., & Day, A. (1988). Percutaneous automated diskectomy in athletes. *The Physician and Sports Medicine, 16*(8),61–73.

Modic, M.T., Masaryk, T.J., & Ross, J.S. (1989). *Magnetic resonance imaging of the spine.* Chicago: Yearbook Medical Publishers.

Newschwander, G.E., & Dunst, R.M. (1989). Limb lengthening with the Ilizarov external fixator. *Orthopaedic Nursing, 8*(3),15–21.

Pearson, R.L., & Perry, C.R. (1989). The Ilizarov technique in the treatment of infected tibial nonunions. *Orthopaedic Review, 8*(5),609–613.

Pipino, F., (1986). The present-day value of simple displacement osteotomy in surgical treatment of osteoarthritis of the hip. *Orthopedics, 9*(10),1369–1378.

Pyka, W.R., & Nagel, D.A. (1988). Use of the Ilizarov external fixator for tibial lengthening: Case report. *Contemporary Orthopaedics, 17*(2),15–21.

Rockwood, C.A., Jr., Green, D.P., & Bucholz, R.W. (1991). *Rockwood & greens fractures in adults* (3rd ed.). Philadelphia: Lippincott.

Rodts, M.F. (1987). Surgical intervention for adult scoliosis. *Orthopaedic Nursing, 6*(6),11–16.

Sherk, H. (Ed.). (1989). *The cervical spine.* Philadelphia: Lippincott.

Simon, M.A., (1986). Limb-salvage treatment versus amputation for osteosarcoma of the distal end of the femur. *The Journal of Bone and Joint Surgery, 68A*(9),1331–1337.

Sladen, A. (1986). Postoperative respiratory therapy. *Surgical Rounds for Orthopaedics, 9*(11),39–46.

Spetzler, B., & Anderson, L. (1987). Patient-controlled analgesia in the total joint arthroplasty patient. *Clinical Orthopaedics, 215,*122–125.

Stewart, J.R., & Thorne, R.P. (1986). Complications of metrizamide (Amipaque) myelography. *Orthopaedic Nursing, 4*(4),53–55.

Stoller, D.W. (1989). Magnetic resonance imaging of the spine and joints. *Orthopaedic Review, 8*(2),4–20.

Strickland, J.W. (1986). Flexor tendon injuries—Part 2. *Orthopaedic Review, 15*(11),701–721.

Strickland, J.W. (1986). Flexor tendon injuries—Part 1. *Orthopaedic Review, 15*(10),632–645.

Tibone, J.E., (1986). Surgical treatment of tears of the rotator cuff in athletes. *The Journal of Bone and Joint Surgery, 68A*(6),887–891.

Weinstein, J.N., & Wiesel, S.W. (1990). *The lumbar spine.* Philadelphia: Saunders.

Willin, J., Anderson, J., Toomoka K., & Singer, K. (1990). The natural history of burst fracture at the thoracolumbar junction. *The Journal of Spinal Disorders,* 3(1),39–46.

Wittert, D.D. (1986). Rotator cuff tears. *Orthopaedic Nursing,* 5(4),17–25.

# 13

# *REHABILITATION PRINCIPLES AND PRACTICES*

To be alive connotes the ability to use one's body to obtain, to use, and to dispose of raw materials, energy, and communications. Life connotes movement within and through one's environment for these energy exchanges.

Movement is relative to a person's ability and capacities to perform the required functions. Many persons have some degree of disability, incapacity, or immobility that limits their freedom for living and moving.

This chapter focuses on the aids for increasing mobility as goals for health and nursing:

- To regain = mobility by overcoming immobility
- To retain = ability by overcoming disability
- To maintain = capacity by preventing incapacity
- To attain = habilitation (living) through rehabilitation

## ACTIVITIES OF DAILY LIVING

Daily living activities include eating, breathing, transferring or moving from place to place, dressing, eliminating, and communicating. Each of these activities requires musculoskeletal functions, abilities, and repetitive movements. Orthopaedic conditions and trauma may result in a functional disability or handicap. Adaptation to that deficit requires living with that disability or handicap.

The processes that facilitate that adaptation are referred to as rehabilitation. Habilitation constitutes outfitting—clothing or dressing—and rehabilitation implies regaining some or all of these abilities.

## CONCEPT OF REHABILITATION

Rusk defined rehabilitation as a dynamic, active program with the ultimate long-term goal of returning a functional individual to his/her environment. Achievement of that goal may involve the use of alternate tissues to perform a function that can no longer be performed by the original tissues or structures. Included in the long-term goal of rehabilitation are shorter-term goals designed to prevent, eliminate, reduce, or circumvent disability. Rehabilitation requires teams of personnel who perform activities with one or more aids during appropriate intervals according to the particular needs of the disabled individual. Mutual consent and determination of goals provide the soundest bases for goal achievement.

Primary or secondary effects from an injury or disease require rehabilitative efforts. Primary effects include loss of a part or an entire extremity; loss of motor functions, sensory perceptions, or abilities; and alteration in organic functions or reserves. Secondary effects may include muscle atrophy, contractures, osteoporosis, pressure ulcerations, urinary calculi, pneumonia, phlebothrombosis, and alterations in psychological functioning. These are generally the effects of immobility and are frequently referred to as the "hazards of immobility." Rehabilitative efforts are designed to prevent further loss from the primary injury, to avoid secondary effects, and to substitute for primary structural or functional loss to regain mobility for daily living.

## REHABILITATIVE PRINCIPLES AND ACTIVITIES

Multiple activities and aids are used for rehabilitation, including exercises, temperature variations, sound waves, massage, electro- or hydrotherapy, and mobility or ambulatory aids. Psychological, vocational, and occupational counseling are also rehabilitation activities.

### Exercises

Rehabilitative exercises use the principles of time and repetition to increase strength of contraction, tone, or precision. Exercises are performed to increase range of motion, to overcome effects of disuse or atrophy, to increase speed of reaction, and to increase elasticity or stretch of muscle fibers. Energy requirements and expenditure of effort by the patient correlate with the various types of exercises, including *active* exercises, performed unassisted; *active-assisted*, performed with assistance of a therapist; *resistive-active*, performed against resistance provided by weights, devices, or a therapist; *passive*, performed without active patient participation; and *selective, special*, performed by the patient to increase the strength of muscles used in sitting, ambulating, breathing, and coughing. Each type of exercise, the number of repetitions, and the effort expenditure are determined and performed to meet the individual needs of the patient. Physical therapists generally assist with the design, execution, and evaluation of the exercise program and are invaluable team members during rehabilitation. Nurses participate actively in this phase of the patient's rehabilitation by encouraging active exercise participation, performing passive range-of-motion exercises, observing and recording patient's reactions to the exercise regimen, and cooperatively coordinating daily care activities to assure that the patient will be available and present at the scheduled exercise sessions (see Fig. 13.1).

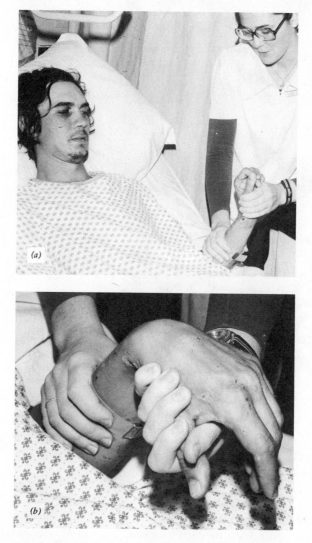

**Figure 13.1** Active-assisted exercises to wrist and fingers. (a) Wrist dorsiflexion; (b) wrist plantarflexion;

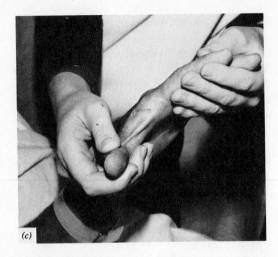

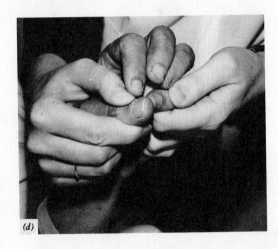

**Figure 13.1 (continued)**
(c) extension and abduction
of the thumb; (d) flexion of
thumb and fingers;

## Applications of Moist or Dry Heat and Cold

Therapeutic uses of moisture, heat, or cold, and combinations of these therapies are commonly employed in orthopaedic care. Knowledge of the rationale for the particular therapy and its effects on the tissues is vital to the effective use of moist or dry heat or cold.

*Principles in the Use of Warm or Hot Applications.* Primary and secondary effects of heat occur over time: for the first 20 to 30 minutes after application vasodilation occurs with its corresponding increased circulation, followed thereafter by the reflex vasoconstriction and slowing of circulation possibly as the body attempts to regain homeostasis. These alternating effects can result

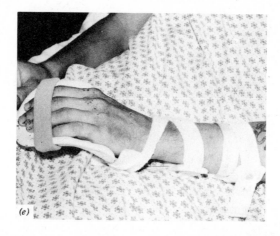

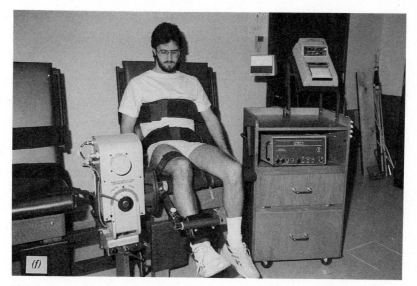

**Figure 13.1 (continued)** (e) splint to maintain proper position; (f) patient doing active strengthening exercises using Cybex machine.

in injury to cells from prolonged applications of heat. Cell injury can be avoided by shorter (less than 20 minutes) periods of application followed by a period of rest to permit cell and vascular recovery. Temperatures vary from warm to very hot (90–115°F), according to the purpose, length, and site of application. Temperatures must be carefully measured to prevent tissue injury or burning. Awareness that children, spinal-cord injured, and older persons have altered skin and temperature tolerances is also vital knowledge for safe care (see Table 13.1).

**Table 13.1** Therapeutic Uses of Heat

| Primary Effects of Heat | Purpose(s) | Type of Application |
|---|---|---|
| Vasodilation | Increase circulation and improve tissue oxygenation; hasten removal of irritants and wastes | Hot-water bag or bottle; infrared lamp; heating pads |
| Muscle relaxation Relief of pain | Decrease in muscle spasm Decreased edema and spasm, increased removal of wastes | Whirlpool bath; diathermy Heating pads, hot packs, paraffin "baths" |
| Remove external debris, drainage, and necrotic tissues; hasten suppuration | Cleanse area; heal area by removal of inflammatory products, wastes, or localizing inflammation | Moist, warm compresses (wet to dry compresses); Hubbard tank bath; whirlpool; sitz bath |
| Provide heat or warmth locally and/or systemically | Warm body and tissues; assist drying as with casts | Hot-water bottle; heat cradle; heating pad |

Policy statements of some health care agencies discourage or do not permit use of electric heating pads unless demurrers for use/injury are signed and the heat-selector indicators are set to allow only use of low heat. Nurses should use caution that—where heating pads are permitted—the covers are kept dry, the cover is secure over the pad, and the pad is not bent, because this could impair overall function. Covers should be of soft absorbent flannel or cotton and be changed when they become damp. Electric circulating water pads should be carefully monitored for correct temperature, for skin reactions following application, and for dryness of covers. Moistness may cause skin maceration and increase tissue or cell injury instead of relieving inflammation. Covers over hot-water bags or bottles should be dry to prevent untoward tissue reactions (see Fig. 13.2 and Table 13.1).

Loss of heat from the skin is slowed by the application of oils, petroleum jellies, and heated paraffin. Skin temperatures remain higher because of the slower heat loss; therefore temperatures for the application of heat through oils, paraffin, or other petroleum substances should be lower to avoid cell or tissue injury.

When using any application of heat, both the structure and the function of the enclosed and surrounding tissues must be considered to prevent fatigue or incorrect pressure or positioning in, on, or around the areas being treated.

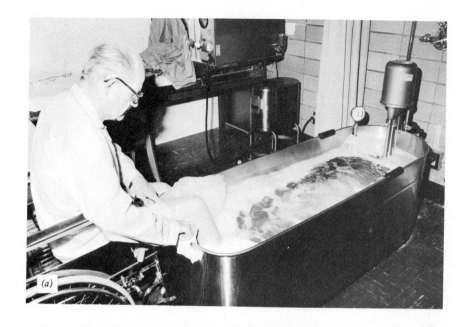

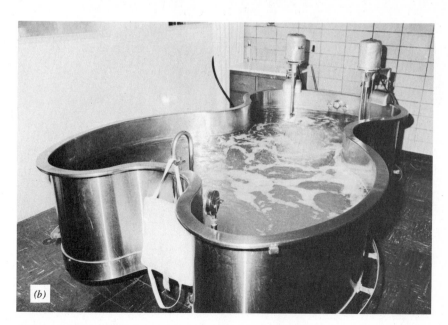

**Figure 13.2** (a) Patient immersing stump in whirlpool to clean wound and increase circulation to the stump; (b) Hubbard tank filled and ready for a patient;

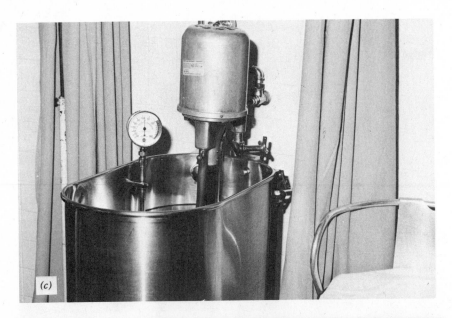

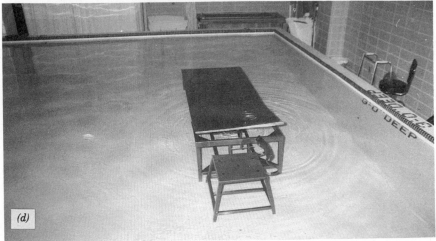

**Figure 13.2 (continued)** (c) whirlpool tank for upper extremity treatment; (d) swimming pool for strengthening exercises.

Conditions causing decreased circulation—such as diabetes, neuropathies, and sensory deficits—result in altered responses and/or sensations of temperature. Care must be taken to use lower temperatures, shorter period for application, and possibly an alternate treatment to avoid injury. Applications of heat may be used prior to massage, or prior to drainage of abscesses. Heat increases blood supply to hasten healing in those instances.

*Principles in the Use of Cold Applications.* Secondary effects of cold applications result from reflex actions causing vasodilation; therefore, cold applications should be intermittent with periods of "recovery" time between applications to prevent tissue damage. Temperature, type, and duration of the cold application depend on the age of the patient (children, spinal-cord injured, and older persons have altered responses), purpose of the application, and underlying condition of the tissues to be treated (see Table 13.2).

**Table 13.2** Therapeutic Uses of Cold

| Primary Effects of Cold | Purpose(s) | Type of Application |
|---|---|---|
| Vasoconstriction | Decrease circulation to decrease bleeding | Ice bag; hypothermia; iced irrigations |
| Decrease circulation | Decrease tissue metabolism and decrease edema formation | Ice bags; cool bath with wet cloths or towels; cold compresses |
| Decrease temperature | Slow metabolism or suppuration (decrease inflammation) | Temperature sponge bath (alcohol in water); ice bags; hypothermia |
| Decrease pain | Anesthesia to area | Hypothermia; ice to lower sensitivity |

Temperatures of the cold application vary from 5–15° lower than body temperature. As the cold is transmitted through the walls of the ice bag and hypothermia blanket, the cold absorbs some heat from the environment; therefore the cold applied to the skin and underlying tissues gradually absorbs the skin temperatures. This heat absorption melts the ice in an ice bag and causes moisture accumulation from condensation and perspiration, resulting in loss of effectiveness of the "cold." Cold applications should not have melted water or damp or wet covers, and they should not be left unattended for so long that they warm up from tissue or environmental heat. Frequent replacement may be required to maintain the desired degree of cold. Damp covers on ice bags must be changed, and condensation or perspiration must be removed. The patient's skin should be dried and checked for signs of excess vasoconstriction, such as pale, bluish, or mottled areas, and also secondary vasodilation, such as erythema (red areas). Ice bags should usually remain in place for 30 minutes, be removed for 10–15 minutes, and then be reapplied. This pattern should be followed for the entire time the ice bag is needed.

Ice should never be applied directly to uncovered skin. The resultant vasoconstriction could cause tissue anoxia severe enough to cause cell death and tissue slough. Cloth or rubber buffers the cold from ice, as does water. "Slushy" ice water can be used for immersion of a finger, hand, or foot to decrease bleeding or edema in injuries from sports and other minor injuries. The injured part is immersed for 10–20 seconds, removed for 1 minute, reimmersed for 10–20 seconds, then removed; this pattern is repeated for 5–10 minutes. The pattern of immersion-removal plus the water-buffered cold allows tissue recovery combined with the therapeutic effects of the cold to lessen bleeding and edema. This technique is useful for the first aid of strained or sprained fingers and for foot or ankle injuries during the first hours after injury. The application can be repeated several times during the first 24 hours after the injury.

Use of hot or cold applications for orthopaedic conditions is a daily experience for thousands of person at home or in therapy clinics or departments in hospitals, nursing units, or extended care facilities. Indeed, thermal applications are vital in order to decrease the immediate and eventual effects of injury, degeneration, or disease. Specific uses for heat or cold are shown in Tables 13.1 and 13.2.

## Ambulatory Aids

Persons with conditions affecting the hips, pelvis, or lower extremities often require temporary or permanent assistance to aid ambulation and increase mobility. Such assistance is provided by the use of walkers, crutches, canes, wheelchairs, and braces.

*Walkers.* Constructed of aluminum or metallic alloys, walkers are lightweight aids strong enough to withstand prolonged use. Newer-style walkers are easily foldable for storage or ease in transporting. Heights are adjustable for individual needs. The use of a walker facilitates partial weight-bearing or full nonweight bearing. Before using a walker, the patient should understand the specific amount of weight bearing permitted or nonweight bearing to be maintained, and how to use and care for the walker. Demonstrating the technique to be used for a particular patient is beneficial, because techniques vary for nonweight bearing versus partial weight-bearing. For both walking activities, the assistant supports the patient to prevent loss of balance, tipping, or uneven balance on the walker. The affected limbs should be referred to as left or right leg, knee, side, and such, not as "good" leg or "bad" leg, as those words are physiologically and psychologically distressing to many persons (see Fig. 13.3).

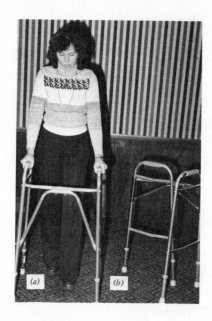

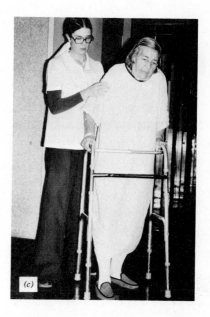

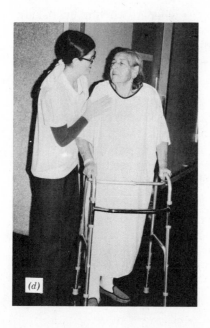

**Figure 13.3** (a) Patient using walker; (b) partially closed walker showing foldability; (c, d) patient ambulating with assistance of therapist.

## Procedures

### ASSISTING A PATIENT TO AMBULATE WITH A WALKER (WITH NONWEIGHT BEARING ON ONE EXTREMITY)

- Instruct the patient to place hands on the nurse's shoulders and to lift self to a standing position while the nurse helps lift the patient. It is vital that the nurse or assistant use proper body mechanics to help lift the patient by placing one knee in front of the patient's unaffected leg to brace the patient's knee if necessary to prevent buckling of the knee, placing the hands under the patient's axillae or at the waist, and shifting the weight from the forward to the backward foot and standing straight as the patient rises. Caution the patient to keep the hands on the nurse's shoulders and to take deep breaths to help stabilize the blood pressure and oxygenation. Also remind the patient to keep all the weight on the unaffected extremity.

- Place the walker in front of and close to the patient.

- Instruct the patient to lift and move the walker forward 8–10 inches. Support the patient around the waist or under the arms while the patient begins to walk.

- Instruct the patient to put all the body weight on the wrists and arms (elbows must be straight to absorb weight) and to step forward with the unaffected leg (Use "right" or "left" leg when instructing the patient. Avoid referring to "good" or "bad" leg.) Remind the patient not to put weight on the affected leg. Continue to monitor the patient's color, breathing, overall strength, or complaints of pain as indication of ability/inability to continue to walk at this time.

- Have the patient bring the affected leg forward by bending the knee and "stepping" to bring the affected leg even with the opposite leg. The affected leg should *not* precede the opposite leg *when no weight bearing is permitted on that leg*. If it should be ahead, weight could inadvertently be borne on it during the next step forward. Thus, each time the affected leg and foot come forward, the step should only be enough to bring the foot up to the unaffected one.

- Have the patient repeat the movements with each step: Move the walker forward; transfer all weight to wrists and forearms with elbows straight; step forward with unaffected leg without allowing any weight on the affected leg; and step forward with affected leg and foot.

Ambulation when partial or touch-down weight bearing is permitted is similar to that given for nonweight bearing, but either limb can be advanced initially. Partial weight-bearing more closely approximates normal walking; joints and muscles are used as normally for walking except that less weight is placed on the affected limb. Personnel should attend patients when using a walker until they are assured that the patient's understanding and strength are sufficient for safe solo ambulation. Observing unaccompanied patients on their excursions may reveal a need for attendance and/or additional or continued reminding about the amount of weight permitted or the distance covered. One of the pleasures of being a member of the health profession is assisting patients in regaining mobility with a walker after trauma to a foot, leg, knee, or hip, then "graduating" to the use of a cane or crutches, and finally to unassisted walking and moving when possible.

*Crutches.* Persons using one or two crutches as aids for ambulation are seen every day. Types of crutches vary, from axillary to forearm extensions and holds (see Fig. 13.4). The user's proficiency varies with age, condition, degree or extent of injury, musculoskeletal functions, and so on. Use of crutches may be a temporary aid for persons with sprains, in casts, or following surgical treatments; or crutches may be routinely and continuously used for those with congenital or acquired musculoskeletal anomalies, neuromuscular weakness, or paralysis; or they may be used after amputations.

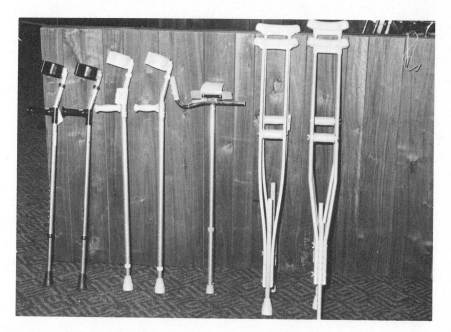

**Figure 13.4** *Various types of crutches for patients with various injuries and varying muscle strengths.*

*Gaits for Crutch Use.* The use of two-, three-, or four-point "gaits" is dependent upon the type of injury, presence, and usability of the lower extremities. "Point" refers to the tip of the crutches or the foot, each tip or foot counted as one point (see Figs. 13.5 and 13.6).

The *two-point gait* is used by persons with partial weight-bearing limitations and for those with bilateral lower extremity amputations (with or without prosthetic replacement). Two-point gait involves advancing one crutch with the opposite extremity so they make a simultaneous "point" or touch. One crutch is always advanced with the opposite extremity or side.

The *three-point gait* is frequently used when partial or full nonweight bearing is desired. Both crutches and the affected extremity are advanced; weight is then borne on the wrists and crutches while the unaffected (normal) extremity is advanced. The patient should be cautioned to walk slowly, to take small, even-sized steps, and to rest periodically. While resting, care should be taken that undue pressure is not placed on axillary tissues by dropping

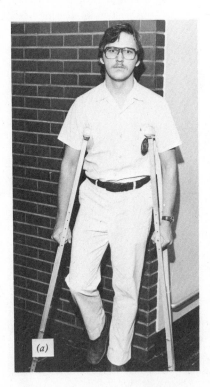 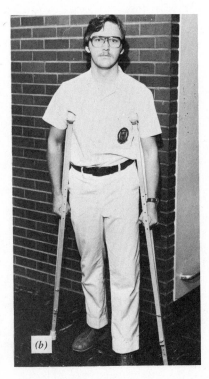

**Figure 13.5** Crutch gaits: (a) three-point gait; (b) two-point gait. (One foot and crutch are moved simultaneously.)

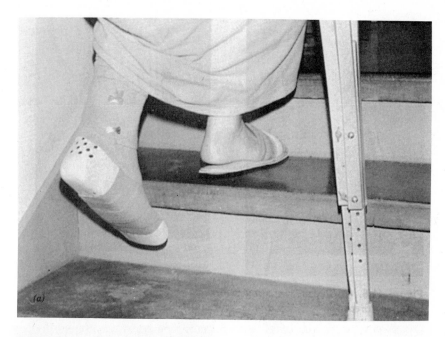

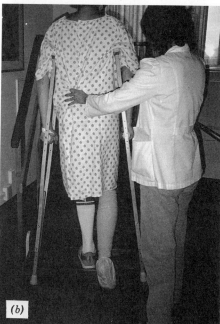

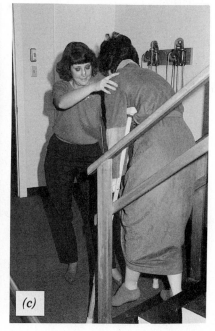

**Figure 13.6** (a) Patient ascending stairs with both crutches in one hand; (b) Patient ascending stairs with a crutch in each hand and assistance of therapist; (c) Patient descending stairs with one crutch in each hand and assistance of a physical therapist.

shoulders to rest axillae on crutch crosspieces. Pressure on axillary vessels and nerve pathways is reflected to the forearm and hand, causing numbness, tingling, or circulatory changes that may be temporary or permanent, depending on the extent of injury.

Several variations of the three-point gait are commonly used for persons with varying degrees of weight restriction, muscle strength, and/or paralysis. One variation uses only one crutch until full strength is regained and the crutch use is discontinued. Generally, when only one crutch is used, it should be used on the unaffected side to bear the body's weight when the normal extremity is advanced. Another variation of the three-point gait is the swing-through gait used by persons with lower extremity paralysis. Both extremities equal one point; with the knees fully extended both legs are swung forward together, and the crutches are advanced by lifting the shoulder girdle muscles while bringing the crutches ahead simultaneously. A final variation of the three-point gait is the tripod gait, which involves bringing forward one crutch, then the second crutch, followed by pulling or dragging the body forward up to the crutches. This gait is very tiring and requires strong shoulder, arm, and abdominal muscles to move the paralyzed lower extremities forward.

The *four-point gait* most nearly approximates the normal arm-leg, swing-step movements used in walking. It is accomplished by advancing first one crutch, then the opposite foot, second crutch, and second foot. Crutch advancements and steps should be equal in size and even in rhythm for pacing and comfort.

*Rising from a Sitting to Standing Position with Use of Crutches.* Placing the crutches in an easily accessible location is the first requirement to their use on rising. Accessible sites are at the back or side of the chair or upright against a near cabinet or wall. The handrests of the crutches may be used as a bracing area while rising if the chair is solid and heavy enough to preclude tipping if only one arm would be used with the crutches for bracing while rising. If the chair is lightweight, both armrests should be used for even bracing while rising, then the crutches placed for ambulating. When sitting down or rising, the patient should be carefully instructed to use either both armrests or one armrest and both crutches together as one rest to maintain balance. Balance can be lost or chairs can be tipped from uneven or one-sided pressure.

*Walking Up or Down Stairs.* Patients should be instructed on correct techniques for negotiating stairs or steps. Two methods are safe, and the patient's comfort and skill may be decisive in which one the person will use routinely (see Fig. 13.6).

*(1)* The technique of using one crutch on each side requires sound teaching, practice, and a relatively uncluttered or unpopulated stairway. The person ascends the stairs by placing both crutches sufficiently away from the step to prevent catching the toes as he/she steps up with the unaffected foot; then the

person brings both crutches, the affected foot, and the body upward simultaneously. Each succeeding step is negotiated in a similar fashion: first stepping up with the unaffected foot, then bringing the crutches, affected limb, and body up. Descending stairs is accomplished by reversing the movements. To descend, the person places both crutches on the next step, moves the affected limb forward, then steps down to the crutches by lowering the body and the unaffected foot. Descending stairs is more threatening for most persons on crutches, because they fear falling downward. Very careful instruction, secure holding by the instructor, and clear visibility and visual acuity facilitate crutch walking and provide comfort and security to the learner.

(2) With one or both crutches in the same hand, stairs may be negotiated using the banister as a "crutch." As with all crutch-walking techniques, the crutches must be securely braced in the hand, within the arm-axillary area, and firmly placed on the step to prevent their slipping, sliding, or falling, which could cause the person to lose balance or fall.

Crutch walking is very advantageous as a means to increase a person's mobility. It can be safe and viable when precautions are taken to be certain that the person, crutches, and environmental conditions provide assurances for safety, skill, and comfort.

## Canes

Depending on musculoskeletal need, a person can use one or two canes for ambulation. The canes may be wooden or metallic. If metallic, the cane may be triangular or quadrangular "pointed" for greater support. Metallic canes are heavier than their wooden counterparts and are frequently adjustable, which is not possible with wooden canes. When canes are unilaterally used, they are most commonly used opposite the weak or injured side and are advanced forward with the uninjured or unaffected limb. Canes primarily increase the person's security and balance by increasing the base of support. Canes also absorb or take the body weight when necessary for mobility during partial weight-bearing periods. Instruction for use of cane-assisted ambulation is required to assess the person's balance, strength, and confidence. Muscle-strengthening exercises such as knee-and-foot flexions and walking in parallel bars help the person increase strength and confidence before using a walker, crutches, or a cane. Rubber tips on the ends prevent slipping when using any of the aids. Teaching to lift rather than slide the aid lessens the possibility of catching the tips, which could cause the user to lose balance, trip, or fall (see Figs. 13.7, 13.8, and 13.9).

## Wheelchairs

Wheelchairs are available in several materials and can be equipped with multiple parts to provide safety and comfort. Wooden wheelchairs are gener-

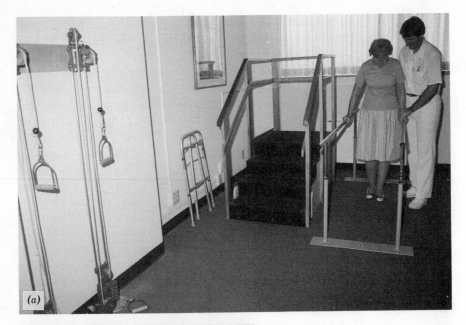

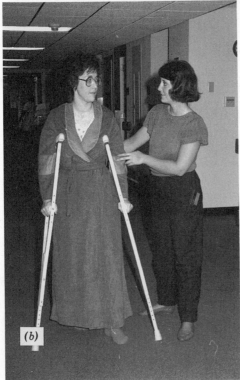

**Figure 13.7** (a) Patient using parallel bars under supervision of nurse; (b) patient using crutches under supervision of physical therapist.

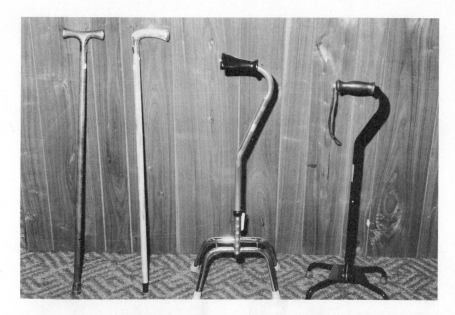

**Figure 13.8** *Various types of canes. The two canes on the right are heavy and more difficult to use than the two on the left.*

ally being replaced with lightweight metal chairs equipped with detachable or removable arm or leg rests, straps, or supports. Easily opened or closed pressure-sensitive straps facilitate opening or closing by persons with weakened muscles or those with limited hand, arm, or finger movements or use. Use of the better-equipped chair also eases transfer into or from the wheelchair or bed, as well as allowing easy movement of the chair from place to place. Motorized chairs provide additional mobility for many persons; brake levers are easily applied or released; wheels turn freely with tires that leave no marks on floors; canvas seats provide strong, firm, yet soft support for long-term use. Special cushions that contain special gels or air are also available (see Figs. 13.10 and 13.11).

Additional safety features of some wheelchairs include leg straps, belts for maintaining upright sitting positions, and removable trays or rests for individual uses. Wheelchairs can be adjusted for individual heights; leg-rest lengths are also adjustable. Special chairs can be built for unusually tall or short persons. Chairs are also available with reclining or removable backs, but use of these features may require the assistance of others.

Techniques for transferring to and from a wheelchair and for propelling or stopping the chair generally require special training, special rooms, and qualified personnel for teaching persons with paralyzed or nonusable musculoskeletal tissues. Usually those persons requiring such specialized training are neurologically injured following spinal-cord injuries.

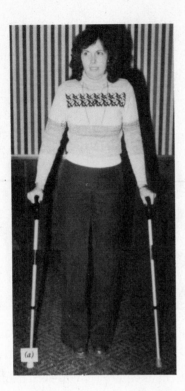
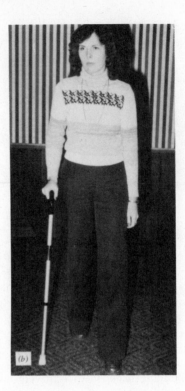

**Figure 13.9** (a) Patient ambulating with two canes and (b) using one cane, carried in the hand opposite the weak limb.

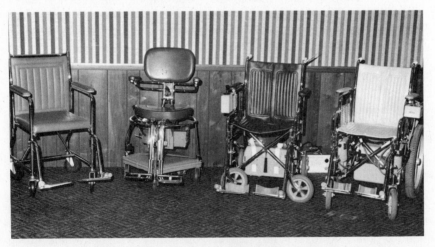

**Figure 13.10** Types of wheelchairs with detachable belts, straps, or pads. Some are motorized.

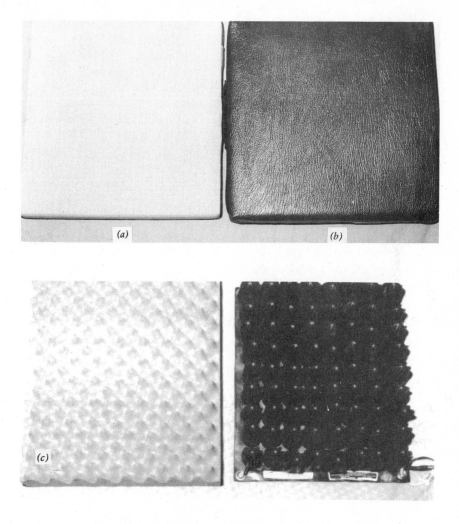

**Figure 13.11** (a) Foam-filled pad for wheelchair or bed; (b) Water-filled pad. (c) Foam pads with alternating peaks and valleys to change pressure areas. (d) Inflatable pad to alternate pressure areas.

Many members of the health team participate with the patient in the rehabilitative activities. Assistance with transfer techniques and muscle retraining exercises requires the specialized skills of physical therapists. Occupational therapists and vocational counselors participate in the planning, training, and perfection of skills for home or job as well as using individualized programs of crafts to regain or use alternate muscles for returning to home and society.

Members of the rehabilitative team must contend with the social attitudes and prejudices toward handicapped persons. Family members may desert the patient during the long and frequently stressful period of rehabilitation. The postrehabilitation roles of the handicapped person will of necessity be changed or modified, sometimes to such a degree that family roles can no longer be maintained, because family members become anxious or feel vulnerable in the presence of the handicapped person. Thus, counseling must incorporate all family members as well as the handicapped person in order to make the interpersonal social adjustments helpful, hopeful, and mutually satisfying within the limits attainable.

## Braces

Braces assist movement or maintain immobility in the tissues involved. Braces may be applied to incorporate one or more joints, depending on the rationale governing the use of the brace.

Braces may be constructed of metal bars with leather straps, heavy canvas with metallic inserts, softer polyethylene foam collars, or combinations of metal, canvas, muslin, or foam. Neck braces hold the cervical vertebrae rigid following whiplash or fracture injuries. Chest and abdominal braces hold the thoracic and lumbar vertebral column to correct scoliosis, kyphosis, or lordosis. Lumbar braces hold lumbar and sacral tissues following spinal surgery and fusions. Leg braces hold the thigh, leg, and foot in functional positions for weight bearing and ambulation; and shoulder, arm, and hand braces are used as support for healing, to decrease pain, or to maintain mobility when desired. Flexor-hinge splits are used wherever joint mobility is desired, such as in the knee, wrist, or elbow (see Figs. 13.12, 13.13, and 13.14).

## Utensils

"Utensils" for eating, self-care, and recreational, occupational, and vocational activities aid daily living for handicapped persons. Curved, hinged, or extra-long handles, straps, and personalized utensils help handicapped persons negotiate eating, dressing, and bathing, as well as engage in recreational, vocational, artistic, and other individually adapted activities (see Figs. 13.15 and 13.16). Availability of utensils and educational aids can be determined through discussions with physical and occupational therapists.

## ECONOMIC AIDS FOR REHABILITATION SERVICES

Although federal aid for selected categories of physical conditions has been provided since 1798, only since World War I has federal legislation been

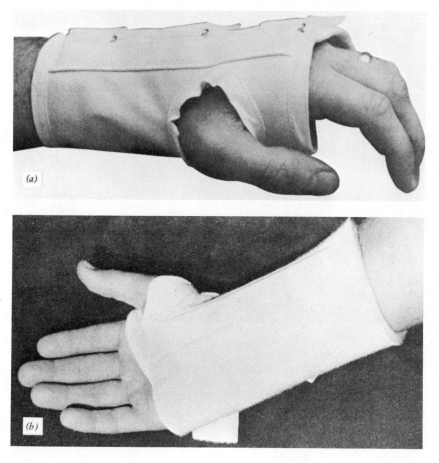

**Figure 13.12** (a) Wrist cock-up splint, adjustable to desired angle; (b) Wrist and palm splint, also adjustable.

passed, primarily for rehabilitation of disabled veterans. Since then, the concept of rehabilitation has been broadened to incorporate civilian and veteran alike, regardless of source or type of disability. Social Security, Medicare, and Medicaid legislation provide primary or supplemental funds for rehabilitation of handicapped persons. The Department of Vocational Rehabilitation provides vocational, occupational, financial, and counseling services for aiding resocialization of rehabilitated persons. Efforts are directed toward returning not only physically handicapped but all handicapped persons to their maximal capacities. Offices in all major cities offer rehabilitation services.

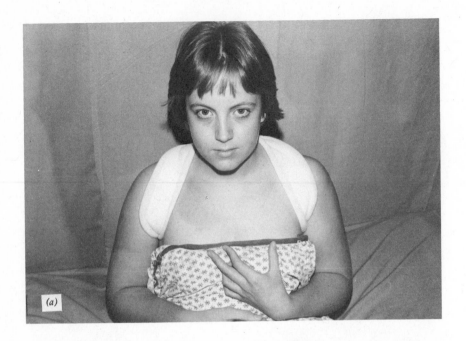

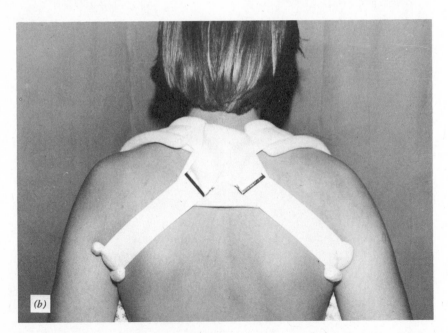

**Figure 13.13** (a) Anterior and (b) posterior views of a commercial "figure of eight" support for immobilization of a fractured clavicle. Note axillary padding to prevent pressure to brachial plexus.

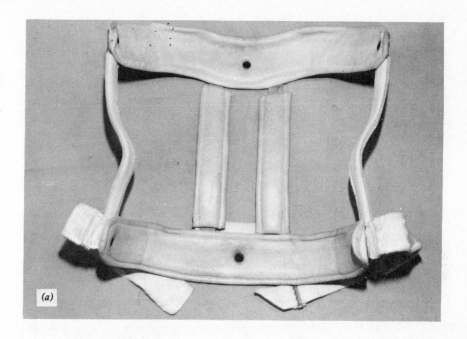

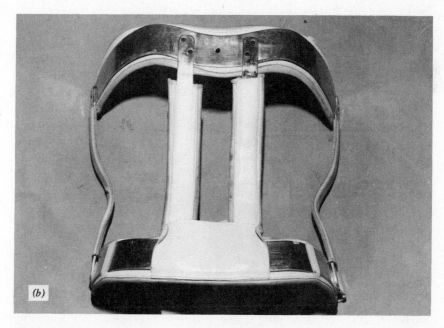

**Figure 13.14** (a) Anterior and (b) posterior views of a metal-reinforced back brace;

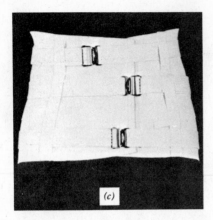 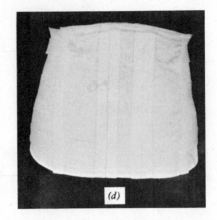

**Figure 13.14 (continued)** (c, d) canvas back support.

**Table 13.3** Principles of Body Mechanics

Posture is Maintained by "Putting on the Internal Girdle"

- Abdominal muscles are contracted giving a feeling of upward pull, while gluteal muscles are contracted giving downward pull.
- Contracting the shoulder girdle backward while pulling the vertebral column "straight" within the normal curves also are good postural habits.

Use of "Proper" Muscles and Stance Can Prevent Injury

- Use the longest and strongest muscles of the back and thighs whenever possible for lifting, carrying, or pulling activities. When these muscles are used in conjunction with the internal girdle muscles, fatigue and injury are avoided.
- Working close to an object prevents muscle strain from unnecessary reaching (stretching).
- Placing feet apart provides a broad base of support, which aids stability.
- Slide, roll, push, or pull rather than lift objects to reduce the energy needed to lift against the pull of gravity.
- When lifting, bend knees, put on the internal girdle, and come close to the object to be lifted. Use the strong leg muscles to help in lifting. Do not lift from a standing, stooping position, which arches the vertebral column. This position puts unnecessary strain on all muscles involved.

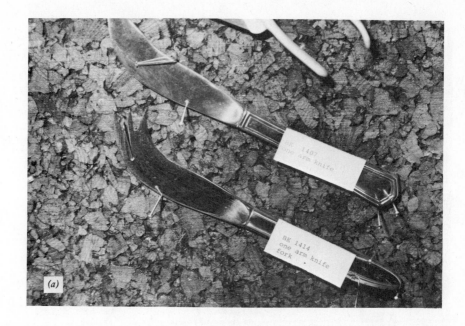

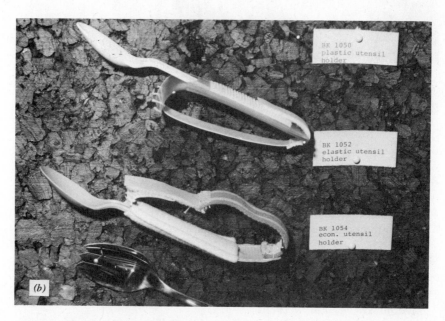

**Figure 13.15** (a, b) Various utensils to assist persons with weakened muscles to eat unassisted;

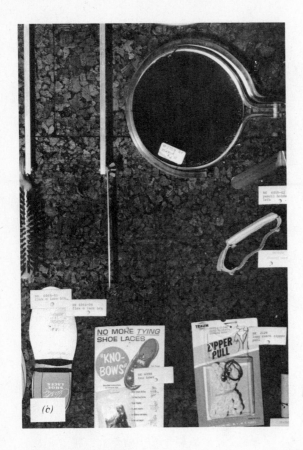

**Figure 13.15** (c) types of equipment to assist persons with self-care and dressing.

## BIBLIOGRAPHY

Ball, G.V., & Koopman, W.J. (1986). *Clinical rheumatology.* Philadelphia: Saunders.

Banwell, B.F., & Gall, V. (Eds.). (1988). *Physical therapy management of arthritis.* New York: Churchill Livingstone.

Buchanan, W.W. (1989). Managing arthritis in elderly patients. *Journal of Musculoskeletal Medicine* (Suppl), 4(3),516–17.

Frontera, W.R., & Adams, R.P. (1986). Endurance exercise: Normal physiology and limitations imposed by pathological processes, Part 2. *The Physician and Sports Medicine, 14*(9),108–120.

Hald, R.D., & Mellon, M.B. (1989). Taping and wrapping of common sports injuries. *Journal of Musculoskeletal Medicine, 6*(1),78–101.

Hicks, J.E. (1989). Exercise for patients with inflammatory arthritis. *Journal of Musculoskeletal Medicine, 6*(10),40–56.

Hukins, D.W.L., & Mulholland, R.C. (Eds.). (1986). *Back pain.* Manchester, England: Manchester University Press.

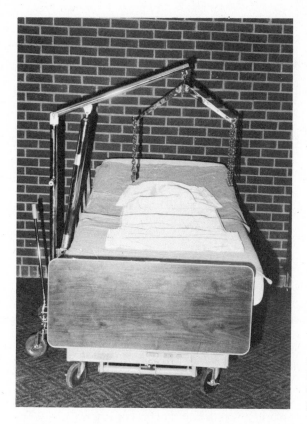

**Figure 13.16** Porta-lift used to transfer patients. Lifts such as this may also contain a scale to weigh patients.

Koszuta, L.E. (1986). Water exercise causes ripples. *The Physician and Sports Medicine, 14*(10),163–167.

Melvin, J.L. (1989). *Rheumatic disease in the adult and child: Occupational therapy and rehabilitation* (3rd ed.). Philadelphia: Davis.

Moskowitz, R.W., & Haug, M.R. (1986). *Arthritis and the elderly.* New York: Springer.

Mourad, L. (1991). *Orthopedic disorders.* St. Louis: Mosby-Yearbook.

Schumacher, H.R., & Gall, E.P. (1988). *Rheumatoid arthritis.* Philadelphia: Lippincott.

Sculco, T.P. (Ed.). (1985). *Orthopaedic care of the geriatric patient.* St. Louis: Mosby-Yearbook.

Tollison, C.D., & Kriegel, M.L. (1988). Physical exercise in the treatment of low back pain II: A practical regimen of stretching exercises. *Orthopaedic Review, 17*(9),913–923.

Zarandona, J.E., Nelson, A.G., Conlee, R.K., & Fisher, A.G. (1986). Physiological responses to hand-carried weights. *The Physician and Sports Medicine, 14*(10),113–120.

# 14

## COMPLICATIONS ASSOCIATED WITH ORTHOPAEDIC TRAUMA, DISEASES, AND SURGERY

A complication is an undesirable outcome of an injury or disease. Complications related to orthopaedic trauma and to common orthopaedic conditions can occur despite all efforts to prevent them.

Complications associated with orthopaedic conditions are the focus of this chapter, and are organized according to the tissues involved.

Complications related to bone union include:

- *Nonunion:* failure to achieve callus formation at the fracture site (generally not a nonunion until 7–9 months or longer postfracture) (see Fig. 14.1)
- *Malunion:* bone union in a nonanatomic position (see Fig. 14.2)
- *Delayed union:* prolonged time period for evidence of callus bridging across fracture site (generally declared after 5–7 months, depending on the specific bone and type of fracture)
- *Refracture:* recurrence of a fracture at or near the initial site of the original fracture
- *Pseudarthrosis:* a "false" joint forming at the fracture site. Pseudarthrosis frequently results from presence of muscles or other tissues between the fractured bone fragments, which prevents adequate formation of callus.
- *Joint Fusion:* bone union and joint structures healing with joint stiffness or fusion if an injury or fracture is through or within a joint. It is a complication if the fusion is not the desired form of healing.

Nurses caring for patients with a failure of proper bone union must assess neurovascular functions, degree or extent of mobility limitation, use and type of ambulatory aid, presence, type, and intensity of pain, and effects of the specific complication on the patient's ADL, employment, and self-concept.

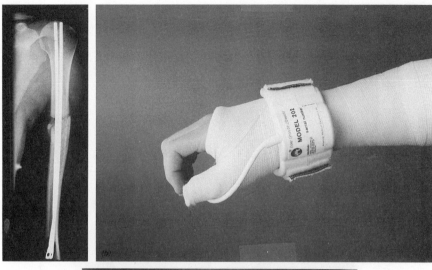

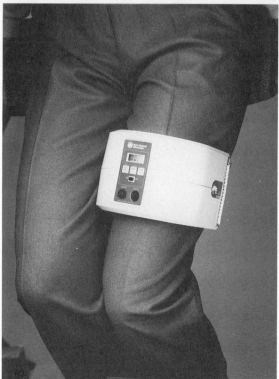

**Figure 14.1** (a) Nonunion of fracture of humerus with bone grafts and intramedullary rods. (b, c) Electrical bone stimulators used to enhance bone union.

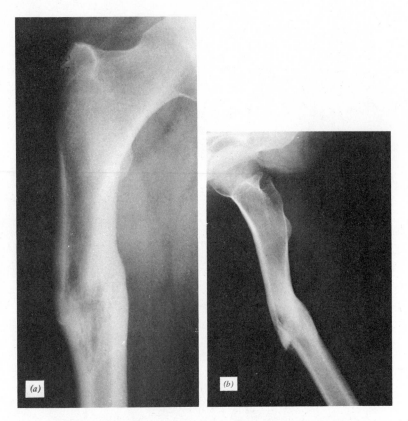

**Figure 14.2** Malunion of a midshaft femoral fracture. (a) Anterior view showing apparent good position. (b) Oblique view showing malunion of proximal fragment. No treatment was required as callus was sufficient for weightbearing.

Nurses must also clarify, as needed, explanations regarding the proposed specific treatment(s) for the conditions. Treatments may include open reduction with internal fixation with plates and screws, nails, pins, or bone grafts (see Figs. 12.16 and 12.17). A cast or brace may be needed, or even a joint replacement. Use of an electrical bone stimulator enhances bone healing in many instances of delayed union (see Fig. 14.1b, c). The aim of these treatments is to achieve satisfactory bone union, relieve pain, and assist the patient to regain usual roles, responsibilities, and social activities.

Two complications are related to circulatory compromise following orthopaedic trauma. These are avascular necrosis and compartment syndrome.

## AVASCULAR NECROSIS

Avascular necrosis is loss of bone substance due to loss of blood supply to a specific bone. It can occur in any bone after a single incident, or following repetitive traumatic incidents, but the bone most frequently affected is the head of the femur.

The head of the femur receives much of its blood supply through the ligamentum teres (see Fig. 14.3), and from the surrounding hip capsule arteries. With trauma in which the head is twisted or dislocated from the acetabulum, the blood supply is disrupted or lost, resulting in time in avascular necrosis. Avascular necrosis may also result from steroid medications injected into a joint or taken orally over long periods. The exact etiology of steroid-induced necrosis has not been determined, but it may be related to altered lipid metabolism during steroid therapy (see Fig. 14.3).

Avascular necrosis initially affects the cartilage covering the bone. Because cartilage has no intrinsic blood supply, disturbances in circulation lead to deterioration of the joint or bone cartilage followed by weakening or deterioration of the subchondral bone and, eventually, loss of joint surfaces. The process of avascular necrosis occurs over time with few symptoms to alert the person that the process is happening. As the destruction continues, it produces intermittent, then constant pain on weight bearing, limitation of motion in or around the involved joint, and eventual loss of function resulting from posttraumatic arthritis of the joint.

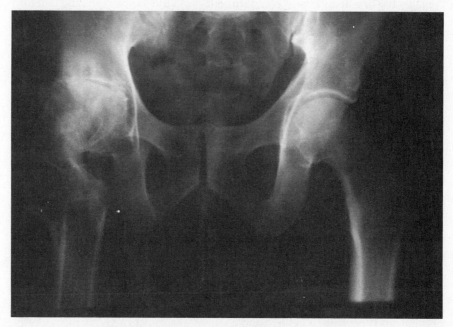

**Figure 14.3** Avascular necrosis of head of femur.

Avascular necrosis of the navicular or lunate bones of the wrist occurs due to the repetitive trauma from striking the heel of the hand on cash register keys or other machinery. Avascular necrosis of those bones is referred to as Kienbock's disease. Legg-Calve-Perthes disease involves avascular necrosis of the capital epiphysis of the femur in young children (ages 5–12), and Kohler's disease is avascular necrosis of the tarsal navicular bone.

Treatments for avascular necrosis include replacement of the affected bone with a prosthesis. Occasionally, for avascular necrosis of the head of the femur, a total joint replacement may be performed if the cartilage on both sides of the joint has become devitalized or degenerated. Prosthesis and total joint replacements have been discussed in Chapter 12.

## COMPARTMENT SYNDROME

Compartment syndrome is a marked increase in tissue pressures that affect tissue and cellular perfusion and can lead to severe tissue damage. It arises when the circulation and functioning of tissues within a closed space are compromised by increased pressure within that space. A compartment contains arteries, veins, muscles, and one or more nerves (see Fig. 14.4). Compartments are formed or limited by the fascia that cover muscles with arteries, veins, and nerves traversing the muscle mass. Extremities are more susceptible to the development of compartment syndrome than other tissues because of the fascial coverings. The forearm contains the dorsal and volar compartments, and the leg contains the anterior, lateral, superior posterior, and deep posterior compartments. Increased tissue pressures can occur in one or more compartments at the same time.

The amount of pressure needed to produce compartment syndrome depends on multiple factors, including the duration of the pressure elevations, vascular tone, local blood pressure, and the metabolic rate of the tissues. Pressure rises may vary from normal 15–30 mm Hg to rises of 60–70 mm Hg. Such elevated pressures *must* be relieved within 4–6 hours, and no longer than 12–24 hours, or nerve and muscle ischemia will result in permanent functional losses and development of Volkmann's ischemic contracture (see Figs. 14.5 and 14.6). The extent of muscle damage is usually proportional to the duration and severity of the ischemic process. Muscle necrosis is reversible, if circulation can be restored before fibrous replacement has occurred. Compartment syndrome can develop in tissues damaged by injury, fractures, burns, and other soft tissue trauma.

*Volkmann's ischemic contracture* is the deformity resulting from an injury to an extremity in which markedly elevated tissue pressures cause a profound reduction in arterial perfusion and, therefore, tissue ischemia. Ischemic changes lead to cellular dysfunction; marked edema; color changes, proceeding at times to cyanosis; pain in increasing amounts and severity; shortening of and spasms primarily in flexor muscles; nerve pressure indicators of increasing numbness, tingling, and "pins and needles"; and changes in ability to actively move digits. If the increased tissue pressure is not relieved, the affected extremity will

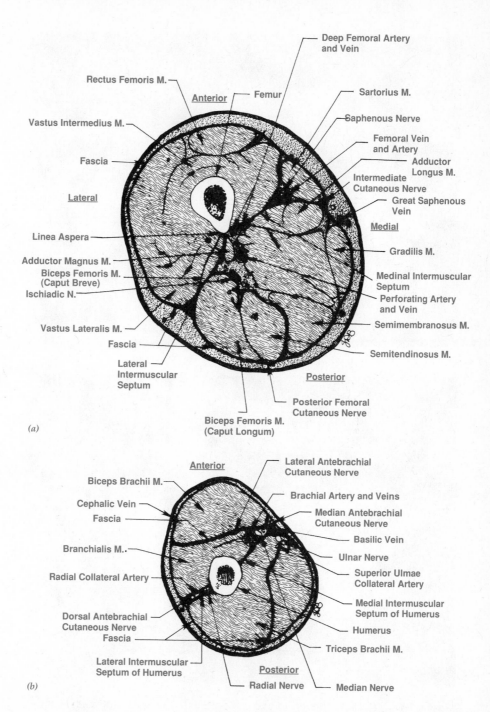

**Figure 14.4** (a) Compartments of the thigh and (b) of the upper arm.

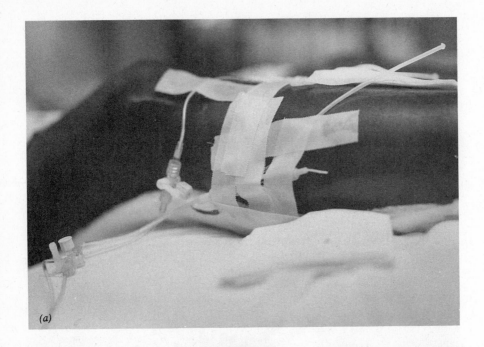

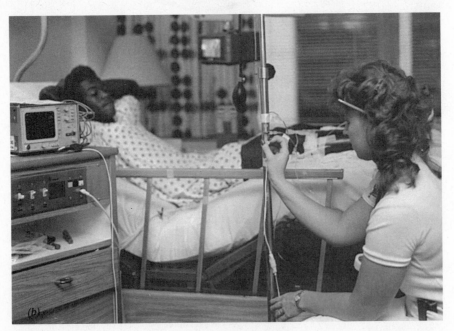

**Figure 14.5** (a) Wick catheters in two compartments in the leg; (b) nurse measuring tissue venous pressure by the Wick catheter method.

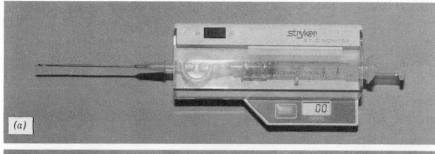
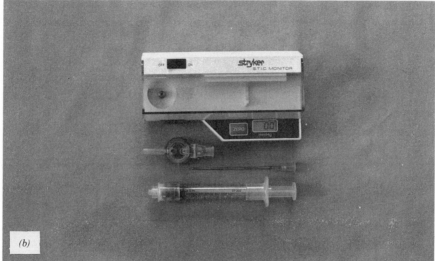

**Figure 14.6** (a, b) Stryker tissue pressure monitor (used with permission of the Stryker Corporation). Technique for measuring tissue pressures: Eject small amount of saline from pre-filled syringe. Prep skin area with antiseptic for needle insertion. Burn on-off switch on. Press zero button to obtain digital readout. Physician inserts needle into compartment being checked and injects less than .3 ml. saline into tissues. Read indicator for amount of tissue pressure. Remove needle and syringe. Hold site until drainage stops.

develop claw hand (or foot) deformity with markedly flexed fingers or toes, hard leathery skin, and limitation of joint movements (see Fig. 14.7). Twelve or more hours of total ischemia are required to produce such contractures.

Compartment syndrome as a forerunner of Volkmann's ischemic contracture does not need to result in a nonfunctional or limited-functional limb if immediate and continuous care is provided. The medical treatment is a fasciotomy, a surgical opening of the fascia covering the specific compartment. The fascia is opened the length of the muscle, which permits the edematous muscle to bulge into the opening. Release of the constricting fascia should result in increased circulation to the muscle, with a subsequent return of venous pressures to normal ranges and to normal tissue perfusion and oxygenation. The operative

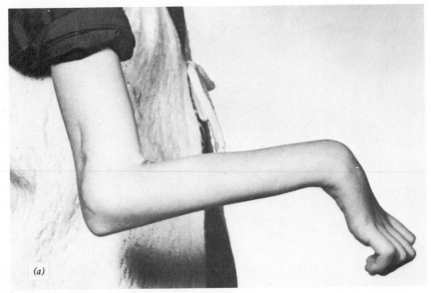

(a)

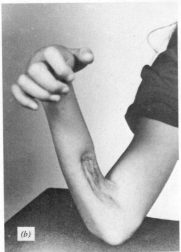

(b)

**Figure 14.7** (a, b) Volkmann's ischemic contracture following supracondylar fracture of the humerus. Fasciotomy was unsuccessful in restoring circulation to the muscles, leading to atrophy and contracture of the forearm and wrist.

wound is left unsutured and is closed in 7–10 days after the muscle edema has abated. The fascia can be closed with direct suturing, or a split-thickness skin graft can be applied to cover the defect or muscle mass.

If a fasciotomy is not done, and if the condition progresses to become a Volkmann's contracture, the patient is faced with multiple treatments; none is completely satisfactory, because devitalized tissues usually cannot be restored to full functions. Some treatments include physical therapy with exercises, whirlpool baths, splints for joints, tendon transfers, joint fusion, and rarely, amputation of the nonfunctional limb.

## COMPLICATIONS ASSOCIATED WITH MUSCLE TISSUES

One major muscular complication of an inflammatory nature is myositis ossificans circumscripta. This condition involves inflammation of muscles caused by increased scarring, with the deposition of calcium in the previously injured muscles. Generally, myositis ossificans circumscripta follows trauma, but occasionally no history of trauma can be traced. Frequently, the hip, thigh, or knee is involved. In myositis ossificans circumscripta there is an overproduction of collagen, which eventually becomes calcified. Sometimes the resulting lesion becomes difficult to differentiate from an osteosarcoma. As the lesion matures, it can be transformed into bone and, if around joints, can produce an ankylosis. It can also cause muscle atrophy (see Fig. 14.8).

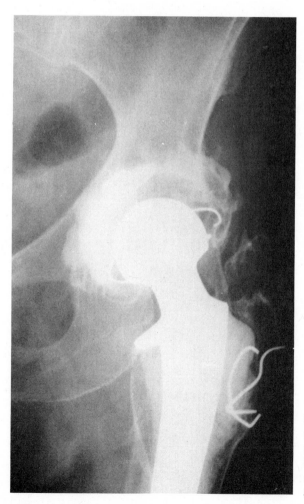

**Figure 14.8** Myositis ossificans secondary to a total hip replacement. Note the excessive calcifications around the acetabulum.

Myositis ossificans secondary to trauma is not to be confused with the condition myositis ossificans progressiva, which is a congenital, hereditary, and sometimes a familial disease in which group after group of muscles, tendons, and ligaments ossify until eventually all active movements are lost and the person dies in respiratory failure.

Observations include measuring the effects of myositis ossificans on patient's ROM, mobility, and, at times, the presence of a muscle mass. Treatments include use of physical therapy programs to increase muscle strength and administration of steroid medications to lessen the inflammatory response. Surgical removal of the calcified mass is occasionally necessary to permit pain-free weight bearing.

## CARPAL TUNNEL SYNDROME

*Carpal tunnel syndrome* is the pattern of edema, pain, paresthesia, and altered functions of the fingers resulting from compression of the median nerve at the wrist (see Fig. 14.9). *Tarsal tunnel syndrome* is a pattern of similar symptoms associated with the ankle, foot, and toes from entrapment of the posterior tibial nerve.

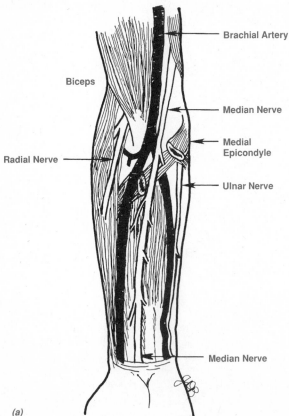

*(a)*

**Figure 14.9** (a) Nerves of the forearm.

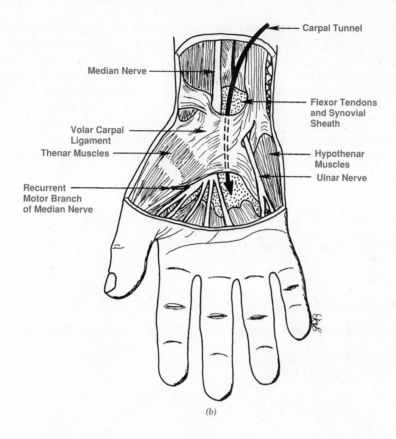

Carpal Tunnel

Median Nerve

Flexor Tendons
and Synovial
Sheath

Volar Carpal
Ligament

Thenar Muscles

Hypothenar
Muscles

Ulnar Nerve

Recurrent
Motor Branch
of Median Nerve

*(b)*

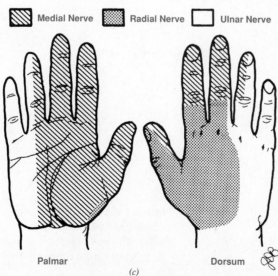

Medial Nerve   Radial Nerve   Ulnar Nerve

Palmar

Dorsum

*(c)*

**Figure 14.9** (b) Volar carpal ligament, which constricts the median nerve and tendon sheath in carpal tunnel syndrome. (c) Sensory distribution of the nerves of the forearm to the fingers.

Carpal tunnel syndrome may occur unilaterally secondary to trauma or bilaterally during the third trimester of pregnancy. Its association with pregnancy has not been fully explained to date, but may be related to altered hormonal balances and fluid retention.

Carpal tunnel syndrome may be partially diagnosed by having the patient place the two wrists against each other in 90° flexion, and hold this position for 1 minute. This test, referred to as Phalen test, is considered positive for the syndrome if the patient develops paresthesia over the distribution area of the median nerve (see Fig. 14.10). Tinel sign is elicited by tapping over the median

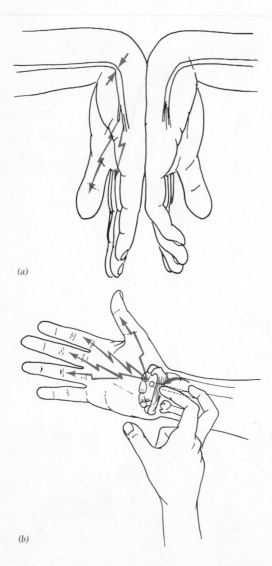

(a)

(b)

**Figure 14.10** (a) Phalen test to detect carpal tunnel syndrome. (b) Tinel sign for detection of carpal tunnel syndrome.

nerve in the volar aspect of the wrist. The sign is positive if there is tingling in the fingers as the median nerve is tapped.

Sensory functions of nerves are integral parts of n-v checks (see Fig. 14.11). Nurses observe or assess for complaints of numbness, tingling, pins and needles sensations, edema, and pain in injured areas. Elevation of the affected part may lessen edema. Effects of anti-inflammatory medications or other analgesics must be determined to note if a change may be needed. A splint may be worn at night to lessen possibility of flexing the affected joint (flexion increases symptoms from decreased circulation or increased pressure). Steroids may be injected into the affected tissues to lessen the inflammation. Surgical decompression of the tendon sheath by release of the constricting ligament is a common treatment for tunnel syndromes. Following release, the patient should regain full functions in 2–3 weeks.

Pressure over some peripheral nerves can cause temporary or permanent neurological complications with evidence noted by deformities, as shown in Figs. 14.12, 14.13, and 14.14. Fortunately, these complications, such as foot drop, wrist drop, waiter's tip hand, and finger deformities, are rare. These complications all involve excessive pressure on the nerves for prolonged periods, resulting in the alteration or loss of function of the parts enervated by the specific nerve or nerves (see Tables 14.1 and 14.2).

| Date | 1/13/92 | | | | | | | | | | | | | | | Comments | Nurse's signature |
|---|---|---|---|---|---|---|---|---|---|---|---|---|---|---|---|---|---|
| Time | 1 PM | 2 | 3 | 4 | 5 | 6 | 7 | 8 | 9 | 10 | 11 | 12 | | | | | |
| Neurovascular checks | | | | | | | | | | | | | | | | | |
| A. COLOR OF TISSUES<br>Pink (normal) = 1<br>Pale = 2<br>Blue = 3<br>Mottled = 4 | 1 | | | | | | | | | | | | | | | | |
| B. TEMPERATURE OF TISSUES<br>Warm (normal) = 1<br>Cool = 2<br>Cold = 3<br>Hot = 4 | 2 | | | | | | | | | | | | | | | | |
| C. EDEMA<br>None = 0<br>Slight = 1<br>Moderate = 2<br>Marked = 3<br>Pitting = 4 | 2 | | | | | | | | | | | | | | | | |
| D. PAIN<br>None = 0<br>Slight = 1<br>Moderate amount = 2<br>Severe = 3<br>Radiating = 4 | 2 | | | | | | | | | | | | | | | | |
| E. CAPILLARY REFILL<br>2-4 seconds (normal) = 2<br>4-6 seconds = 2<br>longer than 6 sec. = 3 | 2 | | | | | | | | | | | | | | | | |
| F. MOTOR FUNCTIONS<br>Active ROM all joints = 1<br>involved<br>Passive only 2<br>Weak = 3<br>Paralyzed = 4 | 1 | | | | | | | | | | | | | | | | |
| G. SENSORY FUNCTIONS<br>Discriminates sharp/dull = 1<br>Decreased sensation = 2<br>Pins and needles = 3<br>Numb = 4 | 2 | | | | | | | | | | | | | | | | |
| H. COMPARED WITH LIKE TISSUES<br>Same = 1<br>Different = 2 (also place letter of check that differs) | D.E.G<br>2 | | | | | | | | | | | | | | | Dr. Taylor informed at 1:15 pm, orders given - see order book | S. Smith RN |

**Figure 14.11** (a) Flow sheet for neurovascular checks.

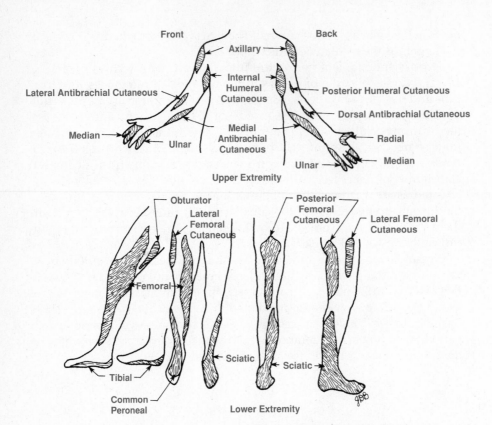

**Figure 14.11** (b) Sensory dermatomes to the upper and lower extremities.

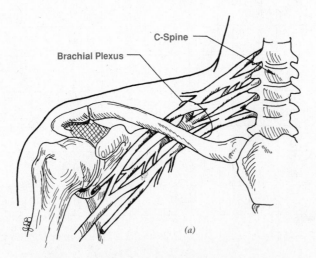

**Figure 14.12** (a) Nerves of the brachial plexus.

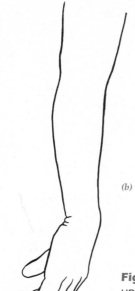

*(b)*

**Figure 14.12** (b) "Waiter's tip" deformity from injury to the upper trunk of the brachial plexus.

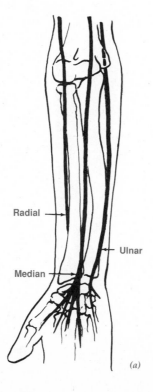

Radial

Ulnar

Median

*(a)*

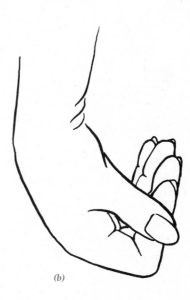

*(b)*

**Figure 14.13** (a) Nerve distribution to the forearm and hand. (b) Wrist drop following injury to the muscles or the radial nerve.

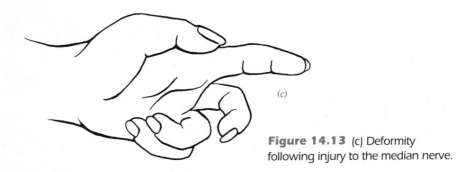

**Figure 14.13** (c) Deformity following injury to the median nerve.

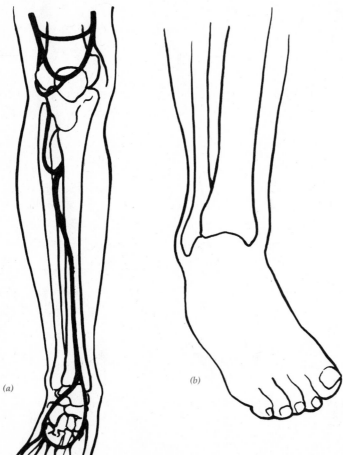

**Figure 14.14** (a) Distribution of the common peroneal nerve in the lower extremity. (b) Foot drop following injury to the peroneal nerve or muscles of the lower extremity.

**Table 14.1** Nerve Plexes with Major Nerves and Anatomical Distributions

| Nerve Plexus | Major Nerves | Anatomical Distribution |
|---|---|---|
| Brachial | Axillary | To surgical neck of the humerus and deltoid and teres minor muscles |
| | Musculocutaneous | To muscles of upper extremity and lateral surfaces of the upper forearm |
| | Median | To muscles of forearm, dorsal surfaces of thumb and index and middle fingers, and palmar surfaces of same fingers and palm |
| | Radial | To muscles on radial side of forearm, thumb, index finger, and half of middle finger, and back of thumb |
| | Ulnar | Muscles on ulnar side of forearm, ring and little fingers, and muscles at base of thumb and dorsum of hand |
| Lumbar | Obturator | To adductor muscles of thigh (except pectineus) and to skin on medial aspect of thigh down to knee and hip |
| | Femoral | To muscles of the anterior thigh, medial and anterior thigh surfaces, medial side of calf, and hip and knee joints |
| | Iliohypogastric | To anterior abdominal wall muscles |
| | Ilioinguinal | To muscles of anterior abdominal wall |
| | Genitofemoral | To skin of scrotum and external genital areas |
| | Lateral Cutaneous | To lateral thigh muscles and skin areas |
| Sacral | Gluteal: | |
| | Superior | To gluteus medius and minimus muscles of buttocks |
| | Inferior | To gluteus maximus muscle of buttocks |
| | Pudendal | To skin around anus, perineum, and urethra, external anal sphincter and perineal muscles |

(continued)

**Table 14.1** (Continued)

| Nerve Plexus | Major Nerves | Anatomical Distribution |
|---|---|---|
| | Sciatic | To posterior muscles of buttocks and thigh, and to hip joint |
| | Tibial | To posterior muscles of calf, medial malleolus and long flexors of toes |
| | Sural | To skin of lateral and posterior calf, lateral sides of foot and little toe, and dorsum of foot |
| | Common Peroneal | Superficial—to lateral side of leg and lateral malleolus, deep anterior surfaces of calf, ankle and long toe extensor muscles, little, second, and great toes |
| Coccygeal | Coccygeal | To coccyx |

**Table 14.2** Nerve Injuries and Resulting Deficits

| Major Nerve Injured | Resulting Deficits |
|---|---|
| Axillary | Paralysis of deltoid and teres minor muscles, leading to inability to abduct and externally rotate arm |
| | Waiter's tip hand deficit occurs in brachial and axillary paralysis |
| Musculocutaneous | No major disability results |
| Median | Loss of movement of middle fingers and wrist and hand pain: carpal tunnel syndrome |
| Radial | Inability to extend wrist, leading to dropped wrist deformity |
| Ulnar | Ulnar neuritis; claw-hand deformity (Klumpke palsy) from injury to lower branches of brachial plexus and ulnar or median nerves |
| Obturator | Inability to adduct thigh to abdomen; loss of sensations to anterior thigh, hip, and knee |
| Femoral | Inability to flex knee and adduct or extend thigh |
| Ilioinguinal | Loss of feeling and ability to contract abdominal rectus muscles |
| Iliofemoral | Loss of feeling over abdomen and groin |
| Genitofemoral | Loss of feeling to scrotum and external genitalia |

(continued)

**Table 14.2** (Continued)

| Major Nerve Injured | Resulting Deficits |
| --- | --- |
| Gluteal | Inability to contract muscles of buttocks to hold body upright, to contract hamstrings, thus to walk without assistance |
| Pudendal | Loss of sensation and continence of external anal muscle; loss of sensation or contraction of perineum and external urethra |
| Sciatic | Paralysis of hamstring muscles and muscles below the knee, leading to inability to bend (flex) knee, and dropped foot |
| Tibial | Inability to flex or extend foot actively |
| Sural | Loss of sensation to lateral and posterior lower calf and lateral foot surfaces; tarsal tunnel syndrome |
| Peroneal | Inability to dorsiflex foot, leading to dropped foot deformity |
| Coccygeal | Coccydynia (pain in the area of coccyx) |

## SHOCK SYNDROMES

Shock is a physiological reaction to trauma and stress. Shock syndrome is a series of changes resulting from decreased peripheral perfusion at the capillary level. Decreased peripheral perfusion leads to inadequate delivery of oxygen and other nutrients to the cells for maintenance of normal cell functions. Individual cells cannot tolerate decreased perfusion for even brief periods.

Table 14.3 lists the types and common causes of shock. The symptoms of shock, in general, are quite similar except for several specific exceptions discussed later. The most commonly noted symptoms are changes in blood pressure, with the systolic pressure readings below 80 mm Hg (a drop of 5 mm Hg in a hypertensive person is considered significant), increases in pulse and respiratory rates, rise in peripheral vascular resistance, and alterations in cardiac output. Changes in the person's sensorium, orientation, and behavior are common, as are skin color changes. Cardiac arrhythmias may occur and urinary output decreases as a sign of decreased renal perfusion. Body temperature changes are common.

Orthopaedic trauma may lead to hemorrhagic, septic, vasogenic (if neurologic trauma is also present), and, at times, cardiogenic shock.

Rapid diagnosis of the presence or state of shock must be made so that corrective measures can be instituted. Routinely, persons in shock, regardless

**Table 14.3** Types of Shock

| | |
|---|---|
| Hypovolemic | Hemorrhage; trauma; burns; dehydration |
| Septic | Gram-negative organisms, including Salmonella, Escherichia coli, Proteus vulgaris, Pseudomonas, and Klebsiella species, or gram-positive organisms, including Staphylococcus aureus and Streptococcus species. Anaerobic organisms including Clostridium welchii and botulinus |
| Cardiogenic | Myocardial infarct; cardiac myopathy; cardiac tamponade |
| Vasogenic | Neurogenic trauma (spinal shock, head injury) |
| Anaphylactic | Allergic reaction or antigen-antibody reaction |

of cause, are given oxygen via mask, nasal cannula, or mechanical ventilation to increase cellular oxygenation. Intravenous fluid replacement with whole blood, plasma, and crystalloids helps restore blood volume to increase capillary perfusion. Monitoring equipment and devices, such as central venous monitors, pulmonary artery catheters, cardiac monitors, arterial lines, and indwelling urinary catheters, are vital for the ongoing, frequent checks of the patient's condition. Additionally, medications such as antibiotics, steroids, bronchodilators, antihistamines, vasoconstrictors, cardiotonics, antipyretics, and analgesics are administered for the specific treatment of a particular type of shock. Prompt treatment is vital to prevent death from shock.

Patients in shock may be in the emergency room, intensive care unit, surgical suite, or nursing unit. Close monitoring over long periods is required to note untoward changes early or as soon as possible to prevent the changes from becoming irreversible. At times, due to such severe injuries, shock leads to multiple organ failure and patient death.

## FAT EMBOLIZATION

Fat embolization is a result of the release of fat molecules from the marrow of a fractured long bone into the bloodstream or from the chemical changes in the blood serum following long-bone fractures. Microemboli or larger emboli travel to the lungs, where they obstruct pulmonary circulation, leading to respiratory changes. Microemboli may also interfere with circulation in other organs. Most commonly, fat embolization occurs 1 to 3 days after a long-bone fracture, but it can also occur at later periods.

Symptoms of fat embolization include a sudden development of shortness of breath, dyspnea, change in mental alertness, disorientation or confusion, sense of foreboding or danger, tachycardia, tachypnea, drop in blood pressure, chest pain, pallor, cyanosis, and appearance of a fine, petechial rash from nipple line on chest, up to neck, on eyelids or conjunctivae. Diagnosis must be made quickly so treatments can be instituted promptly. Treatments include oxygen therapy per mask, nasal cannula or ventilator, intravenous fluids, administration of steroid medications, and use of dextran or low-molecular-weight solutions. Close monitoring is required to note any changes in the patient's condition. Multiple fat embolization can lead to respiratory failure and death (see Table 14.4).

**Table 14.4** Comparisons of Fat and Pulmonary Emboli

| | **Fat Emboli** | **Pulmonary Emboli** |
|---|---|---|
| Pathophysiology | Emboli develop as a result of release of fat molecules from marrow of fractured long bones into bloodstream or from chemical changes in the blood following trauma. There may be multiple micro-emboli or large emboli that obstruct pulmonary circulation and circulation in other organs. | Emboli develop secondary to thrombophlebitis. They become dislodged, travel in the bloodstream through the heart, and become lodged in the pulmonary circulation, causing obstruction. |
| Occurrence | Most frequently 1–3 days after a long-bone fracture but can also occur at later periods. | Frequently 7–10 days after trauma or development of thrombophlebitis, though can occur weeks or months later. |
| Signs/Symptoms | Sudden development of shortness of breath and dyspnea, changes in mental alertness, confusion, sense of danger, tachycardia, tachypnea, chest pain, drop in blood pressure and appearance of fine, petechial rash from nipple line on chest, up to neck, and on eyelids or conjunctivae, pallor or cyanosis. | Same as for fat emboli, except for rash. |
| Diagnosis | History of long-bone fracture; physical examination with presence of petechiae | History of thrombophlebitis; physical examination; arterial blood gases; |

(continued)

**Table 14.4** (Continued)

|  | Fat Emboli | Pulmonary Emboli |
|---|---|---|
|  | over chest, neck, and conjunctivae; chest x-ray; arterial blood gases (pa $O_2$ below 60 mm Hg). | complete blood count with differential; ventilation and perfusion scans; chest x-ray; pulmonary angiography. |
| Treatments | Bed rest; $O_2$ therapy; mechanical ventilation, if needed; external hypothermia, if hyperpyrexic; administration of steroids; heparin therapy; intravenous alcohol; administration of antibiotics; intravenous albumin; intravenous hypertonic glucose with insulin coverage. | Bed rest; $O_2$ therapy; intravenous heparin therapy; antibiotic administration; long-term administration of anticoagulant medications. |

## PULMONARY EMBOLISM

Pulmonary embolism is occlusion of one or more branches of the pulmonary arterial tree with thrombi which may break loose from an area of thrombophlebitis, or arise from tumors or air bubbles in the circulation. Pulmonary emboli may be singular or multiple and can lead to respiratory failure and death if not diagnosed promptly.

Symptoms include sudden, sharp chest pain, shortness of breath, dyspnea, sense of danger or dread, tachypnea, tachycardia, drop in blood pressure, pallor, and change in mental alertness. Pulmonary emboli occur most commonly 7–10 days after thrombophlebitis, although they may occur weeks or months later.

Treatments include bed rest, oxygen therapy by mask, cannula, or ventilator (with multiple emboli); intravenous fluid therapy, administration of heparin intravenously followed by coumadin therapy orally for 6 months or longer, and administration of antibiotics to prevent pulmonary infection. Steroid medications are also administered for their anti-inflammatory effects. Analgesics are administered for pain relief.

Nursing observations of the patient's vital signs, site and type of pain, skin color, orientation, signs of bleeding from gums, urine, or stool, skin cuts, and laboratory data are vital for patient's recovery. Teaching and preparation for self-care and discharge help the patient develop self-sufficiency and independence.

## THROMBOPHLEBITIS

Thrombophlebitis is the presence of a clot and inflammation in a vein. It is a fairly common complication in orthopaedic trauma secondary to bed rest, stasis, and the initial trauma.

Thrombophlebitis causes inflammation in a vein, usually in the calf of the leg, where the stasis and inflammation lead to clot formation, slowing venous circulation. Edema is noted around and distal to the vein blockage, and redness at the site and up the vein channel are common. The patient complains of soreness and pain in the calf. Homan's sign, which is pain in the calf with dorsiflexion of the foot, may be positive. The diagnosis is made from the patient's symptoms, physical examination, and, at times, a venogram or Doppler plethysmography.

Treatments include bed rest, compression with elastic bandages or elastic hose, warm compresses, intravenous heparin therapy, and elevation of the affected extremity.

## PARALYTIC ILEUS

Paralytic ileus secondary to orthopaedic trauma arises from the shunting of blood away from the intestinal tract during the early stages of the stress response. Because the intestines contain multiple microorganisms, infection in the peritoneum is nearly a foregone conclusion in spite of immediate treatments and antibiotic therapy. Peritonitis and abscess formation are common following intestinal rupture. Adynamic or paralytic ileus is a condition of dilation of the small or large intestine, leading to stasis of fluids and gases with increasing distention and stasis. Severe ileus may lead to rupture of the stomach or intestine, spilling contents into the peritoneal cavity (see Fig. 14.15).

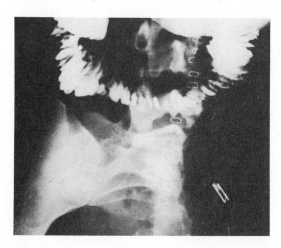

**Figure 14.15** Ileus and bowel obstruction as a result of cast syndrome and compression of the superior mesenteric artery.

Diagnosis of paralytic ileus is made from the patient's history, presence of marked abdominal distention, absence of bowel sounds, complaints of constipation or diarrhea, nausea, and vomiting. The patient may be short of breath due to pressure on the diaphragm, and may have low-grade or spiking temperature elevations.

Nursing interventions include instituting the physician's orders for insertion of a nasogastric tube, keeping the patient NPO, listening for bowel sounds, and measuring the abdominal girth every 4 hours. Vital signs are also measured frequently and intravenous fluids are administered to maintain fluid volumes. Saline irrigations of the nasogastric tube are done to maintain its free flow. Drainage is checked for blood. The patient's overall condition is carefully assessed to note progression or regression of ileus. At times, the patient may require a surgical exploratory laparotomy as one attempt to determine the cause of the ileus, as a thrombus in the mesenteric arterial system may be the cause, with resection of the entire intestinal tract being required. However, the majority of patients with paralytic ileus gradually experience return of peristalsis, bowel sounds, and bowel functions as they regain homeostasis following injury.

## OLIGURIA

Oliguria is decreased urinary output over a period of time, usually 24 hours. Adults should have 30 to 50 ml urinary output per hour, or a total of 720 to 1200 ml per 24 hours as minimal normal amounts.

Orthopaedic trauma can lead to oliguria from direct renal or urinary tract trauma; from blood loss, hypovolemia, or shock; from decreased renal perfusion related to the stress response; or from unknown causes. Oliguria should not be allowed to continue, as permanent renal damage may develop.

Diagnosis of oliguria is fairly easy to make from the hourly measurements of urinary output. Diagnostic studies such as intravenous pyelogram, urinalysis, blood urea nitrogen, creatinine, and x-rays may be done to determine the cause of the condition and its treatments.

Treatments include increasing fluid intake to increase renal perfusion; insertion of nephrostomy tube, ureteral or urethral catheters to relieve obstructions, if present; administration of antibacterial or antibiotic medication to prevent or treat urinary tract infections; administration of diuretic medications or other medications indicated by the results of diagnostic examinations.

Nursing interventions while caring for persons with oliguria include measuring hourly intake and output; monitoring vital signs and weight; observing urine for clarity, odor, color, pH, sugar, and acetone; maintaining bed rest with repositioning every 2 hours if injuries permit; and teaching dietary restrictions when pertinent (see Table 14.5) to prevent development of renal calculi. With prompt diagnosis and proper treatments, oliguria need not progress to irreversible renal problems.

**Table 14.5** Foods High in Calcium, Oxalates, and Foods Which Produce an Acid Ash

| Food | Amount | Calcium (mg) |
|------|--------|--------------|
| *Foods High in Calcium* | | |
| Milk, whole (cow's) | 1 cup (8 oz) | 288 |
| Milk, skim (cow's) | 1 cup | 296 |
| Yogurt (whole milk) | 1 cup | 251 |
| Cottage cheese (creamed) | 1 oz. | 27 |
| Cheddar cheese | 1 oz. | 213 |
| Ice cream (10% fat) | 1 cup | 194 |
| Sardines (canned with bones) | 3 oz. | 372 |
| Kale (cooked) | 1 cup | 206 |
| Broccoli (cooked) | 1 cup | 136 |
| *Foods High in Oxalic Acid (Oxalates)* | | |
| Spinach | | |
| Swiss chard | | |
| Chocolate | | |
| Rhubarb | | |
| Mustard greens | | |
| Dandelions | | |
| *Foods Which Produce an Acid Ash* | | |
| Red meats | | |
| Whole grains | | |
| Cranberries and cranberry juice | | |
| Plums | | |
| Prunes and prune juice | | |
| Eggs | | |
| Cheese | | |

## DECUBITUS FORMATION

Decubitus ulcerations are ulcerations of tissues that develop over and around bony prominences. They may be superficial or deep ulcerations that form as a result of pressure over bony prominences (see Fig. 14.16). Unremitting pressure causes decreased circulation, slow capillary refill, and slowed waste removal.

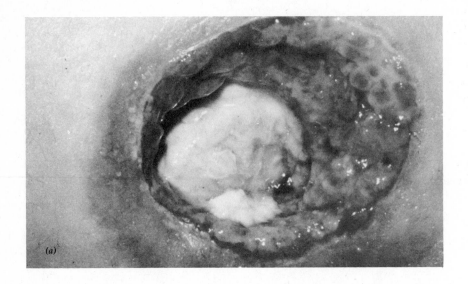

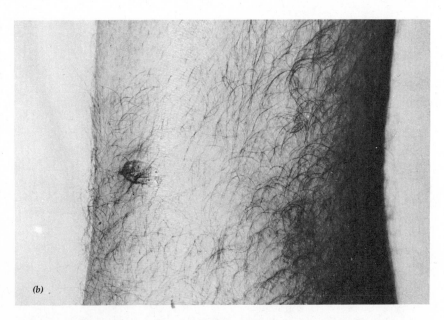

**Figure 14.16** (a) Deep coccygeal decubitus. (b) Pressure decutitus ulcer over tibial prominence from Kirschner spreader bar.

Oxygenation of the tissues is decreased, and if the pressure is not relieved and the circulation restored, inflammatory changes occur with loss of skin and subcutaneous tissue cells. Along with skin and subcutaneous cell loss there is also necrosis of fat cells, development of exudate and drainage, and, eventually, infection, if the ulcer is left untreated and the pressure unrelieved. Decubitus ulcers can cause prolonged morbidity and can lead to septicemia and death.

Prevention of decubitus ulcers is a priority of nursing care for all patients. Preventive measures include turning and repositioning every 2 hours to relieve pressure; massage to surrounding tissues and bony prominences; maintaining hydration and dietary intake with high-vitamin and mineral foods, assisting the patient with ROM exercises to maintain muscle mass and strength, placement on special beds, and ambulating patients when able.

Once a reddened area has developed over a bony prominence, such as over the sacrum, malleoli, elbows, heels, greater trochanter area, shoulder blades, or earlobes, it must be vigorously treated to prevent its progressing to skin breakdown and ulcer formation. Redness is indicative of decreased arterial circulation and arteriole or capillary damage, which can be prevented from progressing to ulceration by relieving pressure in the area and over the prominence. Table 14.6 lists some of the many treatments available for treating decubiti. Some of the variety of special beds are shown in Figs. 14.17, 14.18, and 14.19.

## WOUND INFECTIONS

Wound infections of patients with orthopaedic injuries are severe complications secondary to the degree of trauma, surgical intervention, metallic implants, and susceptibility of weakened patient to development of wound infection. Wound infections in orthopaedic patients are debilitating, prolong morbidity, and predispose to the development of osteomyelitis. The treatments for wound infections and nursing interventions are presented in the discussion of osteomyelitis (see p. 00).

Nurses have vital roles in the prevention of the complications discussed in this chapter, as well as others not covered.

**Table 14.6** Common Treatments for Decubitus Ulcers

| Interventions to Prevent Development of Decubitus Ulcers | |
|---|---|
| Relieve pressure every two hours through turning, when possible, and lifting or shifting weight. Massage around bony prominences gently to prevent capillary trauma. Keep skin surfaces clean and dry. Keep bed linens free of wrinkles. Teach patient how to avoid shearing forces when moving up in bed. Shearing loosens tissues due to the pulling forces. Teach patient to avoid pushing with elbows and heels and to lift self or be lifted off bed when moving up. | |
| **Interventions** | **Rationale** |
| 1. Active movements of muscles and joints | Increase circulation and maintain muscle mass to provide padding over and around bony prominences. |
| 2. Massage around site | Massage fosters removal of cellular metabolites and increases circulation. |
| 3. Low-wattage heat lamp to area of pressure | Heat causes vasodilation, bringing blood to area to remove wastes. |
| 4. Use of foam or self-adhering, adhesive-backed pads as doughnuts around the bony prominences, or use of prepared dressings such as Stomadhesive | Foam and adhesive-backed pads protect the prominence and provide a soft surface between the mattress and the patient's skin. The foam or pads are soft and "give," therefore do not increase pressure under their sites. |
| 5. High-protein, high-vitamin, high-iron diet | Positive nitrogen balance is needed for cellular growth and regeneration; vitamins A, B, and C are required for cellular growth and wound and skin healing. Iron increases the hemoglobin/oxygen-carrying activity, thus increasing cellular oxygenation. |
| If decubitus develops: 6. Whirlpool or Hubbard tank bathing | Hastens debridement through action of soap and water pressure; increases circulation in body. |

7. Application of hydrophilic (water-drawing) powder such as Debrisan twice daily, then covered with dry, sterile dressings

Powder contains beads of macromolecules that form a meshwork to absorb tissue fluids and exudates into their structure through their drawing or suction powers. Powder is white on application, but becomes yellow as it absorbs exudate. It can be rinsed off with normal saline and new powder reapplied as needed, usually twice daily.

8. Wet-to-dry dressings: fine-mesh gauze saturated with normal saline or iodophor solutions placed into ulcer, covered with two layers of dry fine-mesh gauze, and taped loosely

Remove debris through capillary action of wet to dry gauze. When removed every 4 hours, provides for debridement and development of clean granulation tissue.

9. Karaya dressings: Karaya powder lightly sprinkled into ulcer, replenished every 4 hours without removal of previous powder; ulcer gently cleansed every 24 hours and powder reapplied every 4 hours

Karaya resin seals pores and keeps contaminants out; resin also "meshes" cells together. Excellent for "weeping" ulcers to heal irritated areas.

10. Hydrogen peroxide irrigations

Peroxide is an oxidizing agent that destroys protein by absorbing an oxygen atom. Cleanses through its water formation and oxidizing pattern.

11. Cleansing with soap, water, saline, iodophor solutions; done with a brush, sponge, or other soft material

Mechanical action removes surface debris to be flushed away; antiseptics act over time.

12. Ointments such as those containing cortisone, antifungal, and antibacterial medications; these medications may be sprayed on in an aerosol rather than ointment form

Cortisone relieves inflammation in the site but can delay healing. Antifungal and antibacterial agents provide an uninfected surface for healing.

(continued)

**Table 14.6** (Continued)

| Interventions | Rationale |
|---|---|
| 13. Use of enzyme ointments containing collagenases | Act as proteolytic agents to "clean up" debris and exudates to provide a healthy surface for healing. |
| 14. Hyperbaric oxygen to ulcer area and body | Lessens ischemia by increasing oxygen pressure above normal pressures to increase oxygenation to local tissues. |
| 15. Use of special beds or pads (see Figs. 14.17, 14.18, 14.19) | Help distribute pressure over larger areas. Used to prevent as well as treat decubiti. |
| 16. Surgical debridement followed by placement of skin grafts | Provides clean, healthy surface for skin graft to adhere to site of decubitus. |

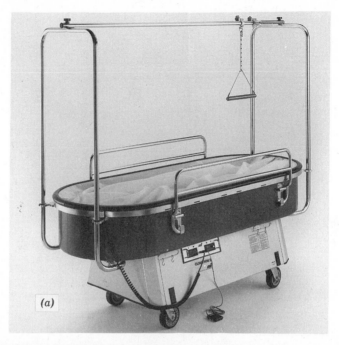

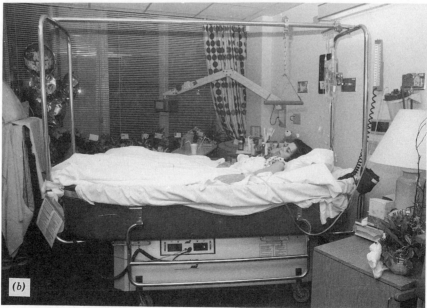

**Figure 14.17** (a) Clinitron bed. (b) Patient in a Clinitron bed. (Used with permission of Support Systems Inc., Charleston, SC.)

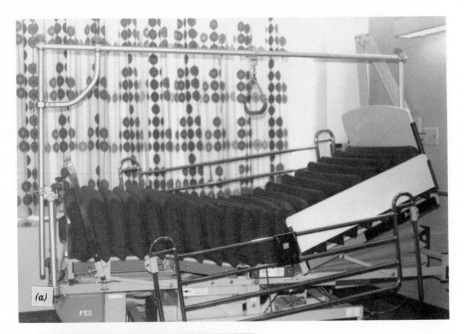

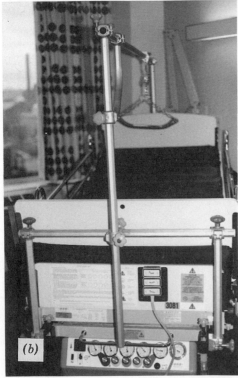

**Figure 14.18** (a, b) Mediscus air fluidized bed. (Used with permission of Therapeutic Patient Systems Inc., Akron, OH.)

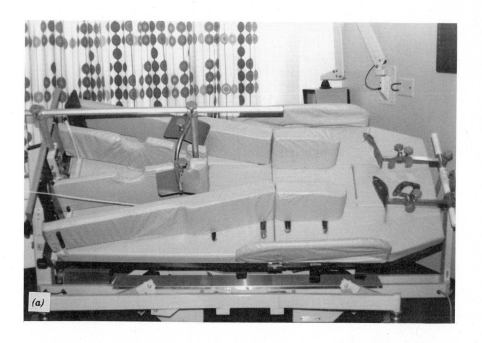

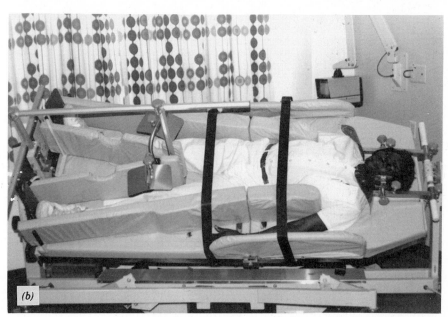

**Figure 14.19** (a, b) Roto Rest Kinetic Treatment Table. (Used with permission of Therapeutic Patient Services Inc., Akron, OH.)

## BIBLIOGRAPHY

Broos, P.L.O., Stappaerts, K.H., Rommens, P.M., Louette, L.K.J., & Gruwez, J.A. (1988). Polytrauma in patients 65 and over: Injury patterns and outcomes. *International Surgery, 73*,119–122.

Epps, C.H., (Ed.). (1986). *Complications in orthopaedic surgery,* (2nd ed.). Philadelphia: Lippincott.

Gerstner, D.L., & Omer, G.E., Jr. (1988). Part II. Peripheral entrapment neuropathies in the upper extremity. *Journal of Musculoskeletal Medicine, 5*(4),37–49.

Kaplan, P.E., & Tanner, E.D. (1989). *Musculoskeletal pain and disability.* East Norwalk, CT: Appleton & Lange.

McCance, K.L., & Heuther, S.E. (1990). *Pathophysiology.* St. Louis: Mosby-Yearbook.

# APPENDIX A
# ANA/NAON NURSING DIAGNOSES*

## NURSING DIAGNOSIS: PAIN

### Assessment Parameters

Assess pain characteristics, including—

Location of pain and areas that are pain-free.

Type, such as burning, stabbing, aching, pressing, and throbbing.

Intensity, such as unbearable, severe, moderate, mild, or painful as measured on a pain scale (e.g., 0 = no pain, 10 = worst possible pain).

Duration, such as minutes, hours, and days.

Pattern, such as constant or intermittent.

Precipitating or aggravating factors, such as movement, cold, stress, specific positioning, and lack of rest.

Alleviating factors, such as rest, massage, relaxation techniques, exercise, specific position, heat, and cold.

Explore the meaning of pain to the individual, including—

Expectation of pain relief.

Previous pain experiences.

Beliefs that certain measures would be effective or ineffective in relieving pain.

Ability and willingness to take an active role in pain control.

*From *Orthopaedic Nursing Practice: Process and Outcome Criteria for Selected Diagnoses*, American Nurses' Association and National Association of Orthopaedic Nurses, 1986.

## NURSING DIAGNOSIS: PAIN MANAGEMENT DEFICIT

### Assessment Parameters

Assess the individual's perception of and beliefs about the causes, consequence, and treatment of pain.

Explore what relief measures the individual has tried, and evaluate their effectiveness.

Assess the individual's expectation of relief.

Evaluate the individual's ability and willingness to take an active role in pain management.

## NURSING DIAGNOSIS: IMPAIRED PHYSICAL MOBILITY

### Assessment Parameters

The nurse assesses the individual's—

Ability to turn, transfer, or walk.

Functional range of motion.

Muscle strength.

Coordination.

Gait pattern.

Comfort level.

## NURSING DIAGNOSIS: KNOWLEDGE DEFICIT REGARDING MOBILITY SKILLS

### Assessment Parameters

The nurse assesses the individual's knowledge and skill regarding—

Appropriate exercise.

Body mechanics.

Gait or ambulation techniques.

Activity restrictions.

Assistive devices.

Safety measures.

The nurse identifies the individual's preferred learning style, such as one-to-one or group learning activities, audiovisual aids, or printed materials.

The nurse assesses the individual's ability and readiness to receive information and learn psychomotor skills.

## NURSING DIAGNOSIS: SELF-CARE DEFICIT

### Assessment Parameters

The nurse assesses the musculoskeletal capabilities required for self-care activities, such as motion, muscle strength, coordination, sensation, and imposed restrictions (cast, brace, traction, or bed rest).

The nurse assesses the individual's participation in self-care.

The nurse assesses the availability of support persons to assist with the individual's self-care.

## NURSING DIAGNOSIS: ACTIVITY INTOLERANCE

### Assessment Parameters

The nurse assesses the individual's usual and desired activity pattern.

The nurse assesses the individual's knowledge of energy conservation measures.

The nurse assesses the type and duration of activity that produces fatigue.

The nurse determines the presence of factors that increase energy demands, such as an inefficient walking mechanism (stiff knee, ankle, or hip; the use of a cane, walker, or crutches; or the presence of casts or braces), recent surgery, or other health problems.

The nurse assesses the availability and willingness of significant others to assist in activities of daily living.

## NURSING DIAGNOSIS: HIGH RISK FOR SKIN BREAKDOWN

### Assessment Parameters

The nurse assesses the individual's skin color, turgor, temperature, and condition.

The nurse assesses the individual's movement and sensation.

## NURSING DIAGNOSIS: HIGH RISK FOR INEFFECTIVE COPING

### Assessment Parameters

The nurse assesses the individual's usual coping style and its effectiveness, including—

The individual's recognition of methods he or she used in dealing with past life crises.

The individual's perception of the present problem.

The nature and frequency of statements regarding the individual's evaluation of his or her strengths, support systems, and life experiences.

The individual's perception of his or her ability to cope with unexpected changes and/or uncertainty.

# APPENDIX B
# PATIENT EDUCATION
# GUIDES

There are several ways to teach a patient, including verbal and visual techniques. The more senses that are involved in teaching, the more likely the patient will remember and implement the change desired. Patient education guides greatly enhance the probability the patient will be able to complete the necessary change in health-related behavior. These guides augment the verbal instruction given in a clinical setting, whether that be a hospital, clinic, or doctor's office. During verbal instruction, the patient may be anxious or unable to focus and, therefore, may not be able to remember instructions given. These guides give concrete information, in hand, that will help trigger the patient's memory.

When writing patient information guides, remember to keep them simple and short. A patient may not read multiple pages or pages that are in small type. Write instructions using simple language. Stay away from medical jargon and phrases that patients may not know. Keep paragraphs short. Generally, write for a 12- to 13-year-old level.

The following are examples of teaching sheets that may be copied for your practice or used as a format.

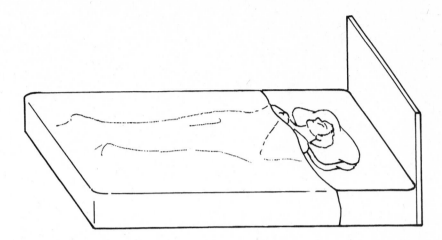

## PATIENT EDUCATION GUIDE: RELAXATION

Relaxation is a healthy way to release muscular tensions which contribute to pain sensations. It is effective because the brain can only interpret one strong signal at a time. Therefore, if you are concentrating on relaxation, you are less likely to be able to interpret pain signals.

Relaxation also enables you to be aware of what situations cause you to be tense and gives you some control of your body's reactions during these situations.

### The Art of Relaxation

To begin relaxing, lie in a quiet room in a comfortable position. Uncross your legs and put your arms at your side.

Concentrate on your breathing and close your eyes. Breathe slowly and deeply.

Focus on a past experience that was relaxing, such as watching the ocean waves, lying in a field with tall waving grass, lying in a hammock, etc. (Others find that clearing the mind of any thought is more relaxing. Do whichever is most helpful for you.)

Now you are ready to begin relaxing your muscles. If you have difficulty knowing if your muscles are relaxed, tighten a muscle and then release. Notice the difference?

Begin relaxing your feet. Wiggle your toes and then let your feet "flop" outward. Concentrate and keep breathing slowly and deeply.

Progress to your calves and thighs. Let all the tension go. When your legs are relaxed your knees will tilt to the side.

Next concentrate on your back. Let your back sink into the bed or chair. Let your shoulders droop down. Think about your breathing. Breathe slowly and deeply.

Now let your shoulders relax and your arms go limp. When your arms and legs are relaxed, they feel very heavy.

You are now ready to relax your face. This takes a great deal of concentration. When you relax your face, think about "letting go" of all the tightness around your eyes, mouth, and cheeks. When you are relaxed your lips will be slightly parted, your cheeks will droop down, and your eyes will be partially closed.

Continue to breathe slowly and deeply.

Don't be discouraged if you find relaxation difficult to do. It is because it is difficult and requires a great deal of concentration, that it may help relieve your pain. Remember, *relaxation improves with practice.*

## PATIENT EDUCATION GUIDE: MYELOGRAM

Your doctor has ordered a myelogram for you. You may have some questions about this examination. This guide was designed to help answer your questions. After you have read it, please feel free to ask any questions you may still have.

What is a myelogram? A myelogram (pronounced my-low-gram) provides a picture of your spinal canal and surrounding soft tissues and is used to locate defects or obstructions. Plain x-rays may also be taken; these show your bones clearly. Both tests provide vital information that your doctor will use to determine a diagnosis for your problem.

Before your myelogram: Your myelogram will require that you be admitted to the hospital temporarily. It may involve your staying in the hospital overnight. If the doctor and you have discussed surgery, your stay will, of course, be longer. Therefore, a nurse from your doctor's office will discuss the best day to schedule your examination with you.

In preparing for your myelogram, we suggest that the day before, you DRINK PLENTY OF FLUIDS, such as water, soda pop, and fruit juices—avoid alcoholic fluids. The fluids will keep you well hydrated.

The day of your myelogram: We ask that you arrive at the hospital 2 hours prior to your scheduled appointment for the myelogram to allow you plenty of time to complete the necessary forms and get acquainted with the hospital personnel. Upon arrival, you will probably be admitted to a holding area for same-day admissions. Here you will be asked to put on a hospital gown. When it is time for your myelogram, you will be transported to the x-ray department by cart. Your family or friends may accompany you to the x-ray unit, where they will wait for you in the lounge until your myelogram is completed.

The myelogram examination: The myelogram is done on the x-ray table; therefore, you will be asked to move from the cart to the table when you reach the x-ray unit. The radiology technician will help you lie on your side or stomach. Your doctor will then clean your lower back with a cool solution and use local anesthesia to numb this area of your back, which may cause a slight burning sensation. Then a contrast solution will be injected into the spinal canal to show during the x-rays. During this part of the test, you may feel a pressure sensation or some discomfort.

Several x-rays will then be taken of the contrast solution as it visualizes the spinal canal. During these x-rays, the x-ray table will be tilted into different positions. You will not fall as the table is moved. The examination takes one hour or less, after which you will be transported by cart to your room. Your family will be informed at the completion of the myelogram and they may accompany you back to your room.

The myelogram procedure causes much less discomfort now than myleograms performed only a few years ago. A very small needle is now used and the contrast solution that is injected no longer needs to be moved.

After the myelogram: You will be asked to stay in bed and rest for 8 hours following the myelogram. You may turn on your side if you like, but you will need to keep your head no higher than 30° elevation of the head of the bed. DRINK PLENTY OF FLUIDS, and you may eat your usual diet.

After you get home: After you are discharged and go home, rest for the first day after the myelogram, then resume your usual activities. CALL YOUR DOCTOR'S OFFICE IF:

- You have persistent headache or vomiting.
- You notice drainage from you puncture site.

Your myelogram is schedule for: _____ at: _____ a.m./p.m.

Please arrive at the hospital by: _____ .

You will be scheduled for preadmission blood work and a history and physical

at _____ Hospital at _____ a.m./p.m.
You should report to Admitting on arrival at the hospital.

## PATIENT EDUCATION GUIDE: IRON REPLACEMENT

Iron can help your body replace blood loss and build hemoglobin. For this reason it is wise to eat food high in iron before and after surgery.

| Foods High in Iron |
| :---: |
| Red meats |
| Organ meats |
| Eggs |
| Green leafy vegetables |
| Dried fruits |
| Whole grains, beans, potatoes, and cereals. |

Foods that are rich in iron include red meats such as beef hamburger, roasts, or steaks, and organ meats such as beef heart, liver, or kidney. Chicken and fish are not as high in iron. Other foods high in iron are eggs, green leafy vegetables such as lettuce or spinach, dried fruits, whole grains such as bread, and legumes such as beans.

In addition to a good iron-rich diet, we suggest that you take iron tablets prior to donating blood for your surgery.

There are several different types of iron preparations that may be purchased without a prescription at your pharmacy. Ferrous gluconate is a reasonably priced iron product and is better tolerated with less stomach upset. (You may also ask your pharmacist for his/her recommendation.)

**TYPES OF IRON TABLETS**

Ferrous gluconate
Ferrous sulfate
Ferrous fumarate

You should begin taking iron as soon as possible and continue for one month after surgery. Follow the directions for dosage on the iron bottle. The usual dosage is one to two tablets two to three times a day. Also, we recommend taking iron with citrus juice such as orange juice because this increases absorption.

Iron may cause some minor problems including diarrhea, constipation, or abdominal cramping. In addition, you may notice black stools. Black stools can be a normal result of taking iron but may also indicate the presence of blood in your stool. Should one of these problems occur, you may decrease the number of times a day you take iron. If these problems continue, please contact our office at _____.

## PATIENT EDUCATION GUIDE:
## MEDICATION INSTRUCTIONS, NONSTEROIDAL
## ANTI-INFLAMMATORY AGENTS

The name of your medication is:

( ) Ibuprofen (Motrin)                    ( ) Sulindac (Clinoril)

( ) Indomethacin (Indocin)               ( ) Tolmetin (Tolectin)

( ) Naproxen (Naprosyn)                  ( ) Piroxicam (Feldene)

( ) Salsalate (Disalcid)                 ( ) Diclofenac sodium (Voltaren)

This medication is used to relieve the symptoms of inflammation and pain associated with disk disease, arthritis, gout, bursitis, or tendinitis. This medication does not cure arthritis or gout, but will help the pain and inflammation if the drug is taken regularly. This may allow adequate symptom relief until the pain episode resolves.

Notify your doctor if you have any of the following side effects:

1. Severe rash or itching of skin
2. Unusual weight gain
3. Swelling of legs or feet
4. Shortness of breath or difficulty breathing
5. Blood in urine or tool or black, tarry stools
6. Nausea, vomiting, stomach pain, or diarrhea

DO NOT take aspirin regularly or consume alcohol while on this medication unless prescribed by your doctor. Doing so may cause stomach upset. Drowsiness or dizziness may occur while taking this medication. For more information about this medication, contact the doctor, nurse, or pharmacist.

*AVOID TAKING OVER-THE-COUNTER MEDICATIONS WITHOUT FIRST DISCUSSING IT WITH YOUR DOCTOR.*

## PATIENT EDUCATION GUIDE: STOOL SPECIMEN FOR OCCULT BLOOD

The hemoccult test is designed to test your stool for the presence of blood. This may be ordered for you as a routine check to follow possible stomach irritation from your medication. The test is a simple procedure:

First write on the front cover of the hemoccult package: your name, age, address, telephone number, and date you collect your stool specimen.

Then collect a stool specimen, using the wooden applicator provided. You may wish to stretch plastic wrap loosely under the toilet seat to catch the stool. Open the front of your hemoccult package and spread a small smear of stool on the A and B windows. Use different parts of the stool for each window. Discard the wooden applicator but do not flush it. Close the cover and mail it back to your doctor's office in the envelope provided. The doctor's office staff will call you only if the test was positive. However, if you are concerned, do not hesitate to call.

DO NOT collect a stool specimen during a menstrual period or if you have bleeding hemorrhoids or blood in your urine.

## PATIENT EDUCATION GUIDE: DRY TO DRY DRESSING

Name _____

Do dressing change _____ times a day or as needed.

Purpose:
1. To protect wound or incision
2. To prevent infection
3. To absorb drainage

Materials needed:
1. Sterile dressings (4 x 3 packets, larger pads)
2. Hydrogen peroxide solution
3. Pair of gloves (sterile)
4. Wastebasket with plastic liner, or plastic bag

Step by step:
1. Gather supplies (plus extra pair of gloves).
2. Wash your hands.
3. Open sterile packages.
4. Remove old dressing and place in plastic bag or wastebasket (touch only outer side of dressings).
5. Look at wound:
    Do you see any changes?
    Do you see pus or infection?
    Do you smell a bad odor?
6. Put on sterile gloves.
7. Clean any drainage from incisional area with hydrogen peroxide swabs (pour peroxide over sterile 4 x 3 dressing).
8. Apply sterile dressing and tape securely.
9. If applicable—wrap with elastic bandages.
10. If you see any changes, call your doctor to report them.

Remember:
1. Wash hands before and after each dressing change.
2. Keep your supplies together.
3. Clean and wipe off table/counter before setting up supplies and after changing dressing.
4. Empty soiled dressings into outside trash can as soon as possible. Do not leave soiled dressings in room.

## PATIENT EDUCATION GUIDE:
## WET TO DRY DRESSINGS

Name _____

Purpose:
1. To remove old or dead tissue from wound
2. To prevent infection
3. To promote healing

Materials needed:
1. _____ dressing/s
2. _____ solution
3. Wastebasket, lined with plastic, or a plastic bag.
4. Clean towel or sheet to place under dressings

Step by step:
1. Gather your supplies.
2. Wash your hands.
3. Spread a clean towel or sheet over your work area.
4. Open sterile packages of dressings and the bottle of solution and place on the clean surface.
5. Pour the solution on the sterile dressings to be used for the wet dressings.
6. Remove the old dressing and place in wastebasket.
7. Look at the wound.
8. Squeeze out the excess solution from 1–2 thin dressings and place them on your wound. Use the thinnest dressing possible so that the dressing will dry out between changes.
9. Use a thin layer of dry dressing on top of the wet dressing and apply tape to secure it.
10. Throw away all unused open packages.
11. Wash your hands.
12. Call the doctor if you:
    See pus or increased drainage
    Smell a bad odor
    See increased redness
    Have increased pain at the wound
    Have a fever

Remember:
1. Wash hands before and after each dressing change.
2. Keep your supplies away from the reach of children.
3. Clean and wipe off your work area before and after dressing change.
4. Place soiled dressings in the wastebasket and empty into the outside trash can as soon as possible.

## PATIENT EDUCATION GUIDE: CARE OF A PERSON IN A CAST

Circle correct term or terms:
1. The cast you or your relative has on is called a:
    a. Short arm cast
    b. Short leg cast
    c. Long arm cast
    d. Hanging arm cast
    e. Long leg cast
    f. Spica cast
    g. Body cast
    h. Minerva Jacket
2. It is made of:
    a. Plaster
    b. Fiberglass
    c. Other material:
3. The cast is:
    a. Still damp and only partially set.
    b. Is already set and dry.
4. The patient can:
    a. Turn side to side.
    b. Turn to abdomen.
    c. Walk with weight bearing on cast.
    d. Walk with crutches with *no* weight bearing on cast.
    e. Walk with crutches with partial weight-bearing on cast.
    f. Be up with arm in the cast in a sling.
    g. Be up with leg in cast elevated on pillows.
    h. Other _____

    _____

5. When in bed, the arm or leg in the cast should be elevated on 1–2 pillows to decrease swelling.
6. Apply plastic bags filled with ice cubes to the outside of the cast to decrease bleeding and swelling. Use the ice bags for 24–48 hours, or as the doctor ordered.
7. Help the patient into the shower or bathtub to bathe. Place a large plastic bag (trash bag) over the cast and seal well with tape to keep the cast dry. Do not wash or wet a plaster cast. A fiberglass cast can be dampened or even totally wetted, but must be dried to prevent skin injury. Dry the cast by using a hair drier on low setting.
8. A large plaster cast takes 2–3 days to dry completely. Keep the cast uncovered until it is totally dry. Once dry, the cast can be covered.
9. Check the skin areas above and below the cast, and compare the casted extremity with the other side, for the following:

a. Color—fingers or toes in cast may be pale, but should not be blue, white, or ruddy (dark red).

b. Temperature—fingers and toes should be warm, not cold. Cover toes with a warm sock if they are cool.

c. Swelling—the fingers or toes may be somewhat swollen, but they should not be greatly swollen.

d. Pain—there may be mild to moderate pain in the area that was injured, but the pain should not be severe and the severity of the pain should not be increasing.

e. Movement—all fingers and toes should move freely and without severe pain. Pain should not increase when the fingers or toes move.

f. Sensations—There should be no numbness, tingling, "pins and needles" sensations, or lack of sensation or feeling.

g. Drainage or odor—there may be some bleeding if the patient has had surgery; otherwise there should be no bleeding or drainage, and no odor from under or inside the cast.

h. Compare the extremity in the cast with the opposite extremity. The opposite extremity should be pinker, warmer, without swelling, pain, movement, or sensory changes when compared with the part in the cast.

10. Call the doctor if the area in the cast exhibits any of the following:
    a. Skin is blue or white.
    b. Skin feels cold and doesn't warm up with covering.
    c. Skin is much hotter than nearby skin tissues.
    d. Fingers or toes do not move when patient tries to move them.
    e. Fingers or toes are greatly swollen.
    f. Person has sensations of "pins and needles," tingling, or burning in cast.
    g. There is drainage and/or a foul odor from the cast.
    h. There are breaks or cracks in the cast.

11. The next appointment with Dr. _____ is:
    a. time _____
    b. place _____

12. After the cast is removed:
    a. Skin cleansing: Gently wash the skin with a cloth dampened with Woolite, which contains enzymes to soften the dried, crusted skin. Let the Woolite remain on the skin for about 20 minutes to soften the crusts. Gently wash skin areas to remove the Woolite, flakes and crusts. Do not rub or scrub the skin, which could cause breaks in the skin. After rinsing the skin well, pat it dry gently. Apply a lotion to moisten the skin. If necessary, repeat the skin cleaning the next day and apply a moisturizing lotion.
    b. Soreness or pain: There may be some soreness or weakness of muscles and joints after the cast is removed. The area will have lost weight from

the decreased muscle use. Gradually begin using the muscles and joints as able to loosen them. The doctor may suggest you do some exercises to regain strength in the muscles and joints, and may also suggest you take aspirin or another pain reliever medication for 24–48 hours or longer until pain lessens. It will take twice as long (or longer) to regain full function and strength of the muscles and joints as the part was in the cast. For example, it will take 10–12 weeks or longer if the cast was on for 5–6 weeks to regain full functions.

c. Swelling: The part that was in the cast may develop some swelling with reuse. This is normal. Elevating the part on pillows for 1–3 days to heart level should decrease the swelling. If the swelling persists, call the doctor to see if you need to do anything more to relieve it.

# APPENDIX C
# UNIVERSAL PRECAUTIONS TO PREVENT OCCUPATIONAL/ NOSOCOMIAL TRANSMISSION OF HIV-1*

- Hands should be washed before and after patient contact and after removing gloves.
- Gloves are indicated when soiling of hands with blood or body fluids is likely (for example, venipuncture).
- Masks and protective eyewear are not generally indicated. They are necessary when performing procedures during which splashing or spraying of blood or body fluids is likely.
- Masks may be advisable for patients with undiagnosed pulmonary disease who are coughing, or for patients being treated with mechanical positive pressure who have copious or blood-streaked secretions.
- Gowns are generally not indicated but should be worn if clothing is likely to be soiled with blood or body fluids.
- Food should be provided on regular dishes and served by the usual food service workers.
- Private rooms are not usually needed unless patients are too ill to use good hygiene or have other infections for which private rooms are indicated.
- Articles contaminated with blood or body fluids should be bagged with isolation labels for decontamination and reprocessing.

*Adapted from: Centers for Disease Control. (1987). Recommendations for prevention of HIV transmission in health-care settings. MMWR, 36(2S), 1S-18S.

- Needles and syringes must be handled cautiously. Used needles must not be recapped and must be placed in designated puncture-resistant containers.
- Spills of blood or body fluids should be cleaned with dilute (1:10) solution of sodium hypochlorite (bleach) and water. The bleach solution should be no older than 24 hours.

# GLOSSARY OF TERMS, WITH GENERIC DERIVATIONS

**Abduction**   (L *ab*, from, + *ductus*, drawing away). Moving away from median line.

**Abscess**   (L *abscedere*, to go away). A localized collection of pus in any part of the body, usually the result of disintegration or displacement of tissue.

**Abuse**   L *ab*, from, + *uti*, to use). To use wrongly or to overuse; to misuse.

**Achondroplasia**   (L *a*, absence, + *chondro*, cartilage, + *plasis*, moulding). Absence of growth at the epiphyseal cartilages.

**Adduction**   (L *adducere*, to bring toward). Moving toward median line.

**ADL**   (*activities of daily living*). Customary daily activities of eating, dressing, or clothing oneself, walking or moving, and so on.

**Adynamic**   (Gr *a*, lack of, or *adynamia*, without strength). Without strength or vital powers.

**Affects**   (L *affectus*, state of mind). Emotional reactions associated with an experience; dispositions or states of mind; psychic traumas.

**AIDS**   Acquired Immunodeficiency Syndrome; characterized by a defect in cell-mediated immunity.

**Alarm stage**   Initial stage of the stress response characterized by physiological reactions to a stressor (threat).

**Allograft**   (Gr *allos*, other, + *graphium*, grafting knife). A graft (skin, organ, or other tissue) taken from one individual to be used on another individual.

**Alteration**   (L *alter*, other). (1) An altering; (2) the result of this change.

**A.M. or am**   (L *ante*, before, + *meridies*, noon). Before noon; morning hours.

**Amputation**   (L *amputare; ambi*, around, + *putare*, to prune). Severance of all or part of an extremity or other projecting part.

**Anabolism**   (Gr *anabole*, building up). Process of cell growth and building up of the body substance.

**Analysis** (Gr *analyein*, to resolve, break up). Study of components or variables affecting outcome of action or behavior; study of parts in relation to a whole; separation into parts.

**Anaphylactic shock** Shock condition resulting from an antigen-antibody, allergic reaction; may result from reaction to an insect sting, antibiotic, or other allergen.

**Anesthesia** (Gr *an*, not, + *aisthēsis*, sensation). Lack of sensation or feeling; loss of touch or other sense.

**Anger** (L *angere*, to vex, trouble, strangle). Emotional agitation of unspecified amount aroused by great displeasure; a feeling that can result from injury, mistreatment, opposition; wrath.

**Angiogram** (Gr *angeion*, vessel, + *gramma*, a written record). X-ray film of a blood vessel taken following the injection of a radiopaque substance into the vessel. Technique is used to define the size and shape of various veins and arteries of organs and tissues.

**Angiosarcoma** (Gr *angio*, vessel, + *sarx*, flesh, + *oma*, tumor). Mixed sarcoma and angioma; malignant tumor of blood vessel walls.

**Ankylosing Spondylitis** (Gr *ankylosis*, bound by adhesions, + *spondylos*, vertebra). Rheumatoid, degenerative fusing of the vertebrae resulting in loss of function and position.

**Ankylosis** (Gr *ankylosis*, bound by adhesions). Stiffening or fixation of a joint due to fibrous bands; abnormal immobility and consolidation of a part.

**Anomaly** (Gr *anōmalos*, irregularity). Anything contrary to general rule; an organ or structure that is abnormal with reference to form, structure, or position; a malformation.

**Anterior** (L *ante*, before). Front or foremost surface of body, organ, or part when in the anatomical position; in the front.

**Anterior tibialis** Artery located anterior to, and on the medial and lateral surfaces of, the malleoli.

**Antibiotic** (Gr *anti*, against, + *biosis*, life). Substance produced by living organisms such as bacteria or molds, which can inhibit growth or destroy other microorganisms.

**Antibody** (Gr *anti*, against). Substance formed by the body as a reaction to a foreign agent or antigen. The antibody formed works only against that particular antigen.

**Antigen** (Gr *anti*, against, + *gennao*, produce). Any foreign substance that causes the formation of antibodies as protective substances in the body.

**Antigen-antibody reaction** Reaction or response by an antibody to the presence of an antigen; hypersensitivity response.

**Antiinflammatory** (Gr *anti*, against, + *inflammatio*, inflammation). Substance or medication that reduces inflammation.

**Anxiety** (L *angere*, to vex, trouble, strangle). Normal reaction to that which is threatening to one's body, life-style, values, or loved ones. A troubled feeling; experiencing a sense of dread; distress over real or imagined threats to one's mental or physical well-being.

**Appendicular skeleton**  (L *appendere,* to hang to). Portion of the skeleton containing the bones of the upper and lower extremities, pelvis, and shoulders.

**Apposition**  (L *ad,* to, + *ponere,* to place). Fitting or bringing together one or more parts, as for example, the thumb brought in apposition to one or more fingertips.

**Arteriogram**  (Gr *arteria,* air-conveyor: the arteries were formerly supposed to be air tubes; + *gramma,* a written record). X-ray films taken after injection of a radiopaque substance to define the size, shape, and condition of arteries.

**Artery**  Vessel carrying oxygenated blood from the heart to the tissues.

**Arthritis**  (Gr *arthron,* joint, + *itis,* inflammation). Inflammation of a joint, usually accompanied by pain and often changes in structure.

**Arthro-**  (Gr *arthron,* joint). Pertaining to a joint.

**Arthrodesis**  (Gr *arthron,* joint, + *desis,* a binding together). Surgical fixation of joint by fusion.

**Arthrogram**  (Gr *arthron,* joint, + *graphein,* to write). A picture of a joint following injections of a dye or radiopaque solution.

**Arthroplasty**  (Gr *arthron,* joint, + *plasso,* forming). Operation to reform or restore a joint; to make an artificial joint.

**Arthroscopy**  (Gr *arthron,* joint, + *skopein,* to examine). Direct visualization of a joint by using an arthroscope.

**Arthrotomy**  (Gr *arthron,* joint, + *tome,* cutting). Surgical cutting into joint.

**Articulation**  (L *articulus,* joint). A joint; point of union of two or more bones.

**Aseptic necrosis**  (Gr *nekrosis,* a killing). Death of bone cells without infection or inflammation caused by loss of blood supply.

**Aspiration**  (of a joint or cavity). To drain pus or fluid via a hollow needle.

**Assessment**  An evaluation or assessing; a way or schedule of assessing.

**Ataxia**  (Gr *a,* lack, + *tassein,* order). Loss of coordination; disorganization of voluntary movements.

**Atelectasis**  (Gr *ateles,* imperfect, + *ektasis,* expansion). Collapse or underexpansion of a part of the lung.

**Athetosis**  (Gr *athetos,* without position or place). Pathological state in which movements are useless, uncontrolled, involuntary.

**Atrophy**  (Gr *a,* without, + *trephein,* nourishment). Wasting away or decrease in size of cell, tissue, or organ.

**Autogenous**  (Gr *autos,* self, + *genes,* produce). Self-producing; originating within the body.

**Autologous blood**  Blood donated for donor's own future use.

**Avascular necrosis**  Death of bone cells (and thus bone) due to cessation of a blood supply.

**Avulsion** (L *avellere,* to separate by force). Forceful separation or tearing away of two connected parts.

**Axial Skeleton** (L *axis,* axis). The head and trunk of the body.

**Axilla(-ae)** (L *axillae,* armpit). Armpit(s).

**Back-lying** (L *dorsum,* back). Position of lying in bed on the back.

**Bacteriology** (Gr *baktērion,* a staff, + *logus,* study). Science or study of microorganisms.

**Baker's cyst** A cyst containing synovial fluid; communicating with synovial fluid of a joint.

**Basal cell carcinoma** The most common type of skin cancer, which forms in the lowermost layer of the skin, grows slowly, and seldom spreads. Easily detected and readily cured when treated promptly.

**Bedfast** Confined to bed or rest by disease or physician's order.

**Bed rest** Lying in bed for specific period or as one part of treatment for selected illness.

**Behaviors** Responses to stimuli; can be observed and measured; usual classifications are verbal, nonverbal, psychological, and physiological.

**Benign** (L *benignus,* mild). Mild; not recurrent; not malignant.

**Benign tumor** An abnormal swelling or growth that is usually harmless.

**Bilateral** (L *bi,* two, + *latus,* side). Having two sides, or relating to two sides.

**Biofeedback** (Gr *bios,* life). Program designed to teach a person to control his/her autonomic (involuntary) nervous system functions of relaxing some muscles, lowering blood pressure, slowing heart rate, and regulating skin temperature. The program uses machines monitored by the person, who regulates his/her behaviors to produce the desired responses.

**Biopsy** (Gr *bios,* life, + *opsis,* vision). Surgical removal of a piece of tissue from a living subject for microscopic examination to make a diagnosis.

**Blister** (Dutch *bluyster,* a swelling). A vesicle containing serum; a collection of fluid below the epidermis usually from a burn or excessive friction.

**Blood count** An examination of the blood to count the number of white and red blood cells and platelets.

**Body Image** The subjective picture or image a person develops of his/her physical body and appearance based on personal observations and reactions of others.

**Bone** A specialized form of dense, connective tissue consisting of bone cells embedded in a matrix consisting of calcified intercellular substance; an individual unit of the skeleton.

**Bouchard's nodes** Enlargements and deformities of the metacarpal and proximal interphalangeal joints, seen in rheumatoid arthritis.

**Brace** Any of various splints or devices for supporting a weak or malformed part of body; a device that keeps something firmly in place.

**Breast self-examination** A simple procedure for examining breasts thoroughly; recommended once a month for all women to do themselves. Men should also set schedule for their own breast self-examination (two or three times yearly).

**Brodie's abscess**   An abscess near the proximal end of a long bone usually noted by an abscess cavity surrounded by dense scar tissue. It is considered a form of osteomyelitis and is usually a staphylococcal infection.

**Bryant's traction**   Type of skin traction used for children under 18 kg (40 lbs). Legs are held vertically in extension to treat a fractured femur.

**Buck's extension**   Type of skin traction in which strips of adhesive or foam are applied to the skin, then attached to a rope, pulley, and weight for extension of a limb.

**Bursa**   (L *bursa,* purse). Sac or cavity composed of synovial membrane containing synovial fluid that serves as a cushioning device between tendon and bone, tendon and ligaments, or between two other structures where friction is likely to occur.

**Bursitis**   (L *bursa,* purse, + *itis,* inflammation). Inflammation of a bursa.

**Calculus**   (L *calculus,* pebble). Any abnormal concretion within the animal body, usually composed of mineral salts, stone.

**Callus**   (L *callosus,* hard). The osseous material formed between the ends of a fractured bone; thickening of a horny layer of skin.

**Cancellous**   (L *cancellus,* lattice, grating). Having a reticular or latticework structure, as the spongy tissue of bone.

**Cancellus**   (L *cancellus,* lattice, grating). Osseous plate of which cancellous bone is composed.

**Cancer**   (L, a crab). A large group of diseases characterized by uncontrolled growth and spread of abnormal cells; malignant neoplasms.

**Cane**   (Gr *kanna,* reed). A slender hand-held stick used for support during walking.

**Carcinogen**   (Gr *karkinos,* crab, + *gen,* produce). Any substance that causes cancer.

**Carcinoma**   (Gr *karkinos,* crab, + *oma,* tumor). A form of cancer that arises in the epithelial tissues that cover or line such organs of the body as skin, intestines, uterus, lung, breast.

**Carcinoma in situ**   (L *situ,* position). A stage in the growth of cancer when it is still confined to the tissue in which it started.

**Carpal tunnel syndrome**   (Gr *karpos,* wrist). Pressure on the median nerve at the point at which it goes through the carpal tunnel of the wrist. Causes soreness, tenderness, and weakness of the muscles of the thumb.

**Cartilage**   (L *cartilago,* gristle). A type of dense connective tissue consisting of cells embedded in a ground substance or matrix. Cartilage has *no nerve or blood supply of its own* and is semiopaque.

**Cast**   A solid mold of a part, usually applied in situ for immobilization in fractures, dislocations, and other serious injuries; plastic or fibrous material thrown off in various pathological conditions, the product of effusion.

**Cast-brace**   A form of immobilization consisting of a hinged brace parallel to a joint to permit flexion during healing. The brace is held in plaster casts above and below the joint. The casts hold the fractured bones immobile for healing.

**Catabolism**   (Gr *katabole*, casting down). The destructive phase of metabolism; the opposite of anabolism.

**C.C. or cc.**   Cubic centimeter; equivalent to one milliliter.

**Cell**   (L *cella*, a chamber). The basic structural unit of life, containing a nucleus, cytoplasm, and cell membrane.

**Cellulitis**   (L *cellula*, little cell, + Gr *itis*, inflammation). Inflammation of cellular or connective tissue.

**Central venous pressure**   The venous blood pressure obtained by inserting a catheter attached to a manometer, into the right atrium or superior vena cava via the subclavian or brachial veins.

**Cervical traction**   (L *tractio*, pull). Traction to the cervical vertebrae by means of head halter or skull tongs.

**Charleyhorse**   A pulled muscle with some intramuscular bleeding causing soreness and stiffness.

**Chemonucleolysis**   Process of dissolving a herniated nucleus pulposus by injection of chymopapain, an enzyme that breaks the protein bonds in the nucleus pulposus. Scar tissue forms in the injected area.

**Chemotherapy**   (Gr *chemēia*, chemistry, + *therapeia*, treatment). Treatment of disease by employing chemical compounds to destroy the disease-causing organisms.

**Chondro-**   (Gr *chondros*, cartilage). Prefix referring to cartilage.

**Chondroma**   (Gr *chondros*, cartilage, + *oma*, tumor). A cartilaginous tumor of slow growth; may occur wherever there is cartilage.

**Chondromalacia**   (Gr *chondros*, cartilage, + *malakia*, softness). Softening of the articular cartilage; erosion of any cartilage.

**Chondrosarcoma**   (Gr *chondros*, cartilage, + *sarx*, flesh, + *oma*, tumor). Cartilaginous sarcoma; malignant.

**Chordotomy**   (Gr *chorde*, cord, + *tome*, a cutting). Division of cords, such as nerve pathways, to relieve pain.

**Chronic**   (Gr *chronos*, time). Long and drawn out.

**Chvostek's sign**   Spasms of facial tissues following tap of facial nerve. Spasms due to tetany from hypocalcemia.

**Circulation**   (L *circuitus*, going round). Movement in a circular course, as blood through the arteries, capillaries, and veins.

**Circumduction**   (L *circum*, around, + *ducere*, to draw). Action or wing of a limb, in such a manner that it describes a cone-shaped figure; circular movement of the eye or extremity.

**Claustrophobia**   (L *cluastrum*, a barrier, + *phobos*, fear). Fear of being confined in a closed or confined space.

**Clawfoot** Deformity of the foot characterized by excessively high longitudinal arch usually with dorsal contracture of the toes.

**Clawhand** Deformity of the hand characterized by hyperextension of the proximal phalanges of the fingers plus extreme flexion of the middle and distal phalanges; usually resulting from median or ulnar nerve injury.

**Clinical** (Gr *klinē,* bed). Relating to the study and treatment of disease in human beings by direct observation, as opposed to laboratory research.

**Closed** (L *claudere,* to close or shut). Not open, as in *closed* fracture, having no skin opening.

**Closed fracture** Fracture without an open skin wound.

**Cock-up splint** Splint designed to immobilize wrist in some extension for treatment of wrist conditions.

**Collagen** (Gr *kolla,* glue, + *gennan,* to produce). A fibrous protein which is found in connective tissues of the body including skin, muscles, bone, ligaments, and cartilage. It makes up about 30% of the total body protein.

**Comminuted** (L *comminuere,* to break in pieces). Crushed; broken into pieces.

**Comminuted fracture** Fracture with bone splintered or crushed in more than two pieces.

**Compartment syndrome** Group of symptoms caused by increased venous pressure within an enclosed area or compartment that lead to tissue necrosis if the venous pressure is not decreased.

**Complication** (L *cum,* with, + *plicare,* to fold). A difficulty superimposed on another with or without direct relation.

**Compression** (L *comprimere,* to press together). A squeezing together; state of being pressed together.

**Compression screw** (L *compressio,* a compression, + *escroue,* nut). A cylindrical metallic device that compresses or forces parts together as it is tightened into place in a bone.

**Computed tomogram (CT)** Special x-ray study using specified "cuts" or layers of tissue per picture. Provides a detailed picture of the tissues studied.

**Concept** (L *conceptus,* to conceive). An idea, thought, or opinion; a mental image of a thing.

**Condom** Prophylactic rubber sheath worn on the penis, used in the collection of urine or sperm.

**Congenital** (L *congenitus,* born with). Present at birth, referring to certain mental or physical traits, diseases, and so on.

**Consolidation** (L *consolidare,* to make firm). The act of becoming solid or converting into a firm dense mass.

**Contracture** (L *contrahere,* to draw together). Permanent contraction of a muscle due to spasm or paralysis; fixed resistance to the passive stretch of a muscle.

**Contusion** (L *contundere,* to bruise). A bruise or injury in which the skin is unbroken.

**Convergence** (L *con*, with, + *vergere*, to incline). Coming together of two parts toward the same point; concentration of force or pull to one spot, as, for example, a muscle insertion point.

**Cord lesion level** Level where spinal cord is damaged; not necessarily spot where vertebrae are broken or displaced.

**Core decompression** Process of coring and removing a section of bone or tissue to relieve pressure in the center of the part.

**Coronal** (Gr *korone*, crown). Vertical line through the body to divide it into anterior and posterior planes.

**Cortical** (L *cortex*, rind). Pertaining to a cortex or outer layers of an organ or tissue.

**Cotrel's traction** A type of skin traction to treat scoliosis that uses a combination of head halter and pelvic belt tractions.

**Countertraction** (L *contra*, against, + *tractio*, pull). Pull exerted in the direction opposite the pull of traction.

**Coxa** (L *coxa*, hip). Hip joint.

**Crepitus** (L *crepitare*, to crackle). To rub against, usually at site of a fracture; the grating of a joint.

**Crutch** (Anglo-Saxon *cryce*). Device for aiding a lame or weak person in walking. Usually a long staff with padded crescent-shaped portion at the top for placing under the armpit.

**Crutchfield tongs** Metallic prongs that are inserted into the skull for skeletal cervical traction. Crosspieced hinges give appearance of ice tongs, hence the name "tongs."

**Cyst** (Gr *kystis*, bladder, sac). An abnormal sac that contains a liquid or semisolid material; may be benign or malignant.

**Cytology** (Gr *kytos*, hollow vessel, something that contains or covers, hence cell). Science dealing with the study of living cells.

**Death** Permanent cessation of all vital functions to a cell, tissue, or the entire body.

**Debridement** (Fr *de*, away + *bride*, bridle). Surgical cutting away of dead and foreign tissue from a wound.

**Decubitus** (L *decumbere*, to lie down). Bedsore; a patient's position in bed.

**Degenerative** (L *de*, from, + *genus*, race). Pertaining to or accompanied by degeneration; a worsening of physical or mental powers.

**Dehiscence** (L *dehiscere*, to gape). A breaking or bursting open, as an abdominal wound.

**Delayed union** Fracture not successfully united after lapse of usual amount of time for that type of fracture.

**Dependence** (L *dependere*, to hang down). The mental and physical state of being dependent upon narcotics in order to achieve a feeling of well-being; state of being influenced and determined by, or of being conditional upon, something else.

**Depression of shoulder**   Pulling the shoulder down.

**Dermatome**   (Gr *dermatos,* skin, + *tome,* incision). A skin segment innervated by a spinal nerve segment.

**Diabetes mellitus**   (Gr *diabetes,* passing through, + *mellitus,* honey-sweetened). A disorder of carbohydrate metabolism, characterized by hyperglycemia and glycosuria resulting from inadequate production or utilization of insulin.

**Diagnosis**   (Gr *diagnosis,* a deciding). Identifying a disease by its signs, symptoms, course, and laboratory findings; determination of the nature of a disease.

**Diagnostic Related Groups (DRGs).**   Groups of related medical diagnoses with relevant information used to determine the average length of a patient's hospital stay and the relative costs for treatments.

**Diaphysis**   (Gr *diaphysis,* a growing through). Shaft of a bone.

**DIP joint**   Distal interphalangeal joint (last finger joint).

**Directed blood**   Blood donated by person known to the recipient for use when needed by the patient.

**Disarticulate**   (Gr *dis,* split, + L *articulus,* joint). Amputation or separation through a joint.

**Disc** or **disk**   (L *discus,* flat plate). Rounded circular structure such as an intervertebral or optic disc.

**Disease**   (Fr *des,* difficult, + *aise,* ease). Impairment of bodily health; ailment; sickness.

**Dislocation**   (Gr *dis,* split + *locare,* to locate). The displacement of any part, especially the temporary displacement of a bone from its normal position in a joint.

**Distal**   (L *distalis,* distant). Far, away from trunk; opposite of proximal; farthest from center or median line.

**Divergence**   (L *divergere,* to turn aside). Separation into two or more parts or from a common center; insertion of muscles spread over several joints.

**Dorsalis pedis**   Dorsal artery of the foot, which is a continuation of the anterior tibialis artery.

**Dorsiflexion**   (L *dorsum,* back, + *flectere,* to bend). Movement of a part at the joint to bend the part toward the dorsum or posterior aspect of the body. The toes will point upward.

**Dorsum**   (L *dorsum,* back). Back, i.e., dorsum of leg—back of leg.

**Dunlop's traction**   Type of skin or skeletal traction used to treat fractures of the humerus.

**Dupuytren's contracture**   A progressive, painless thickening and tightening of the subcutaneous tissues of the palm causing the fourth and fifth fingers to bend into the palm and resist extension.

**Dyschondroplasia**   (Gr *dys,* bad, + *chondros,* cartilage, + *plassein,* to form). Abnormality of growth or development of the epiphyseal cartilages.

**Dyscrasia**   (Gr *dyskrasia,* bad mixture). An abnormal state of the body resulting from presence of toxic substances in the blood; now used as a synonym for disease.

**Dysesthesia**   (Gr *dys,* bad, difficult, + *aisthesis,* sensation). Sensation of pins and needles or crawling; decreased sense of touch.

**Dysplasia**   (Gr *dys,* bad, + *plassein,* to form). Abnormality of development or formation of tissue.

**Dystrophy**   (Gr *dys,* bad, + *trephein,* to nourish). Disorder due to defective or faulty nutrition; abnormal growth.

**Ecchymosis**   (Gr *ek,* out, + *chymos,* juice, + *osis,* condition). A bruised or discolored area due to injury to subcutaneous tissues causing extravasation of blood into the area.

**Economic**   (F *économique,* orderly, methodical). Pertaining to the management of one's private business.

**Economics**   (F *économique,* orderly, methodical). A science that investigates the conditions and laws affecting the production, distribution, and consumption of wealth and products; the material means of satisfying human desires.

**Economy**   (F *économie,* household management). The management or regulation of domestic or household affairs.

**Ectomy**   (Gr *ektomē,* removal). Excision of any organ or gland.

**Edema**   (Gr *oidēma,* swelling). Excessive amount of tissue fluid.

**Education**   Learning; the process of training and developing knowledge, skill, mind, character, and so on.

**Effects**   (L *effectus,* accomplishing). Results of an action or force.

**Electromyogram**   (Gr *elektron,* amber, + *mys,* muscle, + gamma, writing). Graphic record of muscle contraction as a result of electrical stimulation.

**Elephantiasis**   (Gr *elephas,* elephant). Condition resulting from obstruction of the lymphatic vessels.

**Elevation of shoulder**   Pulling shoulder up; raising shoulder.

**Embolism**   (Gr *en,* in, + *ballein,* to throw). Obstruction of a blood vessel by foreign substances or a blood clot.

**Emotion**   (L *emovere,* to stir up). Mental state or strong feeling usually accompanied by physical changes in the body such as alteration in heart rate and respiratory activity, vasomotor reactions, and changes in muscle tone.

**En bloc**   (L *en,* in, + *bloc,* trunk). Removal of diseased tissue in one piece or block.

**Endocrine**   (Gr *endon,* within, + *krinein,* to separate). An internal secretion; pertaining to a gland that produces an internal secretion.

**Endoprosthesis**   (Gr *endon,* within, + *prosthesis,* an addition). Replacement of a part inside the body with a substitute part.

**Environment**   Something that surrounds and influences whatever is within its boundaries; e.g., a home is one example of a family's environment.

**Enzyme**   (Gr *en,* in, + *zymē,* leaven). A complex organic catalyst produced in the body capable of speeding up a particular chemical reaction.

**Epidemiology**  (Gr *epi*, among, on, + *demois*, people, + *logos*, study). The study of incidence, distribution, environmental causes, and control of a disease in a population.

**Epiphyseal plate**  (Gr *epi*, upon, + *physis*, growth). Junction of cartilage epiphysis and bone shaft.

**Epiphysis**  (Gr *epi*, upon, + *physis*, growth). The ends of the long bones before ossification is complete; center for ossification at ends of long bones.

**Equinus**  (L *equus*, horse). Plantarflexion, walking on toes; a deformity in which the foot points downward.

**Erosion**  (L *erodere*, to gnaw away). Degenerative destruction; an eating away of tissue by physical or inflammatory processes.

**Esthesia**  (Gr *aisthesis*, sensation). Perception, feeling, or sensation.

**Ethics**  (Gr *ethos*, custom, usage, or character). Moral principles or conduct; the science of ideal human behavior.

**Etiology**  (Gr *aitia*, cause, + *logos*, study). The study of the causes of disease; cause or causes of disease.

**Evaluation**  (Fr *evaluer*, to appraise). To appraise or determine the value of something, such as achievement of goals.

**Eversion**  (L *ex*, from, + *vertere*, to turn). Turning outward of a body part or parts.

**Ewing's sarcoma**  A highly malignant tumor of undetermined cell source.

**Excision**  (L *ex*, out, + *caedere*, to cut). Surgical removal of a diseased part of the body.

**Excoriation**  (L *ex*, out, + *corium*, skin). Break in skin surface, usually covered with blood or serous crusts.

**Exhaustion**  (L *ex*, out, away from, + *haurire*, to drain). State of being exhausted, extreme fatigue or weariness; loss of vital powers; inability to respond to stimuli; third stage of the stress response.

**Exostosis**  (Gr *ex*, out, + *osteon*, bone). A bony outgrowth from the surface of a bone.

**Expected outcomes**  The goals or desired (expected) outcomes of treatments or nursing interventions.

**Extension**  (L *extensio*, pull out). Straightening; opposite to flexion.

**External rotation**  Turn outward; that is, external rotation of the hip—the leg and foot are turned outward away from the "plumb."

**Extracapsular**  (L *exter*, outward, + *capsula*, a little box). Exterior to the capsule of a synovial joint.

**Fasciotomy**  (L *fascia*, a band, + *tome*, incision). Incision into one or more fascia, coverings around muscles, to relieve pressure.

**Fat embolism**  Embolism composed of molecules of fat that are pushed from the bone marrow after fracture trauma; globules of fat obstructing blood vessels.

**Fibroma**  (L *fibra*, fiber, + *oma*, tumor). A fibrous, encapsulated, connective tissue tumor.

**Fibrosarcoma** (L *fibra,* fiber, + *sarx,* flesh, *oma,* tumor). A spindle-celled sarcoma containing much connective tissue.

**Fibrosis** (L *fibra,* fiber, + Gr *osis,* condition). Scarring or scar formation in excessive amounts.

**Fibrous** (L *fibra,* fiber). Composed of or containing fibers. Opposed to osseous (bony) composition.

**Fibrous union** Fractured bone united with soft, not bony, tissue.

**Fissure** (L *fissura,* cleft). Groove or crack in tissue.

**Flaccid** (L *flaccidus,* flabby). Lack of muscle tone, lacking spasticity, loose; flabby.

**Flail chest** Fractures of one or more ribs resulting in excessive, uncontrolled mobility of ribs and their movements with respirations.

**Flatus** (L *flatus,* a blowing). Gas in digestive tract; eructation of air.

**Flexion** (L *flexio,* bend). Bending; opposite to extension.

**Flexor-hinge splint** Lively splint that causes fingers to meet the thumb when wrist is extended.

**Fracture** (L *fractura,* break). A sudden breaking of a bone; a broken bone.

**Gait** (ME *gait,* passage). Style or manner of walking.

**Gatch frame** Bedframe divided into separate movable sections; can be used for raising patient to a sitting or other position.

**Genes** (Gr *gennan,* to produce). Hereditary units of life that control the cell's transfer of a trait or process.

**Giant cell** Cell of large size with multiple nuclei, appearing to be made up of many cells, but not clearly outlined; found in both kinds of marrow. Also found in tissues that are healing around foreign bodies; and in the inflammatory reaction to tuberculosis; type of tumor, usually benign.

**Gibbus** (L *gibbosus,* humped). Hump; humpbacked.

**Glomus** (L *glomus,* a ball). A small round swelling made up of tiny blood vessels and found in a stroma containing many nerve fibers.

**Goal** Objective or aim to be achieved.

**Goal Achievement** Completion of an objective or the end of an effort.

**Goal conflict** Block hindering goal achievement in a given situation or time.

**Goal priority** Classification or ordering of goals according to necessity or desirability for completion.

**Goniometer** (Gr *gonia,* angle + *metron,* measure). Instrument to measure joint movements and angles.

**Gout** (L *gutta,* drop). Paroxysmal metabolic disease marked by acute arthritis and inflammation of the joints. Joints affected may be at any location, but gout usually begins in the knee or foot or big toe.

**Grab bar** A bar, firmly fastened to wall or floor, used as a handhold.

**Granulation** (L *granulum,* little grain). Fleshy projections formed on the surface of a wound that is not healing by first intention.

**Greenstick fracture** Fracture involving only one of the cortices of a bone; occurs in young children or older (elderly) adults.

**Guaiac test**　A chemical test used to detect hidden blood in secretions or excretions.

**Guilt**　The state of having done or believing that one has done a wrong or committed an offense; culpability, legal or ethical.

**Gypsum**　A hydrated sulfate of calcium, $CaSO_4 \cdot 2H_2O$, occurring naturally in sedimentary rocks and used for making plaster of paris for cast use.

**Halo cast**　Cast enclosing forehead, back of head, neck, and shoulders for cervical fracture treatment.

**Halo-femoral traction**　Skeletal traction to the head (skull) and femurs for straightening of scoliosis curvature.

**Hamstrings**　(Anglo-Saxon *haum,* haunch). Muscles at back of thigh that bend the knee and extend the hip.

**Harrington rods**　Metallic implants used in the treatment of scoliosis. May be used singly or bilaterally on sides of and attached to vertebrae to straighten curvature.

**Healing**　(Anglo-Saxon *hael,* whole). The restoration to a normal condition, especially of an inflammation or a wound; to make whole or healthy.

**Health**　State of being well and within limits defined as "normal."

**Heberden's nodes**　Hard nodules or enlargements of the distal joints of the fingers seen in osteoarthritis.

**Hemangioma**　(Gr *haima,* blood, + *angeion,* vessel, + *oma,* tumor). Benign tumor of dilated blood vessels.

**Hematodystrophy**　(Gr *haima,* blood, + *dys,* difficult, + *trephein,* to nourish). A blood deficiency condition such as anemia.

**Hematology**　(Gr *haima,* blood, + *logos,* study). The study or science of the blood and blood-forming tissues.

**Hematoma**　(Gr *haima,* blood, + *oma,* tumor). A tumor or swelling that contains blood.

**Hematopoietic**　(Gr *haima,* blood, + *poiein,* to form). Pertaining to the production and development of blood cells.

**Hematuria**　(Gr *haima,* blood, + *ouron,* urine). Blood in the urine.

**Hemigastrectomy**　(Gr *hemi,* half, + *gastēr,* belly, + *ektome,* excision). Surgical removal of one-half of the stomach.

**Hemipelvectomy**　(Gr *hemi,* half, + *pelvis,* basin, + *ektoma,* excision). Surgical excision of the entire lower extremity from the hip to the foot.

**Hemiplegia**　(Gr *hemi,* half, + *plēgē,* a stroke). Paralysis of one-half of the body.

**Herniated nucleus pulposus**　Rupture or extrusion of an intervertebral disk in one or more directions, such as rupture anteriorly toward the spinal cord; laterally, obliquely, or posteriorly toward the spinous process.

**Heterograft**　(Gr *heteros,* other, + *graftus,* to attach). A graft taken from another individual or animal of different species from the one intended for the graft.

**Histiocytic leukemia**　(Gr *histos,* web, + *kytos,* cell). Reticuloendothelial cell or tissue cell, present in loose connective tissues, which can change into leukemic cells.

**Hodgkin's disease**   A form of cancer that affects the lymphatic system—the network of glands or nodes and vessels that manufactures and circulates lymph throughout the body to fight infection.

**Hoffman apparatus**   A device consisting of transverse (transfixing) metallic rods that fit into a specific frame to hold weak or fractured bones to aid healing. It is one of a group of devices referred to as external fixation devices.

**Homan's sign**   Pain in the calf of the leg when the toe is passively dorsiflexed; an early sign of venous thrombosis of the deep calf veins.

**Homograft**   (Gr *homos*, same, + *graftus*, to attach). A graft of skin, bone, or other tissue taken from an individual of the same species; now called allograft.

**Hormones**   (Gr *hormaein*, to urge on). Chemicals that help regulate the body mechanisms, including growth, metabolism, and reproduction. Hormones are carried throughout the body.

**Horner's syndrome**   Paralysis of the cervical sympathetic nerve trunk leading to constriction of the pupil, partial eyelid ptosis (drooping), and sometimes loss of sweating on the affected side of the face.

**Hyperalimentation**   (Gr *hyper*, above, + L *alimentum*, nourishment). Supplying nutrients above the normal metabolic needs to assist weight gain. The nutrients are administered per vein (usually a large, central vein) if the GI tract is unable to tolerate or contain the nutrients. May be referred to as total parenteral nutrition.

**Hyperextended**   (Gr *hyper*, above, + *extendere*, to stretch out). Extended beyond the normal position; for example, extended beyond 180° at elbow.

**Hypesthesia** or **hypoesthesia**   (Gr *hypo* under, + *aisthesis*). Lessened sensibility to touch.

**Hypophosphatemia**   (Gr *hypo*, under, + *phosphas*, phosphate, + *haima*, blood). Below normal levels of phosphates in the blood.

**Hysteria**   (Gr *hystera*, uterus). Condition occurring in the absence of organic disease characterized by symptoms simulating almost every type of physical disease, and a series of mental manifestations.

**Ileostomy**   (L *ileum*, flank, + Gr *stoma*, opening). A surgical procedure that constructs an artificial opening of the small intestine through the abdominal wall for elimination of body wastes.

**Iliac crest**   (L *iliacus*, pertaining to the ilium). Bony ridges at sides of abdomen; outer portion of pelvis or either side of the ilium.

**Immobility**   Fixedness; motionlessness; incapability of movement.

**Immobilization**   (L *in*, not, + *mobilis*, movable). Fixation preventing any movement of a part or limb.

**Immune**   (L *immunis*, safe). Protected or exempt from a disease. Exempt from a certain disease by vaccination or inoculation.

**Immunity**   (L *immunitas*, to be safe). State of being resistant to noxious agents or organisms due to previous exposure to the same agent or organism.

**Immunoglobulins** Proteins capable of acting as antigens. Five are presently known: IgG, IgA, IgM, IgD, and IgE.

**Immunology** (L *immunis,* safe, + *logos,* study). A branch of science dealing with the body's resistance mechanism against disease or the invasion of a foreign substance.

**Immunotherapy** (L *immunis,* safe, + Gr *therapeia,* treatment). Treatment of disease by stimulating the body's own defense mechanism against the disease.

**Implants** (L *in,* into, + *plantare,* to plant). Plates, screws, nails, or other devices used in a surgical wound.

**Independence** The state of being independent; freedom from the influence, control, or determination of another.

**Infarct** (L *infarcire,* to stuff into). Area in a tissue or organ that undergoes necrosis following loss of blood supply.

**Infection** (L *inficere,* to taint). Condition in which a part of the body is invaded by a pathogenic agent which multiplies and produces effects which are injurious.

**Infectious** (L *inficere,* to taint). Disease caused by growth of a pathogenic organism in the body that may or may not be contagious; producing infection.

**Inference** (L *inferre,* to bring into). A judgment or conclusion arrived at from observations and other data or knowledge.

**Inflammation** (L *inflammare,* to flame within). Tissue reaction to injury. The succession of changes that occur in living tissue when it is injured.

**Input** That which is put in for energy or power.

**Interaction** (L *inter,* between, + *actio,* to do). Observable behaviors (effects) of one person with another or of a person with his/her environment; mutual or reciprocal action or influence.

**Internal fixation** (L *internus,* within). Operative fixation and repair of fractures by placement of metallic implants on or in the fracture site.

**Internal rotation** To turn inward; for example, internal rotation of shoulder (back of hand placed on small of back).

**Interpersonal relationships** Actions between two or more persons; may involve one or more senses and be verbal or nonverbal.

**Intertrochanteric** Between the two bony processes (trochanters) on the upper end of the femur.

**Intervention** (L *inter,* between, + *veni,* to come). An act or action; may be a nursing act or intervention as part of the nursing process.

**Intervertebral disk** Semigelatinous center of the annular cartilage between two vertebrae. Also referred to as nucleus pulposus.

**Intra-articular** (L *intra,* within, + Gr *arthron,* joint). Within a joint.

**Intracapsular** (L *intra,* within, + *capsula,* little box). Within the capsule of a joint such as the hip or shoulder joint.

**Intramedullary**   Within the medullary canal of a long bone; within the spinal cord.

**Intrathecal**   (L *intra,* within, + Gr *thēkē,* sheath). Within the canal containing the spinal cord.

**Intravascular**   Within a blood vessel.

**Intravenous**   (L *intra,* within, + *vena,* vein). Within or into a vein.

**Inversion**   (L *in,* into, + *vertere,* to turn). Turning inward of part or all of a body part, especially parts of the feet, ankles, or fingers.

**Involucrum**   (L *in,* in, + *volvere,* to wrap). Newly formed bone enveloping sequestrum in bone.

**Ischemia** or **ischaemia**   (Gr *ischein,* to hold back, + *haima,* blood). Insufficient blood supply because of obstruction of blood vessels to a part.

**Ischial tuberosity**   (Gr *ischion,* hip). Bony protrusion under buttocks on the innominate bone.

**Isograft**   (Gr *isos,* equal, + *graftus,* to attach). Graft from another individual or animal of the same species.

**Isolation**   (L *isolato,* isolate). Limitation of contacts or movements of person suffering from a communicable disease or one who is a carrier.

**Isometric**   (Gr *isos,* equal, + *metron,* measure). Having equal dimensions; contraction in which lengthening or shortening is prevented; no mechanical work is performed.

**Isotonic**   (Gr *isos,* equal, + *tonos,* tone). Having the same osmotic pressure; having the same tension or tone.

**Joint**   (L *junctio,* a joining). Point of juncture between two bones, usually formed of fibrous connective tissue and cartilage.

**Joint, DIP**   Distal interphalangeal joint; last finger joint.

**Joint, MP**   Metacarpophalangeal joint; joint at base of finger.

**Joint, PIP**   Proximal interphalangeal joint; middle finger joint.

**Keloid**   (Gr *kēlē,* tumor, + *eidos,* form). Scar formation with excessive growth of a surgical wound or from trauma.

**Ketonuria**   (ketone + Gr *ouron,* urine). Presence of ketones in the urine.

**Ketosis**   (ketone + Gr *osis,* condition). Accumulation of ketone bodies, frequently associated with acidosis.

**Kinesiology**   (Gr *kinēsis,* motion, + *logos,* study). The study of muscles and muscular movement.

**Kyphosis**   (Gr *kyphōsis,* a hump). Abnormal increased convexity in thoracic spine; spinal deformity causing a hump on the back.

**Laceration**   (L *lacerare,* to tear). Wound or irregular tear of the flesh.

**Laparotomy**   (Gr *lapara,* groin, + *tome,* incision). Surgical opening of the abdomen; an abdominal operation.

**Lateral**   (L *latus,* side). To the side or pertaining to the side.

**Learning**   (Anglo Saxon *leornian).* The acquiring of knowledge or skill; acquired knowledge or skill, especially much knowledge in a special field.

**Legal**   (L *lex*, law). Lawful; of, based upon, or authorized by law; permitted by law.

**Leiomyosarcoma**   (Gr *leios*, smooth, + *myo*, muscle, + *sarx*, flesh, + *oma*, tumor). Combined leiomyoma (smooth muscle tissue myoma) and sarcoma.

**Lesion**   (L *laesio*, a wound). Any abnormal change in tissue due to disease or injury; a wound.

**Life-style**   Manner of living one's life.

**Ligament**   (L *ligamentum*, a band). Band of strong fibrous tissue joining bones at a joint.

**Limitation**   (L *limitare*, to limit). Condition of being limited.

**Limitation of motion**   Restriction of movement in range of motion of a part or joint, especially that imposed by disease or trauma to joints and soft tissues.

**Lipodystrophy**   (Gr *lipos*, fat, + *dys*, bad, + *trephein*, to nourish). Disturbance or defectiveness of fat metabolism.

**Lipoma**   (Gr *lipos*, fat, + *oma*, tumor). A fatty tumor.

**Liposarcoma**   (Gr *lipos*, fat, + *sarx*, flesh, + *oma*, tumor). Sarcoma with fatty elements.

**Loads**   Internal or external personal deficiencies or weaknesses that exert negative influences (drag) on the person's coping energy or ability.

**Locomotion**   (L *locus*, place, + *movere*, to move). Movement or power of movement from one place to another.

**Locomotor ataxia**   Sclerosis affecting posterior columns of the spinal cord.

**Logroll**   Method of turning a patient to the side during which the spinal column, hips, and shoulders are maintained straight (as a log).

**Lordosis**   (Gr *lordōsis*, bending). Abnormal anterior convexity of the spine (spine bends backward).

**Low back pain**   Pain or discomfort in the lumbar or lumbosacral areas of the lower back.

**Lumbar**   (L *lumbus*, loin). Relating to the lumbar region of the vertebral column.

**Lupus**   (L wolf). Lupus erythematosus. Chronic, systemic, connective tissue disease characterized by pathological changes in the vascular, renal, and pulmonary tissues.

**Luque rods**   Long metallic rods used along the vertebrae to stabilize the bones following a spinal fusion to correct spinal curvatures (scoliosis) or deformities. The rods are wired to the bones at each vertebral segment.

**Lymph**   (L *lympha*, water). A clear fluid that circulates throughout the body, containing white blood cells called lymphocytes, as well as antibodies and nourishing substances.

**Lymphangioma**   (L *lympha*, water, + *angeion*, vessel, + Gr *oma*, tumor). Tumor composed of lymphatic vessels.

**Lymphedema**   (L *lympha, water,* + oidēma, swelling). Swelling as a result of obstruction of lymphatic vessels or lymph nodes.

**Lymph gland**   Tissue that is made up of lymphocytes and connective tissue and produces lymph and lymphocytes (also called lymph node). These glands act as filters of impurities in the body.

**Lymphocyte**   (L *lympha,* water, + *kytos,* cell). Lymph cell or white corpuscle without cytoplasmic granules. They normally number from 20% to 50% of total white cells.

**Lymphogram**   (L *lympha,* water, + *gramma,* a written record). X-ray recording of the lymph channels following injection of radiopaque dye.

**Lymphoma**   (L *lympha,* water, + Gr *oma,* tumor). Malignant growths of lymph nodes or lymph tissues. Tumors included in this group include Hodgkin's disease, lymphosarcoma, and malignant lymphoma.

**Macrophage**   (Gr *makros,* large, + *phagein,* to eat). Cells of the reticuloendothelial system with the ability to engulf particulate substances.

**Magnetic resonance image (MRI)**   The picture or diagram produced by the emissions of electromagnetic waves released from atoms in the nucleus of a cell that have been exposed to a magnetic field.

**Malignant**   (L *malignans,* acting maliciously). Resists treatment, thus grows worse; virulent; cancerous.

**Malignant tumor**   A tumor made up of cancer cells. These tumors continue to grow and invade surrounding tissues; cells may break away and grow elsewhere.

**Muscle tone**   A state of readiness maintained by the muscles in the body; a steady state of contraction.

**Malnutrition**   Lack of necessary or proper nourishment or absorption of foodstuffs.

**Malunion**   (L *malum,* bad, + *unio,* oneness). Union of fragments of fracture in faulty position; broken bone that has united in an incorrect position.

**Mastication**   (L *masticare,* to chew). Chewing.

**Medial**   (L *medialis,* middle). Inside, near middle; opposite of lateral.

**Median line**   Imaginary line through exact center of body.

**Melanoma**   (Gr *melas,* black, + *oma,* tumor). A pigmented, highly malignant form of cancer of the skin. The tumor may vary in color from nearly black to almost white.

**Meningitis**   Gr *mēninx,* membrane, + *itis,* inflammation). Inflammation of the spinal cord or brain coverings.

**Meniscus**   (Gr *meniskos,* crescent). Intraarticular fibrocartilage of crescent shape, found in certain joints, especially the lateral and medial menisci (semilunar cartilages) of the knee joint.

**Metabolism**   (Gr *meta,* change, + *ismos,* state of). The sum of all the physical and chemical changes that occur in an organism; it involves *anabolism* and *catabolism.*

**Metacarpal** (Gr *meta,* change, + L *carpalis,* wrist). Pertaining to the bones of the hand.

**Metaphysis** (Gr *meta,* change, + *phyein,* to grow). Wide portion of end of long bone adjacent to epiphysis; contains growth zone; portion of child's bone where growth activity occurs.

**Metaplasia** (Gr *meta,* change, + *plassein,* to form). Conversion into a form that is abnormal or not normal for that tissue.

**Metastasis** (Gr *meta,* change, + *stasis,* stand). Process by which cells break away and spread to other places in the body by way of the lymph and blood systems and start new growths.

**Methacrylate** A polymer that, when mixed with a solvent, becomes pliable. Used as a "glue" for holding artificial materials for joint replacements.

**Minerva** Goddess of the hunt whose head, neck, and chest-enclosing armor (mail) is the basis for the naming of minerva casts.

**Mitosis** (Gr *mitos,* thread). Process of cell reproduction by which new cells are formed.

**ML or ml** (L *milli,* thousand). One thousandth of a liter; equal to a cc.

**Mobility** (L *mobilis,* moving). Readily movable; changeable; fluidity or ease in movement.

**Mobilization** (L *mobilis,* move). Allowing mobility after treatment by immobilization.

**Moral** (L *moralis,* manner, custom, habit). Excellence in what pertains to practice or conduct; right and proper.

**Motivation** (L *movere,* to move). Provided with a force or reason for action.

**Motor** (L *motus,* moving). Causing motion; a part or center that induces movements, as nerves or muscles.

**MP joint** Metacarpophalangeal joint; joint at base of finger.

**Multiple myeloma** A neoplastic disease characterized by the infiltration of bone and bone marrow by myeloma cells, forming multiple tumor masses. Usually progressive and generally fatal.

**Muscle** (L *musculus*). A type of tissue, composed of contractile cells or fibers, which effects movement of an organ or part of the body.

**Muscle atrophy** Wasting away of muscle tissue because of disuse or paralysis.

**Myelitis** (Gr *myelos,* marrow, + *itis,* inflammation). Inflammation of spinal cord or of the bone marrow.

**Myelocyte** (Gr *myelos,* marrow or spinal cord, + *kytos,* cell). A large cell in red bone marrow from which leukocytes are derived.

**Myelogram** (Gr *myelos,* spinal cord, + *gramma,* a written record). Roentgenographic inspection of the spinal cord via radiopaque medium injected into the intrathecal space.

**Myositis** (Gr *mys,* muscle, + *itis,* inflammation). Inflammation of muscle tissue.

**Myositis ossificans** (Gr *osteon,* bone). Muscle inflammation marked by ossification (deposits of calcium) in the muscles.

**Myxoma**  (Gr *myxa*, mucus, + *oma*, tumor). A tumor composed of mucous connective tissue similar to that present in the embryo or umbilical cord.

**Nail**  A rod made of metal, bone, or solid material used to attach the ends or pieces of broken bones. May be placed within the medullary canal of the bone or into the cortical layers of bone; e.g., intramedullary nail or hip nail.

**Narcotic**  (Gr *narkētikos*, benumbing). Producing stupor or sleep.

**Natal cleft**  (L *natus*, birth, + *clift*, crevice). Crease between buttocks.

**Necrosis**  (Gr *nekrosis*, deadness). Death of bone cells or other areas of tissue surrounded by healthy cells; a gradual degeneration.

**Need**  A condition requiring relief; a lack of something desired or useful.

**Neoplasm**  (Gr *neos*, new, + *plasma*, formation). Any new abnormal growth of cells or tissues; may be benign or malignant.

**Nerve**  (Gr *neuron*, sinew). A bundle or group of nerve fibers outside the central nervous system that connects the brain and spinal cord with various parts of the body. Nerves conduct afferent impulses centrally from receptor organs and efferent impulses peripherally to effector organs.

**Neuralgia**  (Gr *neuron*, sinew, + *algos*, pain). Severe, sharp pain along the course of a nerve.

**Neurapraxia**  (Gr *neuron*, sinew, + *apraxia*, nonactive). Cessation in function in a peripheral nerve without degenerative changes leading to eventual recovery of function.

**Neurasthenia**  (Gr *neuron*, sinew, + *astheneia*, weakness). Condition of generalized weakness or exhaustion.

**Neurilemma**  (Gr *neuron*, sinew, + *eilēma*, husk). Thin, membranous sheath enveloping a nerve fiber.

**Neurilemmoma**  A firm, encapsulated fibrillar tumor of peripheral nerves.

**Neuritis**  (Gr *neuron*, sinew, + *itis*, inflammation). Inflammation of nerve tissue or nerves, usually associated with a degenerative process.

**Neuroblastoma**  (Gr *neuron*, sinew, + *blastos*, germ + *oma*, tumor). A malignant hemorrhagic tumor composed principally of cells resembling neuroblasts that give rise to cells of the sympathetic system, especially adrenal medulla. Occurs chiefly in infants and children.

**Neurofibroma**  (Gr *neuron*, sinew, + L *fibra*, fiber, + *oma*, tumor). A tumor of connective tissue of a nerve, including medullated layer of a nerve fiber.

**Neuroma**  (Gr *neuron*, sinew, + *oma*, tumor). Nerve tumor or tumor along the course of a nerve.

**Neurosis**  (Gr *neuron*, sinew, + *osis*, disease). Disorder of thought processes without demonstrable disease; contact with reality is usually maintained.

**Neurotmesis**  (Gr *neuron*, sinew, + *tmēsis*, rupture). Nerve injury resulting in complete loss of function of the nerve.

**Neurovascular**  (Gr *neuron*, sinew, + *vasculus*, a small vessel). Concerning both the nervous and vascular systems.

**Nidus**  (L nest). A focus of infection.

**Nonnarcotic**  (L *non*, not, + *narcos*, stupor). Substance that does not produce a stupor or insensibility to pain.

**Nonunion**  (L *non*, not, + *unio*, joining). Failure of broken bone fragments to heal and unite.

**Norepinephrine** or **noradrenaline**  Hormone produced in the adrenal medulla that produces marked vasoconstrictor effects.

**Normal**  (L *normalis*, according to pattern). Standard; performing regular functions; natural; regular.

**Nosocomial infection**  (Gr *nosos*, disease, + *komeion* to care for). Infection acquired in a hospital.

**Nucleus pulposus**  (L *nucleus*, little kernel). Semigelatinous center within the annular cartilage between two vertebrae.

**Nursing**  Activities of nurses to assist persons to recover and regain healthy states; activities to assist persons to remain healthy, independent, and well.

**Nursing diagnosis**  Statement of an actual or potential problem of a patient determined or decided upon following assessment.

**Nursing process**  Interactions between nurse and patient in which the behavior of each affects the other and both are affected by the factors within the environment (situation).

**Nursing process methodology**  System for practicing nursing consisting of observing, measuring, and analyzing data; planning, implementing, and evaluating care within a nurse-patient situation.

**Nutrition**  (L *nutritio*, nourish). Total of the processes involved in the taking in and utilization of food substances by which growth, repair, and maintenance of body activities as a whole or in any of its parts are accomplished.

**Oblique**  (L *obliquus*). Slanting, diagonal.

**Observation**  Gathering of data through observing, measuring, and making judgments; fact that is being noted or seen; taking notice of.

**Obstipation**  (L *obstipatio*, obstruction). Obstinate or extreme constipation due to an obstruction.

**Obstruction**  (L *obstructio*, to build against). An obstacle or thing that impedes.

**Occult**  (L *occultus*, hidden). Concealed; obscure.

**Ochronosis**  (Gr *ōchros*, yellow, + *nosos*, disease). Metabolic condition characterized by dark pigmentation in the ligaments, cartilage, fibrous tissues, skin, and urine.

**Ogilvie's syndrome**  Obstruction of the colon secondary to abdominal or pelvic trauma

**Oliguria**  (Gr *oligos*, little, + *ouron*, urine). Diminished amount of urine formation.

**Oncology**  (Gr *onkos*, mass, + *logos*, study). Study of tumors; has become a specialty branch of modern medicine.

**Open fracture**   External skin wound leading to break (fracture) in bone.

**Open reduction**   Restoration of bone position under direct vision through surgical incision and operation.

**Orthopaedics** or **orthopedics**   (Gr *orthos,* straight, + *pais,* child). Branch of medical science that deals with prevention or correction of disorders involving locomotor structures of the body, especially the skeleton, joints, muscles, and fascia.

**Osgood-Schlatter disease**   Epiphysitis (inflammation) of the tibial tubercle.

**Ossification**   (Gr *osteon,* bone, + *facere,* to make). Conversion of tissues to bone.

**Osteo-**   (Gr *osteon,* bone). Combining form indicating relationship to a bone.

**Osteoarthritis**   (Gr *osteon,* bone, + *arthros,* joint, + *itis,* inflammation). Chronic, destructive process in articular cartilage, with overgrowth of bone and spur formation leading to impaired function; degenerative joint disease.

**Osteoblast**   (Gr *osteon,* bone, + *blastos,* germ). A cell of the mesenchymal cells which aids in bone formation.

**Osteochondritis**   (Gr *osteon,* bone, + *chondros,* cartilage, + *itis,* inflammation). Inflammatory reaction affecting bone and cartilage.

**Osteoclast**   (Gr *osteon,* bone, + *klan,* to break). Multinuclear cell concerned with the absorption and removal of unwanted bone tissue.

**Osteocyte**   (Gr *osteon,* bone, + *cyte,* cell). Bone-forming cell.

**Osteogenesis imperfecta**   (Gr *osteon,* bone, + *genesis,* reproduction, + *imperfecta,* incomplete). A genetic disorder noted by defective development of abnormally brittle and fragile bones that can be easily fractured by the slightest trauma.

**Osteogenic sarcoma**   Sarcoma composed of osseous tissue containing variously shaped cells.

**Osteoma**   (Gr *osteon,* bone, + *oma,* tumor). A benign bony tumor; a bonelike structure that develops on a bone or, occasionally, at other sites.

**Osteomalacia**   (Gr *osteon,* bone, + *malakia,* softening). Failure of calcification of osteoid tissue, resulting in bending of the soft bones; softening of the bones, so they become flexible and brittle.

**Osteomyelitis**   (Gr *osteon,* bone, + *myelos,* marrow, + *itis,* inflammation). Infection of bone or bone marrow caused by pathogens.

**Osteopenia**   (Gr *osteon,* bone, + *penia,* want). Condition of less than normal amounts of bone substance in the body.

**Osteopetrosis**   (Gr *osteon,* bone, + *petra,* stone, + *osis,* disease). Excessive calcification causing spontaneous fractures; marble bones.

**Osteophyte**   (Gr *osteon,* bone, + *phyton,* plant). Outgrowth of bone that is rough and irregular. A synonym for bone spur.

**Osteoporosis**   (Gr *osteon,* bone, + *poros,* a passage, + *osis,* condition). Condition in which bones become demineralized, soft, and spongy.

**Osteotomy**   (Gr *osteon,* bone, + *tome,* incision). Surgical opening of bone or cutting through a bone.

**Ostomy** (L *stoma*, mouth). Surgical procedure that creates a stoma, or artificial opening. An ostomate is someone who has had this form of surgery.

**Otorrhea** (Gr *ōtos*, ear, + *rhoia*, to flow). Discharge from the ear.

**Output** Yield or product; that which is produced.

**Overbed** (AS *ofer*, over). Something across or over a bed, such as an overbed table.

**Pain** (L *poena*, a fine, a penalty). Discomfort, distress, or suffering, due to provocation of sensory nerves.

**Pallor** (L *pallidus*, pale). Lack of color; paleness.

**Palliative treatment** (L *palliatus*, cloaked). Providing relief from symptoms of a disease but not directly curing the disease; alleviating pain.

**Palmar** (L *palma*, hand). Front, palm side of hand.

**Palpation** (L *palpare*, to touch). Detection procedure using the hands to examine organs without the aid of instruments.

**Paraplegia** (Gr *para*, beyond + *plēgē*, stroke). Paralysis of legs and lower body, motor, and sensation functions.

**Paroxysm** (Gr *paroxysmos*, irritation). Sudden, periodic attack or recurrence of symptoms of a disease; a sudden spasm or convulsion of any kind.

**Pars articularis** (L *partes*, part, + *articularis*, articulation). Region of lamina between facets above and below vertebral body.

**Partial weight bearing** Limiting amount of weight on lower extremities and joints when walking or standing.

**Pathology** (Gr *pathos*, disease, + *logos*, study). The science that studies the nature, cause, and development of disease through examination of tissues and fluids of the body.

**Pattern** (OF *patron*, patron). A group or cluster of behaviors observed or noted over time; anything designed as a sample or configuration.

**Pelvic belt** or **pelvic girdle** "Harness" made of heavy muslin to enclose the abdomen and pelvis for pelvic traction. Long straps from the belt are attached to weights for traction to the pelvis and lower back.

**Pelvic sling** Oblong support made of heavy muslin placed under the pelvis for suspension (like a hammock) and slight compression of the tissues and bones following trauma to the pelvic bones or tissues.

**Perception** (L *percipere*, to perceive). The process of perceiving through the senses; an intuitive process; consciousness; that which is perceived.

**Percussion** (L *percussio*, a striking). Tapping the body lightly but sharply to determine position, size, and consistency of an underlying structure and the presence of fluid or pus in a cavity.

**Percutaneous** (L *per* through, + *cutis*, skin). Through the skin.

**Periosteum** (Gr *peri*, around, + *osteon*, bone). The outer, tough covering of bones.

**Peripheral pulse** Pulse recorded in arteries (radial or pedal) in distal portion of limbs.

**Periphery** (Gr *periphereia*, around). Outermost boundary or outer surface of the body.

**Personality**  (L *personalitas,* mask). The unique organization of traits, characteristics, and modes of behavior of an individual; the mental aspects of an individual.

**Petechiae**  (It. *petecchia,* skin spot). Small purplish hemorrhagic spots on the skin.

**Phantom pain**  (Gr *phantasma,* an appearance). Illusion or sensation of pain following amputation that pain is still present in the removed parts; referred to as phantom-limb pain.

**Phlebitis**  (Gr *phlebos,* vein, + *itis,* inflammation). Inflammation of a vein.

**PIP joint**  Proximal interphalangeal joint; middle-finger joint.

**Plantarflexion**  (L *plantae,* sole of the foot, + *flexio,* bent). Extension of the foot, especially the toes, downward from the ankle; can be referred to as equinus.

**Plaster of Paris**  Gypsum cement, $CaSO_4 \cdot H_2O$, mixed with water to form a paste that sets rapidly; used to make casts, stiff bandages, or splints.

**Plate**  A thin flattened part or portion; flattened process of bone; metallic flat plate attached with screws to the long axis of a bone to hold the bones immobile for healing.

**Platelets**  (Gr *plate,* flat). A small circular or oval disk present in blood, that is necessary for the ability of the blood to clot.

**Pleurisy**  (Gr *pleura,* side). Inflammation of the pleura, the coverings around the lungs.

**Plication**  (L *plicare,* to fold). Braiding, folding, or stitching folds to reduce size of an organ.

**P.M. or pm**  (L *post,* after, + *meridies,* noon). After noon or the afternoon hours.

**Polyp**  (Gr *polys,* many, + *pous,* foot). An overgrowth of tissue projecting into a cavity of the body, e.g., the lining of the colon, nasal passage, or vocal cord surfaces; a tumor with a pedicle.

**Popliteal**  (L *poples,* ham). Concerning the posterior surface of the knee.

**Posterior**  (L *posterus,* coming after). Behind, the back of; hindmost surface or area of organ or body.

**Posterior tibialis**  Branch of the popliteal and peroneal arteries ending in the plantaris lateralis and medialis. Posterior tibialis passes just behind the medial malleolus of the ankle before entering the foot.

**Post position**  Planting or "posting" one's foot on the bed mattress with the knee bent to aid in lifting oneself from the bed. The patient bends the knee, posts or plants the foot firmly on the mattress, grasps the trapeze with both hands to pull the body up, holds the back and affected hip and leg straight, and lifts the body off the mattress by pulling up with the arms and pushing down on the posted foot. The post position may be used following acetabular injuries and total hip replacements to prevent excessive hip flexion.

**Powers**  (L *posse,* to have power). Internal or external personal strengths that exert positive influences on the person's coping energy or ability; ability or capacity to act.

**Primary**  (L *primarius,* principal). First in time or order; principal.

**Primary nursing**   A system for delivery of nursing care in which a registered nurse assumes the primary, 24-hour accountability for the nursing care of a patient or patients.

**Priority**   (L *prior*, former, superior). Quality of being superior in rank, position, or preference; prescribing the order in which things are to be attended to.

**Process**   (L *processus*, going before). A method of action; state of progress of disease; a projection or outgrowth of bone or tissue.

**Prognosis**   (Gr foreknowledge). Prediction of the course of a disease and the future prospects for the patient.

**Progressive systemic sclerosis**   A progressively debilitating disease of collagen-containing tissues which may result in hardening of skin tissues, obstruction of the bowel and progressive atrophy of skin and other tissues; formerly called scleroderma.

**Prominence**   (L *prominens*, project). A projection or protrusion.

**Prone**   Lying face downward; hand with palm turned downward.

**Prosthesis**   (Gr foremost). Artificial replacement for a missing body part, for example, breast form, leg, arm, eye.

**Protocol**   (Gr *prōtokollon*, first notes glued to a manuscript). Standardized procedures followed by physicians so that results of treatment of different patients can be compared.

**Protraction**   (L *protractus*, dragged out). Pulled forward, for example, protraction of the shoulder—scapula moved forward on the chest wall.

**Proximal**   (L *proximus*, next). Near, close to trunk; opposite to distal; end of a bone or limb nearest the trunk.

**Pseudoarthrosis**   (Gr *pseudes*, false, + *arthron*, joint, + *osis*, disease). A false joint caused by tissue between fractured pieces of bone.

**Psychology**   (Gr *psyche*, soul, mind, + *logos*, study). The study of mental processes and their effects upon behavior.

**Pulmonary embolism**   Embolism lodging within pulmonary tissues, the pulmonary artery, or one of its branches.

**Pulse**   (*pulsus*, beating). Throbbing caused by the regular contraction and alternate expansion of an artery; the periodic thrust felt over arteries in time with heartbeat.

**Pyrogen**   (Gr *pyr*, fire, + *gennan*, to produce). A substance that produces fever.

**Quadriceps**   (L *quattuor*, four, + *caput*, head). Four-headed; as a quadriceps muscle, composed of the rectus femoris, vastus lateralis, vastus medialis, and vastus intermedius muscles.

**Quadriplegia**   (L *quattuor*, four, + Gr *plēgē*, stroke). Some degree of impairment in all four limbs. Known variously as tetraplegia.

**Quality assurance**   Process of evaluating nursing care, goals, or expected outcomes and other nursing activities through use of established standards of care.

**Radiation therapy**   (L *radiotio*, radiating). Treatment with radiant energy of extremely short wavelengths that damage or kill cells.

**Radiculopathy** (L *radicula,* radicle, + Gr *pathos* disease). Any diseased condition of the roots of spinal nerves.

**Radioisotope** (L *radius,* ray, + Gr *isos,* equal, + *topos,* place). A chemical element with a different atomic weight than its parent element and which gives off radiant energy.

**Radiological** (L *radius,* ray, + *logos,* study). Pertaining to radiology, the branch of science that deals with roentgen rays, radium rays, and other radiations and their curative properties.

**Radionuclide** A radioisotope which disintegrates by emitting electromagnetic radiations.

**Radiopaque** (L *radius,* ray, + *opacus,* dark). Impenetrable to x-rays or other forms of radiation.

**Radiosensitive** (L *Radius,* ray, + *sensus,* feeling). Capable of being destroyed by radiation.

**Radiowaves** (L *Radius,* ray). Short wave-length waves or rays used in some medical diagnostic or therapeutic procedures.

**Raynaud's phenomenon** or **sign** A condition caused by arterial spasms resulting in cyanotic discoloration, coldness, and sweating of the hands, fingers, feet, or toes. Can be secondary to stress or cold, and is a symptom in persons with rheumatoid arthritis, progressive systemic sclerosis, and workers who use pneumatic air hammers.

**Recovery** (L *recuperare,* to recuperate). Regaining health after illness; to regain a former state of health or just a normal state.

**Reduction** (L *reductio,* leading back). Restoration to normal position, as a fractured bone or a hernia.

**Reflex** (L *reflexus,* bent back). Involuntary muscle response to nerve stimulation. Movement not controlled voluntarily.

**Reflex sympathetic dystrophy** (Gr *dys,* bad, + *trephein,* to nourish). A condition of the upper or lower extremity tissues noted by severe, burning pain, hyperesthesia of the tissues, edema, and color changes of the hand(s) or foot (feet). The condition may arise secondary to trauma, may be associated with pregnancy, or may have an unknown etiology. Muscle atrophy may result from untreated conditions.

**Regional involvement** Spread of cancer from original site to nearby areas; metastasis.

**Rehabilitation** (L *rehabilitare,* to restore). Process of restoring to useful life a person who has been ill or who is handicapped. Accomplished through education and therapy.

**Relaxation** (L *relaxare,* to loosen). To decrease tension or strain; to rid of anxiety or nervousness.

**Relaxation techniques** Series of guidelines or instructions given to aid a person to listen to internal cues and to progressively relax or loosen muscles to become calm, less anxious, and thereby more relaxed.

**Remission** (L *remissio,* remit). Complete or partial disappearance of the signs and symptoms of a disease; or the period during which a disease is under control; lessening of severity.

**Remodeling** Final stage in bone healing following a fracture.

**Replacement (bone)** Bone that is formed in cartilage preceding the definitive bone.

**Resistance** (L *resistentia,* standing back). Total of body mechanisms that interpose barriers to the progress of invasion and multiplication of infectious agents, or damage by their toxic products.

**Resorption** (L *resorbere,* to swallow again). Act of removal by absorption.

**Retention** (L *retentare,* to hold back). Retaining in the body that which does not belong there, or which should be excreted, such as urine, feces, or perspiration; holding in place, as traction or a cast, for healing to occur.

**Retraction of shoulder** Draw shoulders back toward one another.

**Rhabdomyosarcoma** (Gr *rhabdos,* rod, + *mys,* muscle, + *sarx,* flesh, + *oma,* tumor). Malignant tumor of striated muscle.

**Rheumatoid arthritis** (Gr *rheuma,* discharge). Form of arthritis with inflammation of the joints, stiffness, swelling, cartilaginous hypertrophy, and pain.

**Rhinorrhea** (Gr *rhis,* nose, + *rhoia,* flow). Thin, watery discharge from nose; cerebrospinal rhinorrhea is discharge of spinal fluid due to a defect in the cribriform plate.

**Rhizotomy** (Gr *rhiza,* root, + *tome,* a cutting). Cutting or sectioning a nerve root for the relief of pain if performed on dorsal root of spinal nerve.

**Rickets** Abnormal shape and structure of bones caused by vitamin D deficiency.

**Rotation** (L *rotatio,* a turning). Process of turning on an axis.

**Rotator cuff** Encircling muscles of the shoulder comprised of the teres minor, infraspinatus, deltoid, and supraspinatus muscles, which permit the shoulder joint to rotate and turn in a circular fashion.

**Sacral** (L *sacralis, sacrum,* sacred). Pertaining to sacral area of the spinal column and lower back.

**Sacroiliac** (L *sacrum,* sacred, + *iliacus,* hip bone). Area between the sacrum and iliac bones of the pelvis.

**Sacrum** (L *sacrum,* sacred). Bony part at base of the spinal column made of the five fused vertebrae above the coccyx.

**Sagittal** (L *sagittalis,* arrow). Vertical plane through the body dividing it into left and right portions.

**Sarcoma** (Gr *sarx,* flesh, + *oma,* tumor). A form of cancer that arises in the connective tissue and muscles, such as bone and cartilage.

**Schwannoma** A tumor of Schwann's cells, cells of ectodermal origin which comprise the neurilemma.

**Scintigraphy** (L *scintilla*, spark, + Gr *graphos*, written). A scan or diagram produced by "counting" the concentration and sites of accumulation of a radioisotope or radionuclide.

**Sciatic** Pertaining to the hip or ischium; afflicted with sciatica.

**Sciatica** Pain in the leg along the course of the sciatic nerve down the back of the thigh and down the leg.

**Sclerosis** (Gr *sklērosis*, hardening). A hardening or induration of an organ or tissue.

**Scoliosis** (Gr *skoliōsis*, curvature). Abnormal lateral curvature of vertebral column.

**Screw** Metallic implant into bone to hold for healing.

**Scurvy** (L *scorbutus*, scurvy). A disease caused by a deficiency of vitamin C, which results in abnormal formation of teeth and bones and hemorrhagic areas in body tissues, especially in the gingiva.

**Secondary** Next to or following; second in order; produced by a primary cause.

**Self-concept** Mental picture of who or what one perceives oneself to be; includes aspects of body image, perceptions of self as a person or family member, social characteristics, and feelings of worth.

**Sensory** (L *sensus*, a feeling). Conveying impulses from sense organs to the reflex or higher centers; pertaining to sensation.

**Septicemia** (Gr *sēptikos*, putrefying, + *haimia*, blood). Morbid condition from absorption of septic products into blood and tissues or of pathogenic bacteria, which may rapidly multiply there.

**Sequestrum** (L *sequestrum*, something set inside). Dead bone separated from sound bone through process of necrosis.

**Setup** Arrangement of instruments or equipment for a treatment, operative procedure or other technique.

**Shearing force** External pressure that exerts diagonal or oblique pressure on tissues, separating them from underlying tissues, thus causing loss of blood supply.

**Shin splint** Leg pain commonly associated with running but may be caused by tendonitis of the anterior or posterior tibial tendons.

**Shock** Disturbance of oxygen supply to the tissues and return of blood to the heart caused by trauma, hemorrhage, infection, and other conditions.

**Side-lying** Lying on one's side in bed.

**Side plate** Plate attached by screws parallel to the long axis of a bone for treatment of a fracture or bone weakness.

**Skeletal traction** Traction exerted directly on long bones.

**Skin traction** One of several kinds of traction applied to the skin; for example, Buck's extension, head halter, and such.

**Sliding board** Transfer board, bridge board.

**Sling** (Anglo-Saxon *slingan*, to wind). A support for an injured upper extremity or pelvic injuries.

**Spasms**  (Gr *spasmos,* a convulsion). Sudden, often violent, involuntary contraction of a muscle or group of muscles.

**Spasticity**  (Gr *spastikos,* convulsive). State of increase over the normal amount of tension in a muscle; imperfect voluntary control of muscles with stiff jerking movements.

**Spectrum**  (L image). A group of things within a specific class; for example, the spectrum of organisms that may cause disease.

**Spica**  (L ear of grain). Reverse spiral bandage, the turn of which crosses like the letter V; casts using this type turn to encircle an extremity and pelvis.

**Spinous process**  (L *spinosus,* thorn). A piece of bone that protrudes, as in the spine where bones can be felt down the back.

**Spiral**  Coiling around a center like the thread of a screw.

**Spiritual**  (L *spiritus,* breath). Of the spirit or the soul, often in a religious or moral aspect, as distinguished from the body.

**Splint**  (L *splinte,* a wedge). An appliance made of bone, wood, metal, and/ or plaster of paris, used for the fixation, union, or protection of an injured part of the body. It may be movable or immovable.

**Spondylitis**  (Gr *spondylos,* a vertebra, + *itis,* inflammation). Arthritis of the vertebral column; inflammation of one or more vertebra.

**Spondylolisthesis**  (Gr *spondylos,* vertebra, + *olisthanein,* to slip). Forward subluxation of the lower lumbar vertebrae on the sacrum.

**Spondylosis**  Noninfective disease of spine where ankylosis is present.

**Sports medicine**  Planned program of activities to prevent and manage sports-related injuries under the guidance and management of a team of health professionals which includes team physicians, trainers, coaches, nurses, dietitians, physical therapists, physiologists, and others.

**Sprain**  (O.Fr *espraindre,* to wring). Excessive stretch or pull of a muscle, tendon, or ligament (or all) in which there is bleeding and tearing of some fibers. The ankle is the area which is most frequently sprained.

**Staging**  Determining the extent of growth of a cancer so that results of treatment can be compared and prognosis offered.

**Standard of care**  A guide for nursing care containing measurable goals (expected outcomes) and nursing interventions to aid in achieving the goals.

**Strain**  (AS *streon,* offspring). Injury to a muscle or tendon from excessive stretch or pull.

**Strategies**  Actions or activities to accomplish goals or objectives.

**Stress**  (Fr *estresse,* narrowness). Abnormal strain; when stress occurs in quantities the system cannot handle, it produces pathological changes; sum of stressors (threats) to a system.

**Stress fracture**  (L *fractura,* a break). Crack or break in a bone caused by repetitive trauma. Most commonly occurs in the tibia or fibula.

**Stressors**  Agents or conditions capable of producing stress.

**Stress response**   Concept developed by Hans Selye to signify the pattern of systemic responses to a threat, both physical and psychological.

**Striated**   (L *striatus*, striped). Striped; marked by streaks or striae.

**Stump**   (ME *stumpe*). The part of a digit or limb remaining after amputation.

**Subluxation**   (L *sub*, under, + *luxatio*, dislocation). Partial dislocation or incomplete dislocation.

**Supine, supinated**   (L *supinus*, bent backward). Face up, palm up; opposite to prone; to turn upward; to rotate the foot and leg outward.

**Sympathectomy**   (Gr *sympathētikos*, sympathy, + *ektomē*, excision). Excision of a portion of the sympathetic branches of a nerve such as the ganglion or plexus of the sympathetic trunk.

**Symphysis pubis**   (Gr *symphysis*, a growing together). Bony part at base of abdomen; junction of the pubic bones in midline in lower abdomen.

**Synapse**   (Gr *synapsis*, point of contact). Point of junction between two neurons.

**Synovial membrane**   (Gr *syn*, together, + *ōon*, egg). The secretory membrane that lines joints and covers structures within them; produces synovial fluid to lubricate joints.

**System**   (Gr *systēma*, a composite whole). An organized grouping of related structures; a group of structures or organs related to each other and functioning together in the performance of certain functions; a group of cells or aggregations of cells that perform a particular function.

**Systems theory** or **approach**   Method or manner of viewing activities, parts, components, units, and boundaries to determine a whole, an objective(s), and performance of the parts related to the whole. Systems theory shows these relationships in terms of the overall objectives or goals of the system.

**Talipes**   (L *talus*, ankle, + *pes*, foot). Deformities involving tarsal joints.

**Tamponade**   (fr *tamponner*, to plug). Condition resulting from accumulation of excess fluid in a sac such as the pericardium.

**Tarsal tunnel syndrome**   (L *tarsalis*, flat surface). The area of the heel and ankle; made up of heel and ankle bones; syndrome made up of pain, soreness, and swelling from constriction of tarsal ligament.

**Tendon**   (L *tendo*, tendon). Fibrous tissue connecting muscle tissue to bone and other parts.

**Tendonitis**   Inflammation of a tendon.

**Tennis elbow**   Obscure, insidious, distressing complaint after playing tennis following a period of muscular inactivity of the arm or following a long duration of play; pain over lateral epicondyle of humerus.

**Tenodesis**   (Gr *tenon*, tendon, + *desis*, a binding). Suturing of the end of a tendon to a point of attachment.

**Tenosynovitis**   Inflammation of the lining of a tendon sheath.

**Tenovaginitis**  (Gr *tendon*, tendon, + *vagina*, sheath). Mild chronic inflammation of the wall of a tendon sheath, prevents free movement of the tendon within the sheath.

**Tetanus**  (Gr *tetanos*, tetanus). A state of sustained contraction of a muscle. Tetanus is also an acute infectious disease caused by the toxin of the tetanus bacillus.

**Therapy**  (Gr *therapeia*, treatment). Treatment of disease.

**Thermography**  (Gr *thermē*, heat, + *graphein*, to write). A technique for measuring the surface temperature of parts of the body to detect underlying disease; used along with mammography and palpation for discovering breast cancer in earliest stage.

**Thoracic**  (Gr *thōrakikos*, chest). Pertaining to chest or thorax.

**Thoracotomy**  (Gr *thorakikos*, chest, + *tomē*, a cutting). Surgical opening of chest cavity.

**Thrombophlebitis**  (Gr *thrombos*, clot, + *phleps*, vein, + *itis*, inflammation). Primarily inflammation of the vein wall, with associated clot that forms on the damaged endothelium.

**Thumb web**  Web between thumb and first finger.

**Tibial Tuberosity**  Part of bone just below and in front of knee joint.

**Tic**  Spasm of muscle; spasm may be tonic or clonic and involuntary; it may be painful.

**Tissue**  (L *texere*, to weave). Collection of similar cells. Four basic tissues in body are: epithelial, connective, muscle, and nerve.

**Tomography**  (Gr *tome*, cutting, + *graphein*, to write). Special roentgenographic technique designed to show detailed images in a selected plane of tissue by blurring images in other planes.

**Tone**  (L *tonus*, a stretching). Normal state of tension maintained by the muscles, organs, or other body tissues.

**Torticollis**  (L *tortus*, twisted, + *collum*, neck). Congenital or acquired stiff neck caused by a spasmodic contraction of neck muscles, drawing the head to one side.

**Tourniquet**  (Fr a turning instrument). A device used in surgery to obstruct blood supply to a part; any constrictor used on an extremity to control bleeding, to distend veins.

**Trabecula**  (L *trabecula*, a little beam). Fibrous cord of connective tissue, serving as supporting fiber by forming septum extending into an organ from its wall or capsule.

**Traction**  (L *tractio*, to pull). Pulling along the length of a limb or part.

**Transaction**  (L *trans*, across, + *actio*, to do). Mutual determination of a goal or goals for care; may be explicitly determined through verbal interactions or implicitly decided from nonverbal interactions (behaviors).

**Transient paralysis**  Temporary loss of sensation and ability to move a part.

**Transverse**  (L *transversus*, across or over). Lying across; crosswise.

**Trauma**   (Gr *trauma*, wound). Injury or damage to body or mind.

**Trendelenburg position**   Position in which bed or table is raised from the foot with the head lower than hips or legs. Position sometimes used in abdominal surgery, in case of shock or low blood pressure.

**Triceps**   (L *tri*, three, + *caput*, head). Muscle that extends the elbow arising from three heads with a single insertion.

**Trigger point**   Spot or site of beginning of pain or muscle spasm. Affected person can usually point or locate the trigger point exactly.

**Trochanter**   (Gr *trochantēr*, a runner). Either of the two bony processes below and on either side of the neck of the femur.

**Tumor**   (L *tumor*, a swelling). A swelling or enlargement; an abnormal mass, either benign or malignant, which performs no useful body function.

**Ulnar border (of hand)**   (L *ulna*, elbow). Same side of the hand as the little finger.

**Unilateral**   (L *unus*, one, + *latus*, side). On one side only.

**Union**   (L *unio*, oneness). Act or state of being united; growing together of severed or broken parts.

**Urostomy**   (Gr *ouron*, urine, + *stoma*, mouth or passage). Surgical procedure that creates a stoma or opening in the urinary tract through the abdominal wall to permit the elimination of urine.

**Valgus**   Bent outward, angulation away from the midline, *refers to the distal segment*. Knock-kneed is genu valgus.

**Values**   (L *valere*, to be strong, be worthy). Returns for something exchanged; the qualities of being excellent, useful, or desirable; worths.

**Variable**   (L *variare*, to change). Changeable or subject to change; inconstant.

**Varus**   Bent inward, angulation toward midline; *refers to distal segment*; genu varus is bowlegged (knee deviates outwardly, and tibia and fibula deviate inwardly).

**Vein**   (L *vena*, vein). Vessel carrying dark red (unaerated) blood to the heart, except for pulmonary vein, which carries oxygenated blood to heart.

**Venogram**   (L *vena*, vein, + *gramma*, a writing). A radiopaque "tracing" of the veins or a portion of the venous system.

**Vesicle**   (L *vesicula*, a small bladder). A blister or sac filled with fluid.

**Viewbox**   Lighted box for viewing x-rays or other radiologic studies.

**Virology**   (L *virus*, poison, + *logos*, study). Branch of biology dealing with study of viruses.

**Virus**   (L *virus*, poison). Tiny parasite that invades cells and uses cell nutrients for nutritive or reproductive needs. Viruses cause many diseases.

**Volkmann's contracture**   Severe, persistent contraction of the forearm and hand due to ischemia from external pressure or crushing injury around the distal humerus and elbow. Muscle atrophy and a clawlike hand result.

**Walker**   A mobile device used to assist a person in walking; consists of a stable platform made of tubing, primarily of lightweight aluminum.

**Weight bearing** Putting one's weight on lower extremities and joints when walking.

**Wheelchair** A mobile chair for weak or disabled persons, mounted on large wheels.

**Work-up** Diagnostic steps or procedures to aid in determining a patient's diagnosis.

**X-ray** Radiant energy of extremely short wavelength, used to diagnose and treat many conditions or diseases; a photograph obtained by use of x-rays.

## BIBLIOGRAPHY

Miller, B.F. & Keane, C.B. (1978). *Encyclopedia and dictionary of medicine, nursing, and allied health.* Philadelphia: Saunders.

Thomas, C.L. (Ed.). (1975). *Taber's cyclopedic medical dictionary* (12th ed.). Philadelphia: Davis.

Urdang, L. (Ed.). (1983). *Mosby's medical and nursing dictionary.* St. Louis: Mosby.

# INDEX

Bold: Page numbers in **bold** type reference non-text material.

## A

Abdomen, flat plate of, **93**
Abdominal reflex, 60
Achilles reflex, 60
Acid ash, foods high in, **491**
Acid phosphatase, studies of, 80
Acromioclavicular injury, 123
Activated partial thromboplastin time, studies of, **87**
Activities of daily living, 437
Adipose connective tissue, tumors, classification of, **203**
Adson test, 62
Alkaline phosphatase, studies of, 80
Allopurinol, 158
Ambulation
    aids for,
        braces, 458, **461**
        canes, 453
        crutches, 449–53
        walkers, 446–49
        wheelchairs, 453, 455–58
Ambulatory aids, physical mobility and, nursing diagnosis, 391–92
Amputation, 417–18
    physical mobility an, 424–25
    self-concept and, nursing diagnosis, 418–19
    stump, wrapping, **423**
Anal reflex, 60
Anemia, gas exchange and, nursing diagnosis, 164–65
Anesthesia
    bowel elimination and, nursing diagnosis, 358–59
    gas exchange and, nursing diagnosis, 356
    injury from, nursing diagnosis, 364–65
Aneurysmal bone cyst, 208–9
    diagnostic procedure for, **205**
Ankle
    examination of, 70
    fracture of, features of, **140**
    ligaments of, **42**
    ranges of motion of, 59
    replacement of, 399–400
    sprain, care of, 114–15
Ankylosing spondylitis
    described, 174
    pathophysiology of, 174–75
Antalgic gait, 57

Anterior drawer test, **71**
Anthrogram, 96
Antinuclear antibodies, studies of, 86
Antistreptolysin (ASO) test, 85
Anturane, 158
Anxiety, injury/mobility loss and, nursing diagnosis, 148–49
Appendicular skeleton, 29
aPTT, studies of, **87**
Arm, upper, compartments of, **471**
Arteriogram, 106
    patient education/preparation for, 106–7
Arthritis. See Osteoarthritis; Rheumatoid arthritis
Arthrodesis, 411–12
Arthropan, 156
Arthroplasty
    joint, 374–76
        patient preparation, 376–77
Arthroscopy, 101
Aspirin, 156
Ataxic gait, 57
Australia antigen, studies of, 86
Avascular necrosis, 469–70
Avulsed fracture, **131**
Axial skeleton, 29

## B

Babinski reflex, 60
Baker's cyst, 127
Band neutrophils, studies of, **77**
Basophils, studies of, **78**
Bed rest
    bowel elimination and, nursing diagnosis, 358–59
    gas exchange and, nursing diagnosis, 356
    skin integrity and, nursing diagnosis, 403–4
Belvor sign, 62
Benemid, 158
Biceps reflex, 60
Blisters, 128
Blood
    diagnostic examinations of, **75–87**
    sugar, studies of, 79
    urea nitrogen, studies of, 79
Body image
    amputation and, nursing diagnosis, 418–19
    calcium, nursing diagnosis, 308–9

    deformities and, nursing diagnosis, 196–97
    inflammation and, nursing diagnosis, 177–78
Body mechanics, principles of, 462
Body planes, 29–30
Body scans, 97
Bone
    anatomy/physiology of, 28–35
    cross section of, **31**
    diseases, metabolic, 231–42
    embryonic development of, 32
    foot, views of, **34**
    formation, regulators of, **234**
    fractures,
        described, 128, 132
        features of, **134–41**
        healing of, 133, 142–45
        illustrated, **129–30**
        nursing process for, 144–49
        types/causes of, **131**
    functions of, 33, 35
    grafts, 340
    humerus, views of, **33**
    infections,
        described, 220
        osteomyelitis, 220–28
    long, described, 30, 32
    major, **29**
    marrow,
        aspiration of, 100
        tumors of, **203**
    resorption, regulators of, **234**
    scans, 97
    scintigraphy, 107
        patient education/preparation for, 107–8
    tumors,
        benign, 203, 208–9
        classification of, **203**
        diagnostic procedures, **205–7**
        malignant, 209–12
        surgical staging system, **204**
        *see also* specific type of tumor
    vertebra, views of, **34**
    *see also* specific name of bone
Bowel elimination, surgical trauma and, nursing diagnosis, 358–59
Braces, 458, **461**
    skin integrity and, nursing diagnosis, 355–56
Brachioradialis reflex, 60

Bragard's sign, medial meniscus tear
   and, 118
Brain, scans, 97
Buck's extension traction, 280
   materials needed for, 287–90
BUN, studies of, **79**
Bunions, nursing diagnosis, 197–98
Bursae, 45
   hip, **46**
   knee, **46**
   shoulder, **47**, 123
Bursitis
   described, 170
   nursing diagnosis, 197–98
   nursing process for, 172–74
   pain and, nursing diagnosis, 173–74
   pathophysiology of, 170, 172
   physical mobility and, nursing
      diagnosis, 172–73
Butazolidin, **157**

**C**
Calcaneus, tarsal bones, fracture of, **140**
Calcium
   body image and, nursing diagnosis
      and, 308–9
   foods high in, **491**
   serum, bones and, 35
   studies of, **84**
Canes, 453
Care
   standards of, 3–4
      impaired physical mobility, 4
      pain, 5–6
Carpal tunnel syndrome, 476–85
Carpus, fracture of, features of, **136**
Cartilage, 41, 43–45
   tumors,
      benign, 203, 208–9
      classification of, **203**
      diagnostic procedures, **205–7**
      malignant, 209–12
Casts
   acute pain and, nursing diagnosis,
      261–63
   application of, 248–53
      materials needed for, 245–48
   body, nursing diagnosis, 355–56
   bowel/bladder elimination and,
      nursing diagnosis, 268–69
   cutting/removing, 275–76
   damp, nursing diagnosis, 253–58
   described, 244–45
   diversional/social activities and,
      nursing diagnosis, 269–70
   gas exchange and, nursing diagnosis,
      259–60, 303–4
   home care needs, nursing diagnosis,
      271–75
   nutrition alternations in, nursing
      diagnosis, 267–68
   petaling a, 250, **251**
   physical mobility, nursing diagnosis,
      258–59
   self-care deficit and, nursing
      diagnosis, 260–61
   skin integrity and, nursing diagnosis,
      263–66

syndrome, 270–71
   walking heels for, **249**
CAT scan, 99
Catheters, urinary elimination alternation
   and, nursing diagnosis,
   392–93
Cells, tumors, classification of, **203**
Cervical spine, ranges of motion of, **59**
Chaddock reflex, 60
Charleyhorse, care of, 113
Chemonucleolysis
   described, 361–62
   surgery for, preparation for, 361–62
Chest, x-ray, **93**
Chloride, studies of, **84**
Choline magnesium trisalicylate, **156**
Choline salicylate, **156**
Chondroblastoma, 208
   diagnostic procedure for, **205**
Chondroma, 208
   diagnostic procedure for, **205**
Chondromyxoma, 208
   diagnostic procedure for, **205**
Chondrosarcoma, 211–12
   diagnostic procedure for, **206**
Chvostek's sign, **62**
Chymopapain, 361
   injury from, nursing diagnosis,
      364–65
Clavicle, fracture of, features of, **141**
Clinitron bed, **497**
Closed fracture, **131**
Colchicine, **158**
Cold, therapeutic use of, 445–46
Collagen, 45, 47
Colsalide, **158**
Comminuted fracture, **131**
Compartment syndrome, 470–74
Compression fracture, **131**
Continuous quality improvement, 6–7
Contusion, defined, 112
Contusions, care of, 111–13
Cotrel-Dubousset rods, 339, **341**
Cotrel's traction, materials needed for, 293
CPK, studies of, **81**
C-reative protein, studies of, **85**
Creatophosphokinase, studies of, **81**
Cremasteric reflex, **61**
Crutches, 449–53
CT scan, 99
Cysts, Baker's, 127

**D**
Decubitus ulcerations
   formation of, 491-93
   prevention interventions, 494–96
Deformities, role performance and,
      nursing diagnosis, 169–70
Deformity
   arthritis related, nursing diagnosis,
      196–97
   body image and, nursing diagnosis,
      196–97
   physical mobility and, nursing
      diagnosis, 196
Degenerative disc disease, described,
   198–201

Delayed union, defined, **466**
Deltasone, **158**
Demographics, impact of, 14–15
Diagnostic examinations
   arteriogram, 106
      patient education/preparation for,
      106–7
   arthroscopy, 101
   blood, 75–87
   bone scintigraphy, 107
      patient education/preparation for,
      107–8
   invasive, 89, **96–100**, 101
   MRI, 102
   myelogram, 104
      patient education/preparation for,
      105
   noninvasive, 88, **93–95**
      patient education/preparation for, 102
   radiologic, 88
   serologic studies, 74
   serum, **75–87**
   urine, 74, 88, **90–92**
Diagnostic related groups, 7
Diclofenac, **157**
Dietitian, 12
Diflunisal, **157**
Disalcid, **156**
Discogram, 99
Dislocation
   defined, 112
   shoulder, 123
Diversional/social activities and, casts,
      269–70, 307–8
Dolobid, **157**
Dorsiflexion, foot, **50**
Drawer test, 62–63, **71**
DRGs, 7
Drop arm test, **62**
Dunlop's traction, 286–87
   materials needed for, **294**

**E**
Echograms, **94–95**
Elbow
   examination of, 68
   injuries to, 125–78
      dislocated elbow, 125–27
   ligaments of, **126**, 179
   ranges of motion of, **58**
   replacement of, 399–400
Electrocardiogram, **93–94**
Electromyogram, **98–99**
Emboli. *See* specific type of emboli
Enchondroma, 208
   diagnostic procedure for, **205**
Eosinophils, studies of, **77–78**
Epicondylitis
   described, 178
   pathophysiology of, 178–80
Eversion, foot, **51**
Ewing's sarcoma, 212
   diagnostic procedure for, **206**
Extension, forearm, **51, 52**
Extremities, sensory dermatomes to, **480**

**F**
Fabere (Patrick) test, **63**

Facial expression, examination of, 68
Factor VIII assay, studies of, **87**
Factor IX, studies of, **87**
Fascia, 39
Fat emboli, 486–88
  gas exchange and, nursing diagnosis, 147–48
  pulmonary emboli, comparisons of, 487–88
  skeletal traction and, 324–27
Fatigue, role performance and, nursing diagnosis, 169–70
Feldene, **157**
Femur
  fractures of, **136–38**
    classifications of, **369**
  head, core decompression of, 410–11
Fenoprofen, **156**
Fernisone, **158**
Festinating gait, 57
Fibroblasts, 32
Fibrosarcoma, 212
  diagnostic procedure for, **206**
Fibrous tissue, tumors, classification of, **203**
Fingers
  examination of, **68**
  ranges of motion of, **58**
  surgery on, **429, 431–32**
Finkelstein test, 63
Fixation devices, external, application of, 314–17
Flexion
  forearm, **52**
  let, **52**
Food
  calcium content of, **237–38**
  purine content of, **240**
Foot
  examination of, **70**
  movements of, **50–51**
  views of, **34**
Forearm, movements of, **51, 52**
Fore-quarter amputation, 418
Fractures
  defined, **112**
  femur, classifications of, **369**
  Ilizarov method and, 425–28
  orthopaedic surgery for, 342–44
  surgical treatment of, 365–74
  *see also* Bone, fractures
Fusion
  spinal, 339, 342
    scoliosis and, 346–48
    spondylolisthesis and, 344–46

**G**
Gaenslen test, **63**
Gaits
  abnormal, **57**
  examination of, **67**
GI distention/obstruction/bleeding, injury potential from, 166–67
Giant cell tumor, 208
  diagnostic procedure for, **206**
Glenohumeral injury, 123–24
Glucose, studies of, **79**
Golfer's elbow, 178

Gordon reflex, **61**
Gout
  described, 239
  pathophysiology of, 239–40
Grafts, bone, **340**
Greenstick fracture, **131**
Groin, pull, care of, 113
Guaiac test, **95**

**H**
HAA, studies of, **86**
Hallux valgus, 193–95
Halo traction, **251**
Hamstring
  pull, care of, 113–14
  reflex, **61**
Hand
  anatomy of, **430**
  movements of, **53**
  surgery on, **429**
Harrington rods, 339, **341**
Haversian canals, 32
Head, examination of, **67**
Head halter traction, 282, **283**
  materials needed for, 294
Health care team
  orthopaedic, 8–9
    dietitian, 12
    occupational therapist, 11
    office nurse, 10–11
    orthopaedic technician, 11–12
    physical therapist, 11
    primary nurse, 9–10
    social worker, 12–13
    staff nurse, 11
Heat, therapeutic use of, 440–45
Hematocrit, studies of, **75**
Hemipelvectomy, 417
Hemoglobin, studies of, **75**
Hepatitis-associated antigen, studies of, **86**
Hind-quarter amputation, 417
Hip
  anatomy of, **379**
  bursae of, **46, 171**
  examination of, **69**
  movements of, **49**
  ranges of motion of, **58**
  total replacement of, 377–81
    exercises for, **387–88**
    postoperative care, 381–82, 384, 393
    turning techniques following, 382–84
Hoover test, **63**
Humerus
  fracture of, features of, **134–35**
  views of, **33**
Hyaline, 43
Hyperextension, forearm, **52**
Hyperthermia, nursing diagnosis, 183–84
Hypophosphatasia, bones and, 35

**I**
Ibuprofen, **156**
Ilizarov method
  fractures and, 425–28
    nursing diagnosis and, 428–29
Immobility
  bones and, 35

bowel elimination and, nursing diagnosis, 358–59
gas exchange and, nursing diagnosis, 356, 401–2
tissue perfusion and, nursing diagnosis, 357–58, 402–3
*see also* Mobility
Immunofluorescence, studies of, **86**
Impacted fracture, **131**
Inactivity, bones and, 35
Indocin, **157**
Indomethacin, **157**
Infections
  bone, 35, 220–28
  hyperthermia and, nursing diagnosis, 183–84
  pain and, nursing diagnosis and, 184–85
  wound, 228–29
Inflammation, signs of, 152–53
Injuries. *See* Trauma
Interpositional arthroplasty, 374
Intravenous pyelogram, 99–100
Invasive examinations, 89, **96–100**, 101
Inversion, foot, 51

**J**
Jaw jerk reflex, **61**
Joints, 47–48
  arthroplasty of, 374–76
    patient preparation, 376–77
  deformities, self-care deficit and, 165–66
  infection in, nursing diagnosis, 182–85, 390–91
  inflammation of, nursing diagnosis, 176–77, 240–41
  movements of, 48–53
  pain and, nursing diagnosis, 192–93
  ranges of motion of, 59–60
  sleep disturbance from, nursing diagnosis, 168–69

**K**
Kernig test, **63–64**
Kidneys
  scans, 97
  tomogram of, 94
Kirschner wire, application of, 311–14
Knee
  anatomy of, **116, 394**
  Baker's cysts and, 127
  bursae of, **46, 171**
  examination of, **69–70**
  fracture of, features of, **138–39**
  ligaments of, **42**
    injuries to, 118–19
  meniscal injuries to, 116–18
  osteochondritis dissecans of, 127
  patella dislocation, 116
  ranges of motion of, **58**
  total replacement of, 393–95
    exercise program following, **407**
    home exercise program, **408**
  trauma to, 115
Knowledge deficit, osteomyelitis and, nursing diagnosis, 227–28
Kyphosis, surgery for, 348–51

**L**

Lachman drawer test, **71**
Lactic dehydrogenase, studies of, **81-82**
Lacunae, **32**
Leg
  examination of, **69**
  movements of, **52**
Leiomyoma, 213
  diagnostic procedure for, **207**
Leiomyosarcoma, 213
  diagnostic procedure for, **207**
Ligaments, **40-41**
  ankle, **42**
  elbow, **126, 179**
  knee, **42**
    injuries to, 118-19
  shoulder, **43, 121, 397**
Linear fracture, **131**
Liver, scans, 97
Logrolling, patients after surgery, 353-54
Long bones, described, 30, 32
Lumbar
  puncture, **97-98**
  spine, ranges of motion of, **58**
Lungs
  scans of, **97**
  tomogram of, **94**
Lyme disease
  described, **181**
  pathophysiology of, 182
Lymphocytes, studies of, 77

**M**

McMurray's test, **64, 71**
  meniscal injuries and, 118
Magnetic resonance imaging, 102
Malunion, **468**
  defined, **466**
Meclofenamate, **157**
Meclomen, **157**
Medial meniscus tears, 118
Mediscus air fluidized bed, **498**
Meniscus, injuries to, 116-18
Metacarpals, fracture of, features of, **136**
Metastatic tumors, bone, 212
Metatarsal bones, fracture of, features of, **141**
Meticorten, **158**
Milgram test, **64**
Mobility
  anxiety and, nursing diagnosis, 148-49
  casts and, 258-59
    nursing diagnosis, 258-59, 298-99
  impaired,
    ambulatory aids and, 391-92
    amputation and, 424-25
    care standards and, 4
    deformity and, 196
    fractures and, 144-45
    joint inflammation/deformityies and, 160-62, 182-83
    nursing diagnosis, 172-73, 359-60, 405-6, 408-9
    osteoarthritis and, 191-92
    osteomyelitis and, 225
    Paget's disease and, 235-36
    tendinitis and, 180-81
    traction and, 298-99, 327-28
    tumors and, 214-15
  *see also* Immobility

Monocytes, studies of, **77**
Motrin, **156**
Mouth, examination of, **67**
MRI, **102**
Muscles, 35-40
  anterior view of, **36**
  complications associated with, 475-76
  posterior view of, **37**
  rotator cuff, **122**
  shoulder, **121, 398**
    views of, **38**
  skeletal, 35
    functions of, 39-40
  spasms, traction and, nursing
    diagnosis, 296-97
  strength ratings of, **59**
  striated, 35
  tumors,
    benign, 213
    classification of, **203**
    diagnostic procedures, 205-7
    malignant, 213
Musculoskeletal
  injuries,
    care of, 111-15
    types of, **112**
  tissues,
    examination of, 67-70
    medications used for, **156-58**
    tests of, **62-66**
Myelogram, **104**
  patient education/preparation for, 105
Myoglobin, studies of, **87**

**N**

Naffziger test, **64**
Nalfon, **156**
Naprosyn, **157**
Naproxen, **157**
Neck
  examination of, **67**
  rotation of, **53**
Nerve
  injuries to, **484-85**
  plexus, nerves associated with, **483**
Noninvasive examinations, 88, 93-95
Nonunion, **467**
  defined, **466**
Nursing
  legal considerations in, 7-8
  process, 1-3
    diagnostic related groups and, 7
  unit,
    demographics and, 14-15
    physical requirements of, 16-26

**O**

Ober test, **64**
Oblique fracture, **131**
Occupational therapist, 11
Office nurse, 10-11
Olecranon, fracture of, features of, **135**
Oliguria, 490
Open fracture, **131**
Oppenheim reflex, **61**
Oppenheim test, **65**
Orthopaedic
  health care team, 8-9
    dietitian, 12
    occupational therapist, 11

    office nurse, 10-11
    orthopaedic technician, 11-12
    physical therapist, 11
    primary nurse, 9-10
    social worker, 12-13
    staff nurse, 11
  nursing unit, 13-14
    demographics and, 14-15
    physical requirements of, 16-26
  surgery,
    amputation, 417-18
    ankle replacement, 399-400
    arthrodesis and, 411-12
    chemonucleolysis and, 361-62
    curve exaggerations and, 346-51
    described, 332-35
    elbow replacement, 399-400
    femoral head core decompression and, 410-11
    finger, 429, 431-32
    fractures and, 342-44, 365-74
    hand, 429
    hip replacement, 377-84
    joint arthroplasty, 374-76
    knee replacement, 393-95
    logrolling patients after, 353-54
    nursing diagnosis, 355-60
    osteotomy, 412-13
    postoperative considerations, 352-53
    preoperative procedures, 335-37
    shoulder replacement, 395-98
    spinal, 337-53
    spondylolisthesis, 344-46
    wrist replacement, 399-400
    *see also* specific type of surgery or disorder
Orthopaedic technician, 11-12
Ortolani test, **65**
Osteoarthritis
  cartilage degeneration and, **188**
  described, 187
  nursing diagnosis, 191-93
  pathophysiology of, 189-91, 194-95, 198
  self-care deficit and, nursing diagnosis, 193
Osteoblasts, 32
Osteochondritis dissecans, 127
Osteochondroma, 208
  diagnostic procedure for, **205**
Osteoclastoma, **205**
Osteocytes, 32
Osteoma, 203, 208
  diagnostic procedure for, **205**
Osteomalacia
  described, 232-33
  nursing diagnosis, 235-39
Osteomyelitis
  described, 220-21
  nursing diagnosis, 225-28
  pathophysiology of, 221-23
  sites of, **222**
Osteoporosis
  bones and, 35
  described, 233
  nursing diagnosis, 235-39
  pathophysiology, 233-35
Osteosarcoma, 208, 209, 211
  diagnostic procedure for, **206**
Osteotomy, 412-13
Oxalates, foods high in, **491**
Oxyphenbutazone, **157**

**P**

Paget's disease
    described, 231–32
    nursing diagnosis, 235–39
    pathophysiology of, 232
Pain
    arthritis and, nursing diagnosis,
        184–85
    bunions, nursing diagnosis, 197–98
    bursitis and, nursing diagnosis,
        197–98
    casts and, nursing diagnosis, 261–63
    comfort alterations, 261–63
        nursing diagnosis, 372–73
    fractures and, nursing diagnosis, 146
    impaired mobility from, nursing
        diagnosis, 363–64
    joint tissue inflammation, nursing
        diagnosis, 163–64, 176–77
    muscle spasms and, nursing
        diagnosis, 192–93
    phantom,
        nursing diagnosis, 420–21
        nursing diagnosis and, 420–21
    sleep disturbance from, nursing
        diagnosis, 168–69
    standard of care of, 5–6
    surgical intervention and, nursing
        diagnosis, 409–10, 415–16
    systemic infection and, nursing
        diagnosis, 184–85
    tissue perfusion, nursing diagnosis,
        226–27
    traction and, nursing diagnosis,
        296–97
    tumors and, nursing diagnosis,
        215–16
Paralytic ileus, 489–90
Parosteal sarcoma, 211
    diagnostic procedure for, **206**
Partial thromboplastin time, studies of, 87
Patella
    examination of, **69–70**
    dislocation of, 116
Patellar reflex, **61**
Pathologic fracture, **131**
Patrick test, 65
Payr's sign, medial meniscus tear and,
    118
Pearson attachment, 311
Pectoralis major, reflex, **61**
Pelvic belt traction, 282, **291**
    materials needed for, 290
Pelvic sling traction, 284, **285**
    materials needed for, 290, 292
Pelvis
    examination of, **69**
    fracture of, features of, **141**
Periosteum, 32
Phalanges, fracture of, features of, **136**
Phalen test, 65
Phantom pain, nursing diagnosis and,
    420–21
Phenylbutazone, **157**
Phosphate, bones and, 35
Physical assessment, 54–56
Physical therapist, 11
Piroxicam, **157**
Plantarflecion, foot, **50**
Platelets, studies of, **78–79**
Pneumonitis, gas exchange and, nursing
    diagnosis, 164–65

Posture, examination of, **67**
Potassium, studies of, **83**
Prednisone, **158**
Primary nurse, 9–10
Probenecid, **158**
Progressive systemic sclerosis, 160
Pronation
    forearm, **53**
    hand, **53**
Prosthesis, displacement of, nursing
        diagnosis, 384–86, 388
Prothrombin time, studies of, **86–87**
Pseudarthrosis, defined, 466
Pulmonary edema, gas exchange and,
        nursing diagnosis, 164–65
Pulmonary emboli, 488
    fat emboli, comparison of, **487–88**
    skeletal traction and, 324–27
Pulmonary function tests, **94**
Purine
    content in foods, **240**
    metabolism, nursing diagnosis,
        241–42
Pyelogram, intravenous, **99–100**

**Q**

Quadriceps gait, **57**

**R**

Radiologic examinations, 88
Radionuclide scans, 107
    patient education/preparation for,
        107–8
Radius, fracture of, features of, **135**
Rash, body image disturbance and,
        nursing diagnosis, 167–68
Raynaud's phenomenon, activity
        intolerance and, 162–63
Red blood cells, studies of, **75**
Reflexes, **60–61**
Refracture, defined, 466
Rehabilitation
    applications for,
        cold, 445–46
        warm/hot, 440–45
    concept of, 438
    exercise and, 438–39
    services, economic aids for, 458–59
Relaxation training, preoperative, 336–37
Replacement arthroplasty, 376
Resectional arthroplasty, 374
Rhabdomyoma, 213
    diagnostic procedure for, **207**
Rhabdomyosarcoma, 213
    diagnostic procedure for, **207**
Rheumatoid arthritis
    body image disturbance and,
        nursing diagnosis, 167–68
    described, 151
    nursing process for, 160–69, 184–85
    pathophysiology of, 154, 159
Rheumatoid factor, studies of, **85**
Rotation, neck, **53**
Rotator cuff
    injuries to, 124–25
    muscles, **122**
Roto rest kinetic treatment table, **499**
Russell's traction, 280, **281**
    materials needed for, 287–90

**S**

Salsalate, **156**

Salter-Harris fractures, **130**
Sandbags, traction and, 294, **295–96**
Sarcolemma, 35
Scaphoid, fracture of, features of, **136**
Scheuerman's Kyphosis, 349
Sclerosis, progressive systemic, 160
Scoliosis, surgery for, 346–48
Senile gait, **57**
Serologic studies, 74
Serum
    amylase, studies of, **82**
    calcium, bones and, 35
    diagnostic examinations of, **75–87**
    glutamic,
        oxaloacetic transaminase, studies
            of, **80**
        pyruvic transaminase, studies of,
            **80**
SGOT, studies of, **80**
SGPT, studies of, **80**
Shin, splints, 127–28
Shock syndromes, 485–86
Shoulder
    anatomy of, **396**
    bursae of, **47**, 123, **172**
    examination of, **67**
    fracture of, features of, **134**
    girdle, illustrated, **120**
    injuries to, 119, 122–23
        acromioclavicular injury, 123
        glenohumeral injury, 123–24
        rotator cuff, 124–25
        separation, 123
        sternoclavicular injury, 124
        subluxation, 123
    joints of, examination of, **68**
    ligaments of, **43**, **121**, **397**
    movements of, **49**
    muscles of, **38**, **121**, **398**
    range of motion of, **58**
    rotator cuff muscles of, **122**
    total replacement of, 395–98
    trauma to, 119–25
Skeletal muscles, 35
    functions of, 39–40
Skeletal traction
    application of, 310–11
    checking, 329–30
    complications of, 330
    described, 310
    discharge planning/teaching, 330–31
    discomfort from, nursing diagnosis,
        323–24
    external fixation devices, application
        of, 314–17
    injury from skeletal pins, nursing
        diagnosis, 320–23
    Kirschner wire application, 311–14
    physical mobility and, nursing
        diagnosis and, 327–28
    pulmonary/fat emboli and, 324–27
    self-care deficit and, nursing
        diagnosis, 328–29
    Steinmann pin application, 311–14
    tissue injury from, nursing diagnosis,
        318–19
Skin integrity
    bed rest and, nursing diagnosis,
        403–4
    braces and, nursing diagnosis,
        355–56
    casts and, nursing diagnosis, 263–66

osteomyelitis, nursing diagnosis, 226
surgical incision and, nursing
diagnosis, 217–18, 421–23
Skin traction
application of, 287–94
bowel/bladder elimination and,
nursing diagnosis and, 305–7
complications of, 309
diversional/social activities and,
nursing diagnosis, 307–8
nutrition and, nursing diagnosis,
304–5
principles of, 278–79
self-care deficit and, nursing
diagnosis, 301–2
skin integrity and, nursing diagnosis,
302–3
tissue injury and, nursing diagnosis,
300–301
types of, 279–87
Buck's extension, 280
Cotrel's traction, 284, 285
Dunlop's traction, 286–87
head halter, 282, **283**
pelvic belt, 282
pelvic sling, 284, **285**
Russell's traction, 280, **281**
Social worker, 12–13
Sodium, studies of, **84**
Spastic gait, 57
Spinal fusion, 339, 342
scoliosis and, 346–48
spondylolisthesis and, 344–46
Spinal stenosis, 198–201
Spinal surgery
fusion, 339, 342
bone grafts, **340**
postoperative considerations, 352–53
Spine
curve exaggerations, surgery on,
346–51
examination of, **68**
Spiral fracture, **131**
Spleen, scans, **97**
Spondylolisthesis, surgery for, 344–46
Sprain
care of, 114
defined, **112**
Staff nurse, 11
Standards of care, 4
impaired physical mobility, 4
pain and, 5–6
Steinmann pin, application of, 311–14
Steppage gait, **57**
Sternoclavicular injury, 124
Strain
care of, 113
defined, **112**
Stress fracture, **131**, 133
Striated muscles, 35
Subluxation, defined, **112**
Sulfinpyrazone, **158**
Supination
forearm, **53**
hand, **53**
Surgery. *See* Orthopaedic, surgery
Synovium, 45
Systemic lupus erythematosus, 159

**T**
Talus, fracture of, **141**
Tandearil, **157**
Tarsal bones, fracture of, features of, 140

Tarsal tunnel syndrome, 476–85
Temporomandibular joint
examination of, **67**
jaw jerk reflex and, **61**
Tendelenberg test, 66
Tendinitis
described, 178
nursing diagnosis, 180–81
pathophysiology of, 178–80
Tendons, 39, 40
Tennis elbow, 178
test, 66
Tenosynovitis
described, 178
nursing diagnosis, 180–81
pathophysiology of, 178–80
Terrible triad injury, 119
Tetanus, 40
Thigh
compartments of, **471**
examination of, **69**
Thomas
sign, 65
splint, 311
Thorax, examination of, **69**
Thrombophlebitis, 489
Thrombosis, deep vein, nursing
diagnosis, 388–90
Thumb, fracture of, features of, **136**
Tibia, fracture of, features of, **139–40**
Tinel sign, 65
Tissue perfusion
immobility and, nursing diagnosis,
357–58, 402–3
surgical trauma and, nursing
diagnosis, 414–15
Toenails, examination of, **70**
Toes
examination of, **70**
ranges of motion of, **59**
Tolectin, **157**
Tolmetin, **157**
Tomograms, 94
Total elbow replacement, 399–400
Total hip replacement, 377–81
exercises for, **387–88**
postoperative care, 381–82, 384, 393
turning techniques following, 382–84
Total joint replacement arthroplasty, 376
Total knee replacement, 393–95
exercise program following, **407**
exercise program for, home, **408**
Total protein, albumin/globulin, studies
of, **83**
Total shoulder replacement, 395–98
Traction
halo, **251**
impaired mobility and, nursing
diagnosis, 298–99
muscle spasms/pain and, nursing
diagnosis, 296–97
sandbags and, 294, **295–96**
skeletal. *See* Skeletal traction
skin. *See* Skin traction
Transverse fracture, **131**
Trauma
elbow, 125–27
first aid measures for, 110–11
knee and, 115–19
management, 111
musculoskeletal injuries,
care of, 111–15
types of, **112**

shoulder, 119–25
surgical, nursing diagnosis, 357–59,
414–15
Triceps, reflex, 61
Trilisate, **156**
TSRH rods, 339, 342
Tumors
bone,
benign, 203, 208–9
diagnostic procedures, **205–7**
malignant, 209–12
surgical staging system, **204**
cartilage,
benign, 203, 208–9
diagnostic procedures, **205–7**
malignant, 209–12
classification of, **203**
described, 202
muscles,
benign, 213
diagnostic procedures, **205–7**
malignant, 213
nursing diagnoses, 214–18

**U**
Ulna, fracture of, features of, **136**
Ultrasound, **94–95**
Unicameral bone cyst, 209
diagnostic procedure for, **205**
Urate deposits, inflammation, 240–41
Urinalysis, **90–92**
Urine
diagnostic examinations of, 74, 88
diagnostic studies of, **90–92**
specimen, securing, 88
urinary catheter and, nursing
diagnosis, 392–93
Utensils, self care and, 458

**V**
Valsalva test, 66
Vascular tissue, tumors, classification of,
**203**
Vertebrae
inflammation of, nursing diagnosis
of, 176–77
views of, **34**
Vitamin D, bones and, 35
Volkmann's ischemic contracture, 470,
**474**
Voltaren, **157**

**W**
Waiter's tip deformity, **481**
Walkers, 446–49
Wheelchairs, 453, 455–58
White blood count
differential, studies of, **76–77**
studies of, **75–76**
Wiltse system, fractures and, **343**
Wound
culture of, 99
infections, 228–29, 493
injury of potential, nursing
diagnosis, 390–91
Wrist
examination of, **68**
fracture of, features of, **136**
ranges of motion of, **58**
replacement of, 399–400

**Y**
Yergason test, 66

**Z**
Zyloprim, **158**